Demographic Research

a free, open-access, expedited, peer-reviewed
journal of the population sciences

Volume 19, Articles 1-10

Book I of Special Collection 7

Childbearing Trends and Policies in Europe

Available in three books:

Book I: Summary and Overview Chapters
Book II: Country Chapters, Albania - Italy
Book III: Country Chapters, Lithuania - Ukraine

All content also available at: http://www.demographic-research.org/special/7/

This book contains a portion of Special Collection 7, "Childbearing Trends and Policies in Europe" which was published in the online journal *Demographic Research* on July 1, 2008. The collection makes public the results of a three-year comparative international project covering 86 percent of the continent's population. All European countries with more than 15 million inhabitants, as well as a number of smaller countries, are included. The goal was to provide readers with an informed portrayal of how almost all aspects of childbearing behaviour and values in Europe have undergone continuous change in recent decades. The four guest editors for Special Collection 7 were Tomas Frejka, Tomáš Sobotka, Jan M. Hoem, and Laurent Toulemon.

Special Collection 7 consists of eight overview chapters and nineteen country studies (approximately 1,200 pages). Full content can be found online as open access material at: http://www.demographic-research.org/special/7/. Due to the immense interest in this project, the editors also decided to provide bound paper copies printed on a demand basis. The content of Special Collection 7 can thus also be obtained in three separate books. The first book contains a preface, summary, and the eight overview chapters. The second book contains the first nine of the country chapter studies (Albania, Austria, Bulgaria, Czech Republic, England and Wales, France, Germany, Hungary, and Italy). The third book contains the remaining country chapter studies (Lithuania, The Netherlands, Poland, Romania, Russian Federation, Slovakia, Slovenia, Spain, Sweden, and Ukraine). Information on how to order bound paper copies is at: http://www.demographic-research.org/info/ordering_a_bound_print_version.htm.

Standing Scientific Review Board Members

Peer Reviewers who contributed to Special Collection 7

Gunnar Andersson
Vladimir Anisimov
Pau Baizán
Gijs Beets
Tommy Bengtsson
Neil Bennett
Laura Bernardi
Alain Blum
Larry Bumpass
Thomas K. Burch
Elwood D. Carlson
David A. Coleman
Henriette Engelhardt
Frances Goldscheider
Joshua Goldstein
Andy Hinde
Vladimíra Kantorová
Kathleen E. Kiernan
Hans-Peter Kohler
Irena Kotowska
Øystein Kravdal
Hill Kulu
Ron Lesthaeghe
Aart C. Liefbroer

Marc Luy
Torkild Hovde Lyngstad
Peter F. McDonald
Clara Mulder
Michael Murphy
Gerda Neyer
Máire Ní Bhrolcháin
Brienna Perelli-Harris
Dimiter Philipov
Harriet B. Presser
Thomas W. Pullum
Jean-Louis Rallu
Marit Rønsen
Robert Schoen
Steve Smallwood
Maria Rita Testa
Elizabeth Thomson
Jacques Vallin
Dirk van de Kaa
Nico van Nimwegen
Andres Vikat
Charles F. Westoff
Frans Willekens
Kryštof Zeman

TABLE OF CONTENTS

Volume 19, Articles 1 – 10

Preface:
Childbearing Trends and Policies in Europe

Jan M. Hoem[1]

The editors of the present Special Collection of the electronic journal *Demographic Research* take pleasure in making the Collection available to the research community and the general public. The Collection's principal focus is the demographic analysis of European fertility trends, their determinants, and public policies modifying childbearing. The collection is the outcome of an international comparative project. It includes nineteen country studies, eight topical overview chapters, and a summary.

Tomas Frejka has acted as the project's *primus motor* and main editor. Tomáš Sobotka, Jan M. Hoem, and Laurent Toulemon have supported him as co-editors. The Max Planck Institute for Demographic Research has provided organisational support.
Initial discussions about this project began in the summer of 2005. By the fall of that year the rationale for the project had crystallised. The following premises served as our point of departure:

- Throughout Europe fertility had reached below-replacement levels;
- Demographers and policy makers were increasingly becoming concerned about possible long-term deleterious consequences;
- A considerable number of investigations concerning fertility trends and their determinants within countries had been undertaken, as well as some international comparative research;
- Comparative surveys on changes in family and fertility attitudes and behavior have been conducted in many countries, and the resulting datasets have been made available.

Despite the value of existing work, we thought that a meaningful contribution could be made if a large number of country studies of childbearing trends and policies were to be executed in a coordinated fashion. This would facilitate international comparability and provide a basis for updating a continent-wide understanding of the situation. We also envisioned that countries might learn from each other's experiences in determining which policies can be applied to reach desired goals.

---

[1] Max Planck Institute for Demographic Research, Rostock, Germany. E-mail: hoem@demogr.mpg.de

Another reflection was instrumental in our decision to embark on this project. We believed that the mechanisms generating childbearing trends in Western European countries, including the Nordic and Mediterranean ones, were reasonably well understood. By contrast, knowledge about the transformations of family formation and childbearing in the formerly socialist countries of Europe was uneven and fragmentary. Our obvious goal was to contribute to a better documentation and understanding of developments across Europe. Thus a project proposal was developed in the fall of 2005, and the project was launched.

The selection of countries was based on the following considerations: We did not strive for complete coverage of all countries in Europe, but rather aimed for a reasonable geographical representation and attempted to include all countries with more than 15 million inhabitants. Our collection contains chapters for countries for which we have managed to find qualified authors who would commit themselves to the demanding task of writing a chapter on the country's recent fertility and family developments at short notice.

The overview chapters cover the following topics:

1. Contemporary levels and trends of fertility in Europe
2. Changing ultimate-parity distribution and family size
3. Birth regulation (contraception and induced abortion)
4. Changing family and partnership behaviour
5. Childbearing during the societal transition in Central and Eastern Europe
6. The diverse faces of the Second Demographic Transition in Europe
7. The rising importance of migrants for childbearing in Europe
8. The impact of public policies on European fertility.

Each of these chapters summarises findings of the country chapters, is set in the framework of the general literature on the given topic, and includes additional analyses.

We adopted a strict regime of peer review with the following elements. First drafts of the country chapters were pre-reviewed by the editors, revised by the authors, submitted to reviewers selected from the journal's Scientific Review Board, revised again, language edited, and were revised once more by the original author(s). Each overview chapter was written by one or two editors, pre-reviewed by other editors, revised, submitted to reviewers, and finally revised again in the light of their comments. (A list of all peer reviewers for the project can be found at the end of this preface.) This whole process was conducted under the time pressure caused by my imminent retirement, which occurred at the beginning of 2008, and the editing work progressed under Tomas Frejka's unflagging supervision throughout. Renee Flibotte-Lüskow has managed the project firmly and with her usual sense of humour. Technical support, language editing, and layout services were organized by staff at the Max Planck Institute.

Because *Demographic Research* has an arrangement with Special Collections, it has been possible to publish this collection in one go in mid-2008, as the first part of Volume 19. The editors chose to use this medium because it gives free online access to all the chapters, because it is unusually cost-effective, and because this was the optimal way to get the material into print so quickly, i.e., within less than three years of the project initiation in the fall of 2005. The material is therefore available fully integrated into the journal from the day of publication, and can be easily accessed at no cost to the reader using the journal's search engine. The Special Collection can be downloaded as open access material, and bound versions are available through a print-on-demand service. We have donated such books to some 50 depositary libraries and research centres.

The editors are impressed by the loyalty with which authors and collaborators have followed instructions and kept deadlines. We want to express our profound gratitude to the country teams of authors and to the reviewers for their collegial spirit and ability to get the job done under very strict time constraints. As emeritus director of the Max Planck Institute, I want to express my great appreciation to Tomas Frejka for initiating the project and firmly leading the work. The editorial team wants to thank the Max Planck Institute for making the resources of the electronic journal available, and for its general organizational support.

Rostock, 1 July 2008.   Jan M. Hoem

Peer Reviewers of country and overview chapters:

Gunnar Andersson
Vladimir Anisimov
Pau Baizán
Gijs Beets
Tommy Bengtsson
Neil Bennett
Laura Bernardi
Alain Blum
Larry Bumpass
Thomas K. Burch
Elwood D. Carlson
David A. Coleman
Henriette Engelhardt
Frances Goldscheider
Joshua Goldstein
Andy Hinde
Vladimíra Kantorová
Kathleen E. Kiernan
Hans-Peter Kohler
Irena Kotowska
Øystein Kravdal
Hill Kulu
Ron Lesthaeghe
Aart C. Liefbroer

Marc Luy
Torkild Hovde Lyngstad
Peter F. McDonald
Clara Mulder
Michael Murphy
Gerda Neyer
Máire Ní Bhrolcháin
Brienna Perelli-Harris
Dimiter Philipov
Harriet B. Presser
Thomas W. Pullum
Jean-Louis Rallu
Marit Rønsen
Robert Schoen
Steve Smallwood
Maria Rita Testa
Elizabeth Thomson
Jacques Vallin
Dirk van de Kaa
Nico van Nimwegen
Andres Vikat
Charles F. Westoff
Frans Willekens
Kryštof Zeman

Summary and general conclusions:
Childbearing Trends and Policies in Europe

Tomas Frejka[1]

Tomáš Sobotka[2]

Jan M. Hoem[3]

Laurent Toulemon[4]

1. Introduction

European fertility early in the 21st century was at its lowest level since the Second World War. This study explores contemporary childbearing trends and policies in Europe, and gives detailed attention to the past two or three decades. We felt motivated to undertake this project because in many European countries, as well as for the European Union as a whole, the overall fertility level and its consequences are of grave concern and draw attention on the political stage. Our account focuses somewhat more on the previously state socialist countries of Central and Eastern Europe, where available knowledge about the impact on childbearing of the momentous political and economic transition that started in 1989 remains relatively scarce.

As family formation and childbearing behaviour are inherent components of societal life, they were influenced and modified by the various political, economic, and social changes that took place in Europe during the past 60 years. There were also profound changes in norms, values, beliefs, and attitudes regarding family and childbearing, and these exerted additional effects on fertility and family trends. To identify such effects, this study pays much attention to the influence of social and family policies on fertility, to the influence of political and economic changes on fertility and family trends, and to the diverse ways changes in values, norms, and attitudes relate to the transformation in family-related behaviour in Europe. In the present chapter, we outline main issues discussed in the subsequent overview chapters, and summarise the main findings of the entire study.

[1] E-mail: Tfrejka@aol.com
[2] Vienna Institute of Demography. E-mail: Tomas.Sobotka@oeaw.ac.at
[3] Max Planck Institute for Demographic Research. E-mail: hoem@demogr.mpg.de
[4] Institut national d'études démographiques (INED). E-mail: toulemon@ined.fr

2. Contemporary fertility levels and trends

During most of the second half of the 20th century, political and economic institutions in Central and Eastern European (CEE) countries differed substantially from those in Northern, Western, and Southern Europe. This created very different environments for family formation and childbearing, which was mirrored in contrasting fertility levels and trends. In the CEE countries, fertility declined in the 1950s and 1960s, while it was relatively high in the rest of Europe, where many countries experienced a baby boom. Conversely, fertility declined rapidly in Northern, Western, and Southern Europe, and was low during the 1970s and 1980s, whereas the CEE countries maintained higher fertility around the replacement level.

The collapse of the authoritarian regimes throughout CEE around 1990 went hand-in-hand with substantial changes in family and reproductive behaviour, expressed in an abrupt decline of fertility to very low levels. In the meantime, a differentiation in childbearing behaviour had taken place in the other parts of Europe. In the countries of Northern and Western Europe, with about one-quarter of Europe's population, fertility stabilised at levels moderately below replacement with total fertility rates (TFRs) between 1.7 and 2.0 births per woman. Fertility continued to decline to very low levels in Southern Europe and in the predominantly German-speaking countries. In the first decade of the 21st century, three-quarters of Europe's population live in countries with TFRs between 1.3 and 1.6 births per woman, namely in the latter two regions and in the CEE countries.

An early childbearing pattern, typical of the baby boom period of the 1950s and 1960s, and retained in Central and Eastern Europe until the mid-1990s, has been replaced by a late pattern characterised by a pronounced delay of entry into parenthood. This secular trend towards later childbearing has contributed greatly to the decline and to the fluctuations in period TFRs. A share of the delayed births was eventually recuperated, especially among childless women, but the extent of recuperation differs by country and region. In Western and Northern Europe, most of the delayed births were recuperated by the time women reached their late twenties and thirties. This recuperation has been notably smaller in the German-speaking countries and in Southern Europe. In most of the formerly state socialist countries, any recuperation of delayed births has been weak so far, especially for second and higher-order births.

3. Change in family size and parity distribution

There were many differences in average family size and in parity distribution across European countries at the end of the 20th century. Nevertheless, the two-child family clearly became the norm. Between 40 and 55 percent of women in the cohorts born in the 1950s and 1960s had two children. Among recent generations, there has been an almost universal increase in childlessness, though this development is not uniform across countries. There were also some incipient signs that the share of two-child families is declining in a number of countries, especially in Central, Eastern, and Southern Europe, where there has been a marked increase in one-child families, and where the share of families with three or more children has continued to decline.

4. Completing the contraceptive revolution

The diffusion of modern contraception has played an important role in giving women control over their reproduction. In tandem with relatively easy access to legal induced abortions, it has affected childbearing behaviour in a number of ways. It has reduced the incidence of unwanted and mistimed pregnancies and births, especially among very young women. It has made it easier for women and couples to postpone their births, and it has provided them with a tool to time pregnancies better than before, and thus to have a more effective control over other life-cycle events, such as education, employment, career development, and marriage. Modern methods of birth control, most recently also including assisted reproduction, constitute major tools for people to have the number of children that best suit their circumstances and reproductive desires. However, historical evidence suggests that the introduction and diffusion of modern contraceptives and relatively easy access to legal induced abortions has had only a marginal influence on fertility levels.

5. The search for explanatory mechanisms

A central issue for all the authors involved in this project is the identification of factors that have generated the respective childbearing trends. In pursuing this goal, we realize that we are faced with a dynamic research situation, and that findings and conclusions may have to be modified as new knowledge emerges. Our starting point is the notion that, under persistent societal norms supporting motherhood, most women will want to have at least one child, given reasonably favourable circumstances.

During the initial decades of the modern welfare state and during the economic growth of the 1950s and early 1960s in the West, marriage was almost universal and fertility was high compared to the low levels of the 1930s. Numerous interacting factors then brought about the precipitous fertility decline of the 1960s and 1970s, and led to the ensuing sub-replacement fertility. The basic demographic mechanism underlying these fertility levels and trends consisted of delayed family formation and childbearing, and only partial subsequent recuperation of delayed births at higher ages in comparison to older generations.

Concomitant with fertility change was a transformation in the character of sexuality, union formation, and family life. Marriage rates declined dramatically, cohabitation and non-marital childbearing increased, and union instability became widespread because non-marital unions are less stable and divorce rates rose. The higher prevalence of the more fragile non-marital unions could have led to lower fertility in itself, but the relationship between changes in family behaviour, living arrangements, and fertility level is by no means straightforward. Early in the 21st century, the unprecedented changes in family life and living arrangements are not closely related to the relatively low fertility on the continent, and much less so in each individual country.

Furthermore, in most of Europe, with the Nordic countries as a partial exception, it became more difficult for young people to establish a separate household in the later decades of the 20th century, and this remains a challenge at the beginning of the 21st. It has become increasingly difficult to find stable employment and to pursue a work career. A secondary or higher-level education has become essential to secure a satisfying job. Ever larger proportions of women have joined the labour force, their status has improved, and they have enjoyed increasing independence. At the same time, the majority of household chores and the upbringing of children have primarily remained their responsibility. Also, housing costs have risen in many countries, making it difficult to secure housing for young people. New risks and uncertainties have emerged alongside changing patterns of partnership relations.

6. Explaining fertility change in Central and Eastern Europe

Developments in the countries of Central and Eastern Europe merit our special attention. During the era of state socialism, the basic demographic mechanism underlying the fertility level and its stability in the CEE countries consisted of almost universal and early marriage, a low age at childbearing with low rates of childlessness, and high rates of first and second births. Societal circumstances underpinning this demographic regime were generated and sustained by social and economic policies that were predominantly pro-natalist in nature. The socialist state and the lack of market forces created a relatively predictable and risk-free environment, and the authoritarian political system limited the range of available options for self-realisation outside the family.

Following the collapse of state socialism around 1990, young people in CEE adjusted to new conditions. This adjustment resulted in rapidly changing forms of family formation and partnership relationships, and in new patterns of childbearing, notably in a precipitous fertility decline. Two major explanations have repeatedly appeared in the literature. One argues that the economic and social crises of the early 1990s were the principal causes of the rapid demographic change. The other explanation claims that the change was essentially produced by a diffusion of western norms, values, and attitudes. Both explanations are supported by valid arguments and contain important insights, but they do not provide comprehensive answers clarifying what generated the new family and childbearing trends. They do not reflect an interpretation that arises frequently in the country chapters, namely that the structural developments involved in the replacement of the state socialist regimes with the economic and political institutions of contemporary capitalism were instrumental in effecting the fertility decline and in inducing later union formation and childbearing. This process was identified as the root cause of the demographic changes and trends during the transition period in Overview Chapter 5. The broader explanation does not deny the validity of the 'crisis' or the 'cultural and ideational' explanations. Both are inherent in the 'root cause' hypothesis. This involves the fundamental change of the societal system from a centrally planned and authoritarian system to a market economy with democratic political institutions, as well as the remarkably rapid rise in tertiary education enrolment rates, continued high female labour force participation rates, and persisting unequal gender responsibilities for child-raising and household maintenance. Arguably, without these and other structural developments, many of the changes in values and attitudes might not have materialised. As political, economic, social, and cultural changes in many CEE countries were closely intertwined and proceeded rapidly, it is practically impossible to isolate the relative importance of specific factors for the transformation observed in demographic behaviour.

7. The Second Demographic Transition

As we mentioned above, the fertility decline and postponement that got underway in the late 1960s and the early 1970s in Northern and Western Europe were accompanied by a transformation in norms, values, and attitudes regarding family life and childbearing. These developments have been termed the Second Demographic Transition (SDT) by Ron Lesthaeghe and Dirk van de Kaa, whose basic proposition is that ideational change in a broad sense (in combination with the 'contraceptive revolution') constituted the main driving mechanism that produced changes in demographic behaviour. The change in family-related values gradually diffused to Southern Europe, and most of its demographic manifestations were observed in the 1990s in the formerly state socialist countries of CEE as well.

More specifically, in most of Europe there has been an increase in the acceptance of intimate relationships among un-partnered individuals, as well as an acceptance of non-family living arrangements and of childlessness, and a positive evaluation of cohabitation as a premarital stage and as an alternative to marriage. Non-marital childbearing has also become widely accepted, especially within stable cohabiting unions, whereas childbearing to single mothers is still mostly regarded as undesirable. At the same time, the family has not become an obsolete institution. On the contrary, family life — though in more diverse forms — continues to be highly and almost universally valued, and parenthood remains at the top of many people's life priorities. What has changed is the motivation for parenthood. Childbearing is less frequently seen as a 'duty towards society' or as an inescapable destiny, and it has increasingly become a result of a planned decision of each couple, who in their decision-making process may consider various potential positive and negative effects of parenthood on their relationship, lifestyle, and economic wellbeing. Parenthood increasingly serves individual self-fulfilment and private joy, but it is also taken very seriously, and there is a considerable emphasis on responsible parenthood and the well-being of the children.

Without a doubt, these changes in norms and values do not take place in isolation from broader economic and social developments; increasing prosperity, rising educational levels, and the rapid spread of labour force participation among women are among the factors that typically accompany the Second Demographic Transition. Several country studies for Central and Eastern Europe included in our project question the validity of the SDT hypothesis as an explanation for the rapid change in demographic behaviour there, and suggest that structural factors were the main generators of these changes. They also show that some of these changes, notably the rise of non-marital childbearing, were initially experienced by disadvantaged population strata in the CEE countries, something that does not fit in the "classical" SDT narrative. This new behaviour has then gradually been adopted by other social groups, and has eventually led to wider attitudinal change.

In our analysis in Overview Chapter 6, we suggest that there appear to be two distinct pathways in the SDT. Along the first pathway, cultural and value changes are driven by economic affluence and are characterised by secular individualism and by an orientation towards personal self-fulfilment as a precondition to large-scale change in family behaviour. The second pathway, typical especially of the CEE countries, may first lead to an emergence of new family behaviour, especially in disadvantaged strata, as a response to changed structural conditions in society. Subsequently, this behaviour gradually becomes accepted and adopted by other social groups, which in turn leads to wider changes in attitudes towards it. This pathway does not conform to the original SDT conceptualisation.

Finally, it is important to note that the experiences of the countries that were forerunners in the SDT process, namely the Nordic and Western European countries, suggest that the second demographic transition does not necessarily lead to the long-lasting decline in fertility to sub-replacement levels, which originally was considered an SDT hallmark.

8. The effects of migration on childbearing

Migration streams to Northern, Western, and Southern Europe have been substantial after 1990, and immigration has become the main source of population growth. An increasing proportion of births in Europe are attributable to immigrants. The question arises whether immigration has had a significant impact on fertility levels.

In general, immigrant women in Europe tend to have higher fertility than indigenous women, in particular shortly after immigration. Typical trends indicate a gradual decline of differentials between immigrants and natives as time since migration increases. Even though immigrant fertility is relatively high, its impact on overall total fertility rates is rather small, mainly because the immigrant population constitutes only a fraction of the total population in most countries. In recent years, immigrants' childbearing raised the TFR in Northern, Southern and Western Europe by three to seven percent, exceptionally by 10 percent.

There are also substantial differences between immigrants and natives in their living arrangements, marriage patterns, and non-marital fertility. Despite these pronounced initial differences, many immigrant groups converge in their fertility behaviour to native women quite rapidly. Especially women who immigrate as children are likely to have fertility levels similar to those of natives.

Experience to date has shown that migration can modify fertility, population size, growth, and structure of European countries. However, a massive amount of immigration would be required to alter substantially contemporary fertility patterns in Europe. On balance, effects of migration could be beneficial by sustaining the size of the labour force and slowing the ageing process. Contemporary economic prosperity and the political stability of most European countries make them attractive destinations for many potential migrants. At the same time, migration is also unstable and is the least predictable component of population change. Furthermore, immigration has become a political question in many countries of Europe, and the lack of will to accommodate and assimilate migrants among the receiving population can be a limiting circumstance.

9. Do public policies affect fertility?

Methodologically, it is difficult to ascertain to what extent individual public policies have had an impact on fertility levels, and how long any such effect has lasted. Depending on the nature of the policies, their impact may have been restricted to influencing mainly the timing of childbearing. To design and recommend policies to modify childbearing behaviour can be even more of a challenge, especially considering that there is a lack of consensus among scholars on the desirability and effectiveness of different policy measures.

Nevertheless, there is evidence that a consistent system of population and family policies can effectively sustain or modify fertility levels in contemporary societies. Total fertility rates have been maintained relatively close to the replacement level in countries where principles of gender equity in the household and in society have been systematically nurtured for extended periods of time, and have been supplemented by wide-ranging societal support for childbearing. Material and structural measures alone, such as paid parental leaves and child bonuses, even when generous, seem to have a limited influence on fertility when they are implemented in a "traditional" male-dominated societal environment. Policy makers need to apply a holistic approach and to use a comprehensive range of policies, which must be sustained over a long period of time to have an appreciable impact on the fertility level.

10. Conclusions and outlook for the foreseeable future

At present, European countries have different levels of low fertility, and there are no signs of a convergence between them. There is also no indication that either childbearing incentives or constraints are likely to change substantially in the near future. In Northern and Western Europe, it is reasonable to assume that fertility will be maintained close to the replacement level. In Southern, Central, and Eastern Europe, some increase in fertility rates may occur, but even so fertility will most probably remain well below replacement. The direction of main trends in family formation and fertility behaviour, values, and attitudes seems reasonably clear. Childbearing and union formation will almost certainly occur later than in previous decades in most countries, the new forms of partnership will probably continue to be practiced, whereas the value attached to the family and parenthood looks likely to remain high. In any case, population ageing will progress to unprecedented levels.

Europe will continue to be attractive to migrants from many other parts of the world, but in the receiving countries there are noticeable pressures, political and popular, to restrict immigration flows. How these countervailing forces will play out is not clear. It is, however, doubtful that migration flows would take on dimensions that would have a sizable impact on national fertility levels in the near future.

At present there is no evidence of coming discontinuities in the basic institutional configurations that affect fertility and family in Europe. Considerable social, political, and economic change, as well as significant alterations in family values, would have to occur to make a real difference in fertility levels. Fertility could possibly be modified by policy measures, but they would have to be durable and of a major dimension to have a long-lasting effect on fertility trends. Unless the institutional environment changes, most European countries, except for those in Northern and Western Europe, may increasingly have to rely on immigration to maintain their population size. Alternatively, they seem to face the prospect of population decline.

Demographic Research: Volume 19, Article 3
research article

Overview Chapter 1:
Fertility in Europe: Diverse, delayed and below replacement

Tomas Frejka[1]

Tomáš Sobotka[2]

Abstract

Early in the 21st century, three-quarters of Europe's population lived in countries with fertility considerably below replacement. This general conclusion is arrived at irrespective of whether period or cohort fertility measures are used. In Western and Northern Europe, fertility quantum was slightly below replacement. In Southern, Central and Eastern Europe, fertility quantum as measured by the period total fertility rate (TFR) and its tempo-adjusted version was markedly below replacement; in many countries it was around 1.5, and in some populations it was as low as 1.3 to 1.4 births per woman. Throughout Europe, a historic transformation of childbearing patterns characterised by a pronounced delay of entry into parenthood has been taking place. This secular trend towards later childbearing has greatly contributed to the decline and fluctuations in period fertility rates. Delayed births were being recuperated, especially among childless women, but the extent of recuperation differs by country and region. All in all, despite a recent upward trend in the period TFR, European fertility early in the 21st century was at its lowest point since the Second World War.

[1] E-mail: Tfrejka@aol.com

[2] Vienna Institute of Demography. E-mail: Tomas.Sobotka@oeaw.ac.at

1. Background

In contemporary Europe, fertility levels and trends are of grave concern—and for good reasons. There was not a single European country in 2005 with a total fertility rate at or above the replacement level (Eurostat 2007)[3]. In the absence of migration, sustained fertility at or below 1.5 births per woman would lead to such a rapidly declining and ageing population that, as a demographic outlook, it "might well be judged unacceptable" (Demeny and McNicoll 2006: 281). The resulting large proportions of the old and very old would signify major burdens for individuals and societies, including costly health care and large pension expenditures. In addition, any influx of immigrants large enough to offset very low fertility levels would be of dimensions likely to make their integration difficult, and could cause serious social and political tensions and problems.

There is a general consensus among scholars that "maintaining fertility at a level that does not fall much below a two-child average – say, around 1.7 – 1.8" (Demeny and McNicoll 2006: 281), would make population ageing and the eventual population decline easier to manage. It is within this framework that the present project has set out to assess and discuss levels, trends, and prospects of childbearing in Europe.

This chapter provides an overview of period and cohort fertility rates in Europe during recent decades, and discusses crucial relevant issues. Section 2 provides an overview of period fertility levels and trends during the past half century. Using period data, Section 3 discusses childbearing postponement, and the extent to which fertility delays lead to distortions in period total fertility rates. Methods that might be used to overcome these distortions are briefly reviewed and adjusted period TFRs for European regions are also presented. Levels and trends in completed cohort fertility rates are discussed in Section 4. In Section 5, childbearing patterns of cohorts that were in different stages of their reproductive periods early in the 21st century are utilized to illustrate the extent of actual recent birth delays and recuperation. Section 6 summarizes conclusions.

---

[3] In this chapter Europe is defined by particular geopolitical boundaries, which include the Asian part of Russia and exclude Turkey and the Transcaucasian countries (Armenia, Azerbaijan, and Georgia).

2. The spread of very low period fertility and the emergence of new fertility divides in Europe

As a consequence of the multiple constraints childrearing imposes on parents, combined with a smaller desired family size and a strong trend towards postponement of parenthood, many European countries have experienced a decline of the period total fertility rate (TFR) to 'very low' (below 1.5), or 'lowest-low' (below 1.3) levels. This process has been particularly rapid during the 1990s, when most post-socialist societies of Central and Eastern Europe joined the latter group during their complex societal transformation (see Overview Chapter 5). In 2002, 16 out of 39 European countries with populations above 100,000 (excluding Turkey) recorded period TFR below 1.3, and 25 countries recorded period TFR below 1.5 (Figure 1). The 'lowest-low' fertility – first analyzed extensively by Kohler, Billari and Ortega (2002) – spread throughout Europe with breathtaking speed, affecting countries with more than one half of the European population by 2002 (Figure 2), up from nil in the early 1990s. This proportion has subsequently declined as the TFR in several large countries (Italy, Russia, and Spain) has bounced back above the threshold of 1.3, or fluctuated around that level. Almost three-quarters of Europeans currently live in societies with a TFR below 1.5, whereas the remaining one-quarter live in countries with a TFR above 1.7 (Figure 2). Although these thresholds are arbitrary, they enable us to identify societies where sustained low fertility might become a serious social and economic problem in the future. In the absence of sizeable immigration, an extended period of several decades of 'lowest-low' fertility would inevitably result in a long-term population decline.[4]

While all European societies currently experience sub-replacement fertility rates, the contemporary European fertility map is characterized by sizeable regional contrasts that have crystallized after 1990 (Figure 3). Larger European regions seem to form relatively coherent units, within which different countries experience similar fertility levels and trends. Countries of Western and Northern Europe (excluding the German-speaking countries) form a 'higher-fertility belt' in Europe, with total fertility rates that are relatively close to the replacement level threshold, ranging in 2006 between 1.7 (the Netherlands and Belgium) and 2.0 (France). Fertility levels in these countries also come close to that of the United States, where period fertility rates have never fallen much below two children per woman, and the period TFR bounced back to 2.10 in 2006

---

[4] A stable population with no external migration experiences an annual population decline of 1.5 percent when total fertility remains constant at 1.3, and of 1.0 percent when it remains constant at 1.5. The former implies a halving time in population size of 45 years, whereas the latter value implies a halving time of 66 years.

Figure 1: **Number of European countries with a period TFR below 1.7, 1.5, and 1.3 in 1970-2005 (out of 39 countries with population above 100,000)**

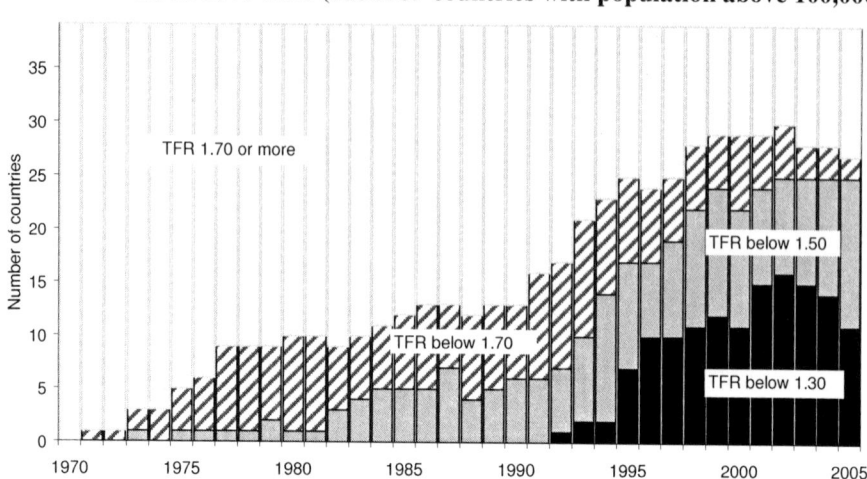

Source: Authors' computations based on Eurostat (2006, 2007) and Council of Europe (2006).
Note: Montenegro counted as a part of the former republic of Serbia-Montenegro.

Figure 2: **Proportion of Europeans living in countries with a period TFR below 1.7, 1.5, and 1.3 (1970-2005)**

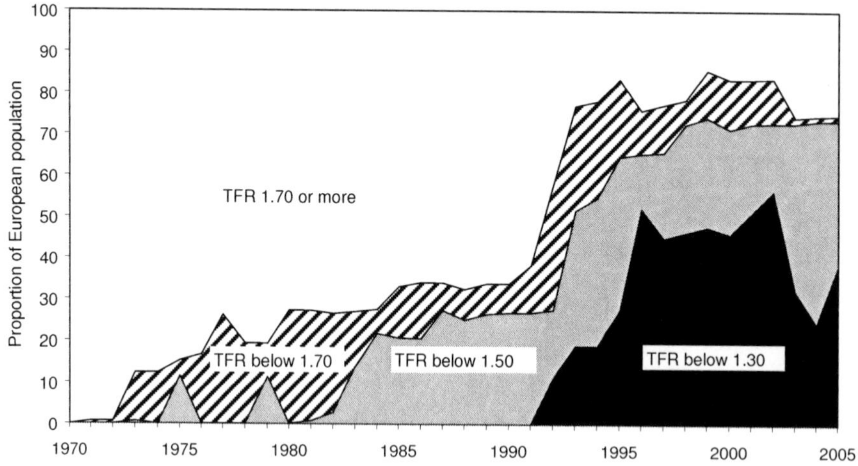

Source: Authors' computations based on Eurostat (2006, 2007) and Council of Europe (2006).

(Hamilton, Martin and Ventura 2007). This 'high' fertility is an outcome of considerable regional, social, religious, and ethnic diversity in fertility patterns (Morgan 1996, Frejka 2004, Lesthaeghe and Neidert 2006). All other regions of Europe have low period TFRs, ranging between 1.2 and 1.5 (several countries and regions of Southeastern Europe, including Albania and Kosovo, constitute an exception). These new regional differences in period fertility gave rise to various explanations of this divide, including those centered on differences in the character of family and gender equality (McDonald 2000, see also Italy chapter), and, more generally, on differences in welfare state regimes and family policies (e.g., France chapter). McDonald (2006) suggests that there is a 'cultural divide' between countries with very low fertility and those with 'moderately low fertility,' where the total fertility rate of 1.5 constitutes a dividing threshold. He further argues that countries with very low fertility should consider policy action to increase fertility rates[5] (see also discussion on fertility policies in Overview Chapter 8).

The argument about a possible cultural divide has an inherent limitation, because it is based on period measures which are influenced by the *tempo effect*—i.e., the distortion caused by shifts in the timing of childbearing[6]—rather than on completed fertility of specific cohorts. Thus, some countries may have experienced a very low period TFR level due to a rapid shift in childbearing ages, rather than because of a very low 'underlying' fertility level. As Figures 6 and 7 indicate, relatively few countries are likely to reach a completed fertility rate below 1.5 in the foreseeable future. Although it is reasonable to expect that the current European divides in low fertility will persist in the next two decades, past experience of sudden shifts and reversals in period fertility suggest that the future may not be entirely free of surprises. Since 1950, the ranking of European regions with respect to their fertility levels has undergone several sharp reversals. The former state socialist societies of Central and Eastern Europe, where fertility trends often run in the opposite direction of trends in other regions of Europe, shifted from being the highest fertility region of Europe in the 1950s, to become the lowest fertility region of Europe in the early 1960s, and then again the highest fertility

---

[5] This call for policy action also rests on a hypothesis of a 'low fertility trap,' formulated by Skirbekk, Lutz and Testa (2006), which posits that, once the fertility level falls below a certain threshold, fertility decline may become self-reinforcing and almost impossible to reverse.

[6] A tempo effect can either inflate or depress period fertility rates. The inflation is caused by an advancement of childbearing, which implies that women are bearing children at progressively younger ages and childbearing schedules of different cohorts overlap to a grater extent than would be the case otherwise. On the other hand, when women postpone childbearing to later ages and the mean age at childbearing (especially at first births) increases, many births that would otherwise have occurred in a given year are put off into the future, and period fertility rates are consequently depressed. This situation is typical of contemporary Europe. Thus, a tempo effect may lead to a considerable divergence between the cohort fertility rates and the commonly used period fertility indicators, such as the TFR (Bongaarts and Feeney 1998, Kohler, Billari, and Ortega 2002, Sobotka 2003).

region by the mid-1980s, and the lowest fertility region by the early 2000s. The relative position of the Nordic countries has also shifted repeatedly, albeit to a smaller extent (Figure 3).

As D. Glass (1937) pointed out at a time when many European countries first experienced an unprecedented decline of period fertility, any evaluation of how serious such observed trends are requires us to reflect on their likely persistence. There is a general agreement among researchers that low fertility (i.e., below-replacement fertility) is likely to persist for the coming decades (e.g., Lesthaeghe and Willems 1999). However, very low levels of the period TFR are typically a result of a combination of quantum and tempo effects, and may thus be a temporary phenomenon in many societies – in this case, 'temporary' could also mean several decades (see also below). Nevertheless, even such a time-limited rapid fall in the period TFR to very low levels has serious consequences for the respective society, as it usually brings a distinct decrease in the number of births. Thus a decline in the period TFR, though limited in duration, can nonetheless affect the future generation size and create imbalances in the age structure of a population.

3. Delayed childbearing and tempo distortions in period fertility rates

Delayed entry into parenthood has become a universal feature of European fertility trends (Kohler, Billari and Ortega 2002; Sobotka 2004a; Frejka and Sardon 2004, 2005, 2006, and 2007). By the early 2000s, practically all European societies, including the countries of the former Soviet Union, experienced the onset of fertility postponement (Figure 4). In many countries of Western, Northern, and Southern Europe, women now enter motherhood at an average age of 28-29 years, up from age 24-25 in the early 1970s. Spanish and Swiss women have become the oldest first-time mothers in Europe (with a mean age of 29.3 in 2005; see the chapter on Spain in this volume). Women in the post-communist countries of Central and Eastern Europe have children at an earlier age, but Central European countries, in particular, have seen an intensive trend towards postponement of childbearing since the mid-1990s (e.g., the Czech Republic chapter). Interestingly, the shift to later childbearing has progressed with a much higher intensity in most parts of Europe than in the United States (Figure 4), which records considerably higher teenage childbearing rates and marked social status heterogeneity in childbearing patterns.

This pronounced delay in childbearing is reflected in the changing age pattern of fertility. Unlike in the U.S., teenage childbearing has become marginal in many parts of Europe, especially in Western, Northern, and Southern Europe (with the notable exception of the United Kingdom, and, to a smaller extent, also Ireland and Portugal), and fertility rates below age 25 have fallen drastically. In many countries, less than one-fifth of births are to women under the age of 25 (Figure 5). In parallel, the peak of childbearing is shifting to ages 30-32 in many populations: in Italy and Spain, women over age 30 contribute almost 60 percent to the overall period total fertility. Whereas the age schedule of fertility is shifting in all parts of Europe, the absolute increase in fertility rates past ages 28-30 differs greatly between countries, indicating wide differences in the pace of fertility recuperation, and contributing greatly to regional heterogeneity in fertility levels (e.g., Lesthaeghe and Willems 1999, see also below). Childbearing rates also increase rapidly at very late childbearing ages (40+), but, all in all, very late fertility still remains rather marginal (Sobotka, Kohler, and Billari 2007).

Figure 3: **Period total fertility rate in major regions of Europe and in the United States, 1950-2006**

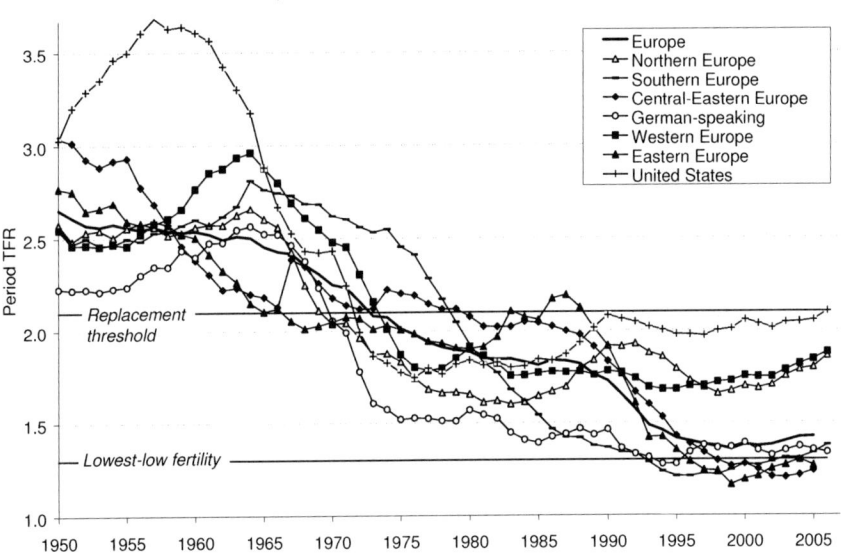

Source: Authors' computations based on Eurostat (2006, 2007), Council of Europe (2006), Festy (1979), Chesnais (1986) and
   national statistical data.
Notes: Data are weighted by the population size of given countries and regions.
Countries are grouped into regions as follows:
Western Europe: Belgium, France, Ireland, Luxembourg, the Netherlands, and the United Kingdom;
German-speaking countries: Austria, Germany, and Switzerland;
Northern Europe: Denmark, Finland, Iceland, Norway, and Sweden;
Southern Europe: Cyprus, Greece, Italy, Malta, Portugal, and Spain;
Central-Eastern Europe: Croatia, Czech Republic, Estonia, Hungary, Latvia, Lithuania, Poland, Slovakia, Slovenia, Bosnia-
   Herzegovina, Bulgaria, Macedonia, Montenegro, Romania, and Serbia & Kosovo;
Eastern Europe: Belarus, Moldova, Russia, and Ukraine.

Figure 4:   Mean age of women at first childbirth in selected countries and regions of Europe and in the United States, 1960-2005 (arithmetic averages)

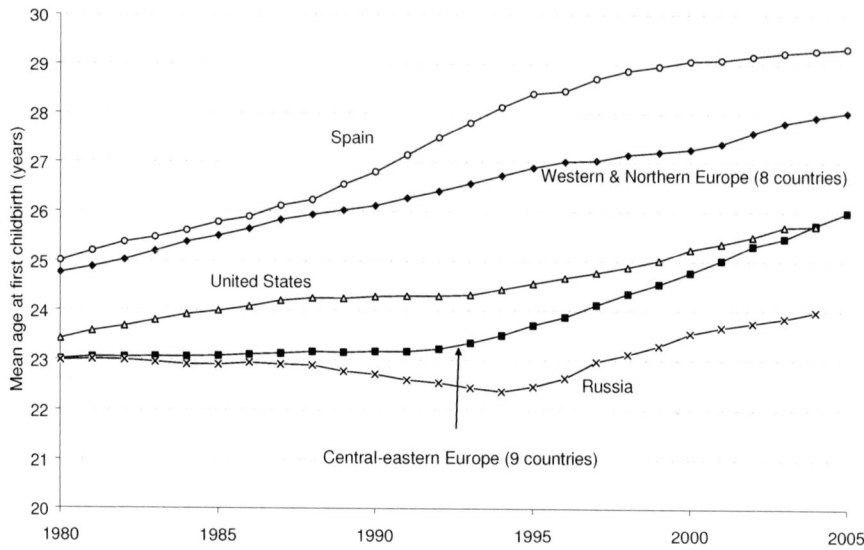

Source: Authors' computations based on Council of Europe (2006), Eurostat (2006, 2007) and national vital statistics data.
Note: See Figure 3 for the specification of regional groupings of individual countries.

The ongoing shift towards later parenthood has led to a reduction in the commonly used period total fertility rates, which does not necessarily reflect underlying changes in the level of fertility. Various methods have been proposed to correct the shortcomings of the conventional TFR, and to provide a measure of the 'underlying' period fertility quantum, undistorted by the changes in fertility timing (e.g., Bongaarts and Feeney 1998, and Kohler and Ortega 2002). Although these adjustments have become increasingly common, a number of researchers have questioned their usefulness and interpretation (e.g., van Imhof 2001, Smallwood 2002, Schoen 2004). The adjustment methods are based on various underlying assumptions, and most of them are considerably more data-demanding than the computation of the ordinary TFR. In particular, the simplest adjustment, proposed by Bongaarts and Feeney, has been criticized for having unrealistic assumptions, of which the most problematic is the assumption that the shape of the fertility schedule by age remains constant when

Figure 5: **Fraction of period total fertility rates contributed by women below age 25 in selected countries and regions of Europe and in the United States, 1960-2004 (arithmetic averages)**

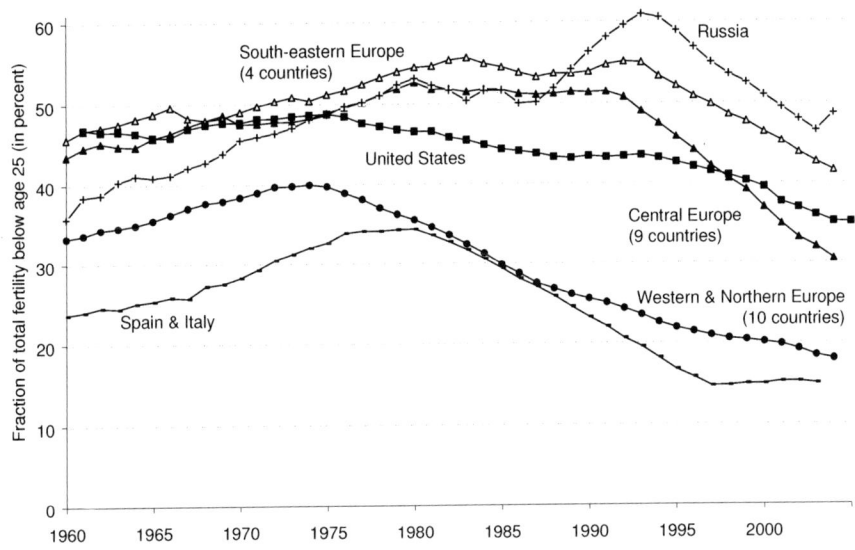

Source: Authors' computations based on Council of Europe (2006) and national vital statistics data.
Note: Regional grouping differs partly from the grouping in Figure 4 as Central-Eastern Europe is split into two regions, Central Europe and Southeastern Europe. See Table 1 below for the specification of regional groupings of individual countries.

childbearing shifts towards later ages, i.e., the premise that, in a given period, women of all age categories 'postpone' or 'advance' births to the same extent.

Despite these shortcomings, the adjusted indicators seem to provide a more realistic picture of current European fertility trends and differentials than the period TFR, especially when the focus is on longer time periods (these indicators often suffer from considerable short-term fluctuations). In addition, they come closer to the completed cohort fertility of women who are in their prime childbearing years at the time of observation (Sobotka 2003). One of the innovative features of this collection is that many country chapters employ various alternative methods of period fertility measurement to evaluate how fertility postponement reduces the values of the observed period TFRs. The methods used range from the Bongaarts-Feeney (1998) adjusted TFR (see chapters on Bulgaria, England and Wales, Lithuania, and the Russian Federation), through the Kohler-Ortega (2002) adjusted fertility index PATFR (a fertility index controlling for parity and age; chapters on the Czech Republic, Poland, and Slovakia), and period parity progression ratios (England and Wales); to a fertility index based on age-specific childbearing intensities for first births, and duration-specific fertility rates for second and higher-order births (Period Average Parity, PAP; chapters on Austria and France).

While the adjustment proposed by Kohler-Ortega is methodologically superior to the Bongaarts-Feeney method; and, while the PAP provides an 'adjustment-free' alternative to the TFR, their computation is data intensive and cannot be provided for a large number of European countries and regions. Consequently, to make a European-wide comparison of the recent levels of period fertility adjusted for tempo effects, we utilize estimates of the Bongaarts-Feeney adjusted TFR for the period 2001-2003 provided by the Vienna Institute of Demography (VID 2006)[7]. These results are grouped in Table 1 for the main regions of Europe and compared to the conventional TFR in 2002, as well as to the Bongaarts-Feeney tempo-adjusted TFR estimated for 1995-2000 (Sobotka 2004b). This exercise confirms that, even if tempo distortions are taken into account, all European regions have sub-replacement fertility, and considerable heterogeneity among countries and regions prevails. In addition, this cross-country variability has increased slightly since 1995-2000 due to the decline in the adjusted TFR in Southern Europe to the low level of 1.43, and due to a lesser decline in Central-Eastern Europe to 1.66.

The 'higher-fertility' regions of Western and Northern Europe (except for the German-speaking countries) retain a stable level of the adjusted TFR above 1.8, with some countries surpassing 2.0 (Ireland, 2.22; Norway, 2.07; France, 2.02). By contrast, some of the 'lowest-fertility' countries, such as Italy, Poland, and Spain, have seen a further drop in the adjusted TFR. Thus, the division of Europe into a group of countries with 'moderately low' fertility, and a group of countries with 'very low fertility,' as suggested by the unadjusted TFR, is also mirrored in the adjusted TFR levels. However, a number of countries do not fit completely in this division. Most countries of Central-Eastern Europe, where the tempo effect is currently the largest in Europe, have reached extremely low TFR levels of 1.2-1.3[8] but only moderately low levels of the adjusted TFR at 1.6-1.7. The estimated tempo-adjusted level of fertility is much lower in the European countries of the former Soviet Union, where it averaged 1.45 (figures for this region are less reliable, however, due to a lack of availability of order-specific fertility data).

---

[7] Displaying the Bongaarts-Feeney adjusted TFR for larger groups of countries also decreases the risk that the adjTFR would be affected by short-term fluctuations and irregularities, and reduces the potential error caused by the violations of the underlying assumptions behind this adjustment method.

[8] Cf. Overview chapter 5, Section 5 *Effects of changing cohort fertility age patterns*, where the extraordinarily low period TFRs around 2000 in Central Eastern Europe are discussed in detail.

Table 1: **Period TFR and the estimated level of tempo-adjusted TFR in main European regions in 2001-2003 and 1995-2000**

	Population size, millions (2002)	TFR (2002)	Adj. TFR (2001–2003)	Tempo effect	Adj. TFR (1995–2000)
Western Europe	149.3	1.75	1.92	-0.17	1.88
Northern Europe	24.3	1.70	1.96	-0.26	1.94
German-speaking countries	97.8	1.32	1.53	-0.21	1.52
Southern Europe	120.4	1.28	1.43	-0.15	1.59
Central Europe	77.6	1.25	1.66	-0.41	1.74
Southeastern Europe	43.7	1.33	1.64	-0.31	1.67
Eastern Europe	205.8	1.25	1.45	-0.19	1.46
EUROPE					
EU-15	378.6	1.49	1.67	-0.18	1.70
EU-12 new (2004 & 2007 accession)	104.1	1.24	1.63	-0.39	1.67
EU-27	482.6	1.44	1.66	-0.22	1.69
Europe	722.0	1.39	1.61	-0.22	1.63

Sources: Authors' computations based on VID (2006) and Sobotka (2004b)
Notes: Data are weighted by population size of given countries and regions.
Regional grouping differs partly from the grouping in Figure 3 as Central-Eastern Europe is split into two regions, Central Europe and Southeastern Europe. Countries are grouped into regions as follows:
For Western Europe, German-speaking countries, Northern Europe, and Southern Europe see notes below Figure 3 above.
Central Europe: Croatia, Czech Republic, Estonia, Hungary, Latvia, Lithuania, Poland, Slovakia, Slovenia;
South-Eastern Europe: Bosnia-Herzegovina, Bulgaria, Macedonia, Montenegro, Romania, Serbia & Kosovo.
Eastern Europe: Belarus, Moldova (excluding Transnistria), Russia (including Asian part), Ukraine.

Overall, tempo-adjusted fertility rates have been remarkably stable in most parts of Europe after 1995, and only Southern European and Central-Eastern European countries have seen a noticeable drop in their adjusted period TFR. In addition, none of the countries analyzed in 2001-2003 and in 1995-2000 had an adjusted TFR below 1.3, which suggests that extremely low levels of the period TFR might represent temporary effects of fertility postponement (Sobotka 2004b). In 2001-2003, the whole of Europe had an adjusted TFR of 1.61, compared with the conventional TFR of 1.39; whereas the European Union (27 countries as of 2007) had an adjusted TFR of 1.66, compared with the conventional TFR of 1.44. This difference indicates there could be considerable scope for a future increase in the conventional total fertility linked to the slowing down of fertility postponement.[9] The recent increase in this indicator in many European countries—including Bulgaria, the Czech Republic, Estonia, Italy, France, the Netherlands, Spain, Sweden, and the United Kingdom—is largely attributable to fertility 'recuperation' among women past age 30, and the declining tempo effect in the TFR. In addition, the increasing size of immigrant populations with higher fertility rates has also played an important role in the observed rise in the TFR in some countries, including Italy, France, Spain, and the United Kingdom (see Overview Chapter 7). However, in each of these countries, 'native' women also experienced rising fertility rates (Dunnell 2007, Héran and Pison 2007, Gabrielli, Paterno and Strozza 2007, Roig Vila and Castro Martín 2007).

On an individual level, later timing of parenthood is associated with lower completed fertility because infertility increases with age, and women have fewer years left to attain their desired family size (Toulemon 2004, see also estimates in the model presented by Billari and Borgoni 2005). However, the aggregate effects of delayed childbearing on completed fertility may still be relatively minor, partly because most women achieve their first pregnancy at an age well before the onset of their infertility,[10] and thus can achieve their childbearing goals (at least from a biological perspective); but also partly because other factors can compensate for fertility-inhibiting effects of later motherhood. Interestingly, two chapters in this book offer a contrasting evaluation of these effects. Whereas the authors of the chapter on Spain argue that the drastic reduction of fertility rates at birth orders three and higher is "primarily the result of the late age at first motherhood," the case of France provides an indication that the shift to a late childbearing pattern does not necessarily reduce completed fertility (France chapter). Together with Sweden, France has one of the highest ages at first motherhood in Europe, and relatively stable levels of the completed cohort TFR, which remains close to the replacement threshold. This evidence indicates that, besides inducing tempo distortions of period fertility rates, the delayed entry into parenthood has so far played only a minor role in the observed shift to low and very low fertility levels in many parts of Europe (see also Overview Chapter 4).

---

[9] It should be noted, however, that the adjusted TFR is—as any other period measure of fertility—changing over time. This limits its usefulness for projecting future trends in the conventional period TFR or cohort TFR. Although one could assume that once the shift towards later childbearing stops, the conventional TFR would increasingly get close to the level of the adjusted measure, some countries may also experience a further decline in fertility quantum (and thus in the adjusted TFR), counterbalancing any increasing effects of the end of fertility postponement (Bongaarts 2002).

[10] Goldstein's (2006) analysis of cohort age schedules of first births concluded that the current populations of developed countries are still far from the (biological) upper age limits of fertility and, consequently, fertility postponement can continue for decades.

4. Completed cohort fertility levels and trends

We now turn to the exploration of cohort fertility, which has the advantage of measuring fertility quantum in an unadulterated way. The problem with completed cohort fertility rates is that these provide information about childbearing behaviour with a certain time lag. In contemporary low-fertility countries, where almost all childbearing is completed by about age 40, the time lag is approximately 10 to 15 years[11]. Nonetheless, trends of total cohort fertility rates (TCFRs) set a historical framework by illustrating long-term trends of the real quantum of fertility, i.e., average parity[12]. The shortcoming of investigations based on TCFRs can be overcome by analyzing cohort fertility patterns of generations that are in the middle of their childbearing years. This is done below in Section 5 of this chapter. Recent studies (e.g., Frejka, Sardon 2004, 2006, and 2007; Sobotka 2004a) have proven that such research can provide useful insights about contemporary fertility behaviour.

Two broad groupings of countries of almost equal size provide an appropriate illustration of long-term cohort fertility trends in Europe during the past half century, namely, (i) Western Europe, and (ii) the former socialist countries of Central and Eastern Europe.[13]

With some exceptions, cohort fertility in Western European countries generally increased among 1920s cohorts, reaching a peak among 1930s cohorts (Figure 6). This was followed by a decline among 1940s birth cohorts, which, in a number of countries, such as France and Sweden, was interrupted among the 1950s cohorts. In other countries, such as Austria, West Germany, and Spain, the descent continued in the cohorts of the 1950s and early 1960s. The outstanding feature is that completed cohort fertility was declining in virtually all Western countries among the cohorts of the early to mid-1960s, i.e., the cohorts finalizing their childbearing early in the 21st century. The one country in which TCFRs did not decline among the 1960s cohorts was Denmark.

The cohort fertility trends in the former socialist countries were even more homogeneous (Figure 7). In most of these countries, the total cohort fertility rates were stable from cohorts of the 1930s through those of the late 1950s. There were a few countries in which cohort fertility was comparatively high among the 1930s cohorts, and in which it declined rapidly from thereon, exemplified by the Slovak Republic and

---

[11] Information provided by total cohort fertility rates (TCFRs) corresponds approximately to the period when the respective birth cohort was in its prime reproductive years. For instance, the TCFR of a 1965 birth cohort in a Western country rendered in 2005 will reflect mainly the level of fertility of the decade of the 1990s; in a former socialist country, the 1965 TCFR reflects mainly fertility levels of the late 1980s.

[12] The use of cohort fertility data is also the appropriate tool to analyse real parity distributions as performed in Overview Chapter 2.

[13] These two broad groups correspond to the sum of the first four and the last three categories in Table 1, respectively.

Poland in Figure 7. Without exception, TCFRs were declining among the cohorts of the 1960s. Preliminary data indicate a continuing descent among the cohorts of the early 1970s (not shown in Figure 7).

   Regional averages of completed fertility of the 1965 cohort ranged from a high of 2.1 in Northern Europe, to lows of 1.6-1.7 in the German-speaking countries and Southern and Eastern Europe (Table 2). A number of countries had TCFRs at 2.0 and above; the larger ones were France (2.03), Ireland (2.19), Norway (2.07), Poland (2.00), and Slovakia (2.04). The lowest 1965 TCFRs were found in Germany (1.51), Austria (1.65), Switzerland (1.66), Italy (1.51), Spain (1.62), Belarus (1.62), Ukraine (1.64), and the Russian Federation (1.65). It is important to realize that all these values

Figure 6:   Total cohort fertility rates, selected Western European countries, birth cohorts 1915-1967

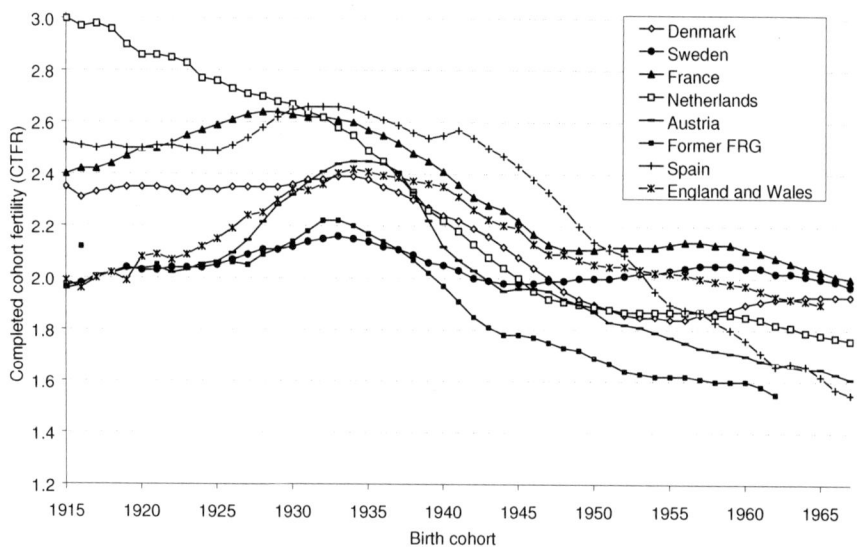

Sources: Observatoire Démographique Européen, Festy 1979, Sardon 1991 and Austria chapter.

Note: The completed fertility rates for cohorts of the 1960s contain estimates for women in their late thirties and forties. The values of the total cohort fertility rates might be moderately underestimated, but the trends depicted in the graph are affected only to a minor extent.

Figure 7: **Total cohort fertility rates, selected Central and Eastern European countries, birth cohorts 1924-1967**

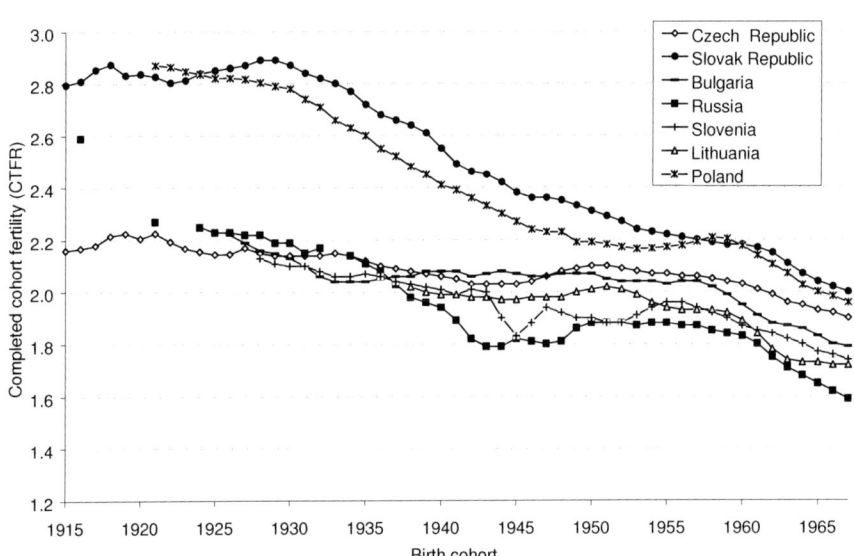

Sources: Observatoire Démographique Européen, Council of Europe (2006), Avdeev and Monnier (1995), Bolesławski (1993), the Czech Republic and Slovakia chapters.
Note: The completed fertility rates for cohorts of the 1960s contain estimates for women in their late thirties and forties. The values of the total cohort fertility rates might be moderately underestimated, but the trends depicted in the graph are affected only to a minor extent.

were within a context of declining trends in the TCFRs. In the Western countries, the 1965 cohort had experienced its main period of childbearing in the early 1990s, when these women were in their mid- to late twenties. In the former socialist countries, women of the 1965 cohort, given their early age pattern of childbearing, lived through the main proportion of their reproductive years in the mid- to late 1980s, i.e., under the conditions of the socialist centrally planned, authoritarian regimes. These were the social and economic conditions which, in most countries, helped to maintain fertility around replacement levels (cf. respective country chapters, see also Overview Chapters 5 and 6).

Table 2:   **Total cohort fertility rate, European regions, birth cohorts 1955 and 1965**

Region	Total cohort fertility rate		Difference between 1955 TCFR and 1965 TCFR	
	1955	1965	Absolute	In percent
Western Europe	2.03	1.92	−0.11	−5.4
Northern Europe	2.07	2.06	−0.01	−0.5
German-speaking countries	1.73	1.61	−0.12	−6.9
Southern Europe	1.94	1.68	−0.26	−13.4
Central Europe	2.04	1.88	−0.16	−7.8
South-Eastern Europe	2.22	2.02	−0.20	−9.0
Eastern Europe	1.87	1.64	−0.23	−12.3

Source: Council of Europe 2006.

Note: Unweighted data. Regional groupings are almost identical to those in Table 2. Data were not available for one or both years for Cyprus, Malta, Moldova, Ukraine, and Bosnia & Herzegovina.

5. Childbearing of cohorts in the midst of their reproductive period

Parenthood postponement has been a crucial factor in fertility trends in the past several decades in the advanced countries (cf. all chapters in this volume, Kohler et al. 2002, Sobotka 2004a, Frejka and Sardon 2004, 2006, 2007). Specific features of timing of births and changes in age patterns of childbearing differ between regions, from one country to another, and between social strata (e.g., by education).

In the latter part of the 20th century and early in the 21st century, the most prominent demographic mechanism determining fertility trends has been the extent to which childbearing postponement has been counterbalanced by birth recuperation. In the Western countries, this process started among the cohorts born during the 1940s (i.e., it started in the late 1960s and the early 1970s). In the former socialist countries, this process was initiated much later, among the cohorts of the 1960s. If the amount of childbearing that was presumably postponed by a cohort early in its reproductive period is fully recuperated when these women are older, cohort fertility trends are stable. Alternatively, if only a portion of the postponed births is recuperated later in the reproductive years, cohort fertility declines. The rate of cohort fertility decline will thus depend on the degree to which delayed fertility is eventually recuperated. At the same time, a thorough understanding of cohort fertility changes helps to explain period fertility trends.

The main objective of the present project is to understand contemporary, i.e., late 20th century and early 21st century, fertility levels and trends. For that purpose, fertility patterns of cohorts that were in the midst of their childbearing years at that time are explored. While such an investigation gives us important insights, it has an unavoidable shortcoming: the younger the cohort is, the less can be currently known about its lifetime childbearing behaviour. Whereas the 1960 cohort was approaching the end of its reproductive years in 2003—the last year for which data were available for all countries at the time of our analyses— the 1970 birth cohort was, for example, only 33 years old, and the 1975 cohort was only 28.

Figures 8 and 9 display developments in three countries—the Netherlands, Spain, and Bulgaria—regarding the interplay of fertility timing and quantum trends. These countries were selected because many of the typical developments occurred here, and can be well demonstrated. Trends in first and second births are studied separately, as they provide clearer insights than the investigation of all birth orders lumped together[14]. Investigation of higher order births could be added, but the additional acquired knowledge would be marginal because of the relatively small proportion of these births. In 1995-1996, first and second births accounted for 84 percent of all births in advanced low-fertility countries (Frejka and Ross 2002), and since then, this proportion has probably increased further.

In the *Netherlands,* about 82 percent of women in the 1960 cohort had become mothers, and the following cohorts were due to reach comparable levels. Women of the 1960s birth cohorts delayed the birth of their first child moderately, but all the delayed first births were recuperated later (Figures 8a and 9a). Women of the 1970s birth cohorts no longer delayed their first births; the curves of the 1970, 1975, and 1980 cohorts are almost identical (as far as the data have been available). As of the mid-2000s, it is not known whether these women will also recuperate all the supposedly delayed first births (compared to the cohorts of the early 1960s), because they are still in the initial stages of their reproductive period. Close to 70 percent of women in the 1960 cohort had a second birth, and the delaying, as well as the recuperating, propensities of subsequent cohorts were similar to first births (Figures 8b and 9b). These processes are reflected in the levels and trends of the period fertility measures by birth order, and of the period TFR. As delaying of parenthood ceased, the TFR increased during the late 1990s from 1.5 in 1996, to 1.7 births per woman in 2000, and remained at that level through 2005.

---

[14] Analyses of the aggregate data and of the birth order data provide complementary information. However, by definition the latter provide more accurate information about childbearing behaviour of women, as two similar aggregate trends of childbearing patterns can be the outcome of different birth order developments.

Figure 8: **Cumulative progression rate to first and second births; birth cohorts 1960, 1965, 1970, 1975, and 1980; the Netherlands, Spain, and Bulgaria**

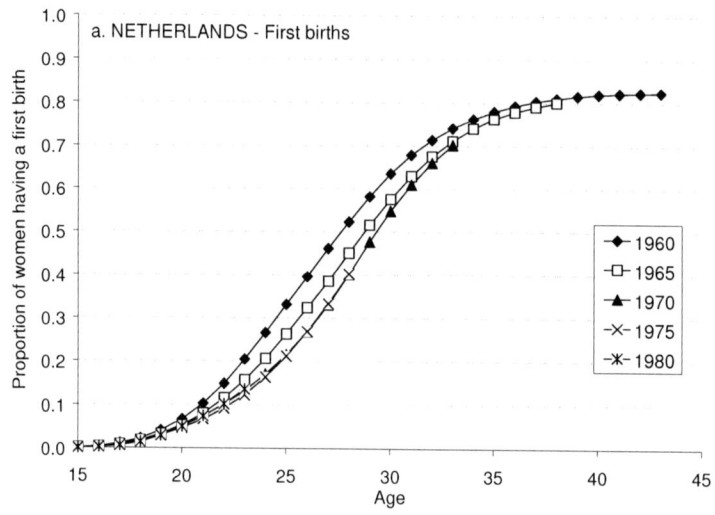

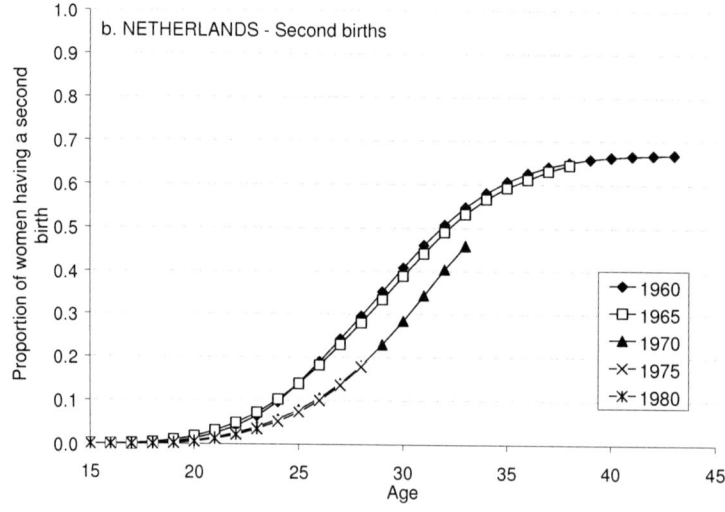

Figure 8: (Continued)

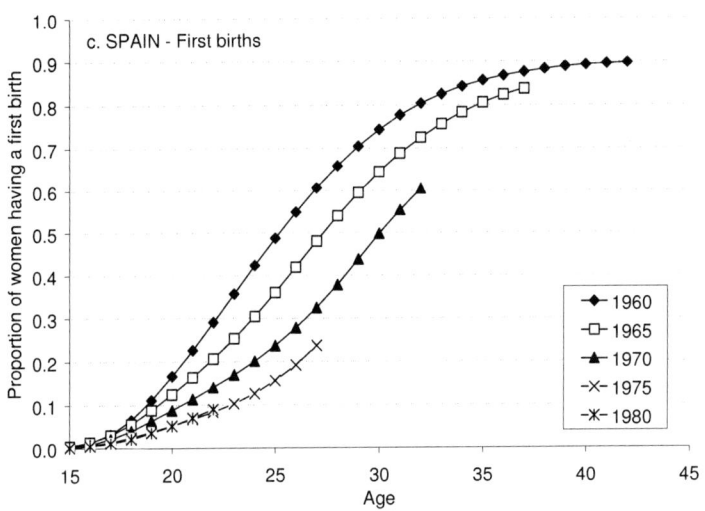

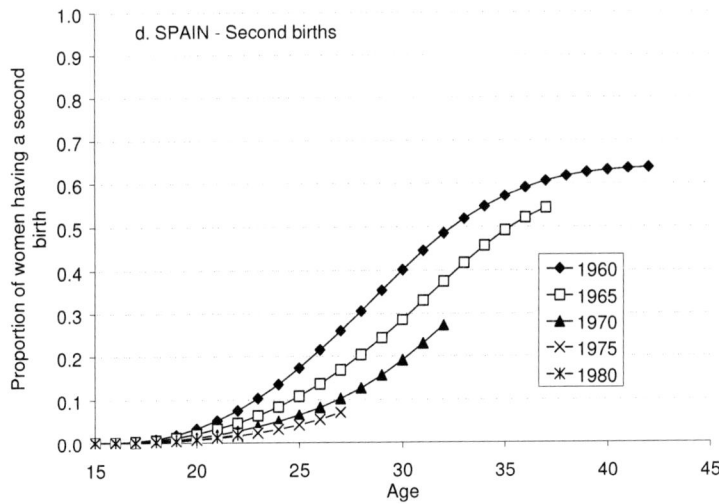

Figure 8:   (Continued)

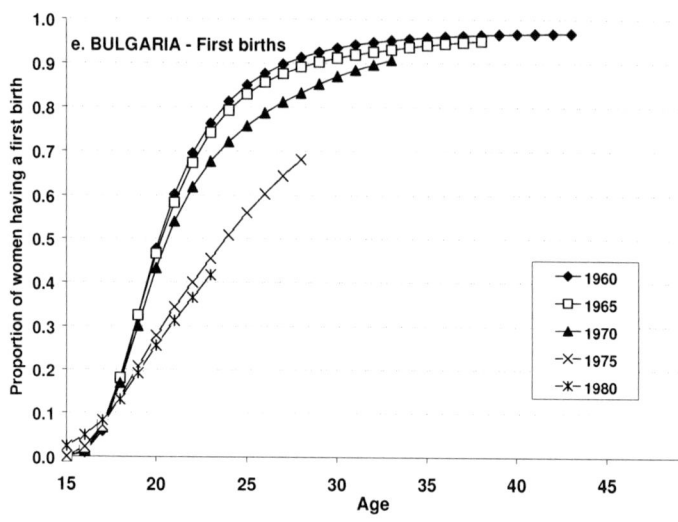

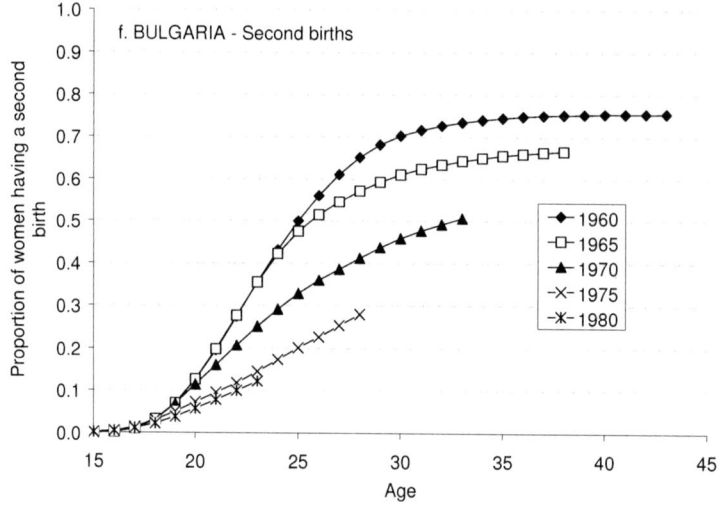

Source: Observatoire Démographique Européen.

Figure 9: **Cumulative change in first and second birth progression rates by age, birth cohorts 1960, 1965, 1970, 1975, and 1980; the Netherlands, Spain, and Bulgaria (benchmark cohort 1960)**

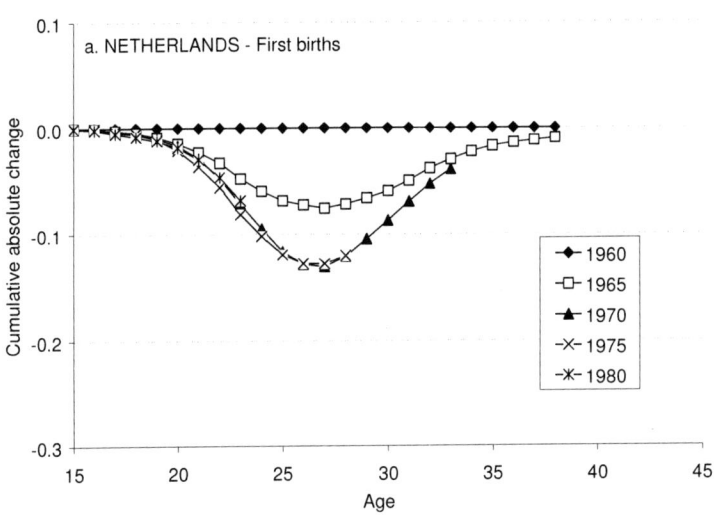

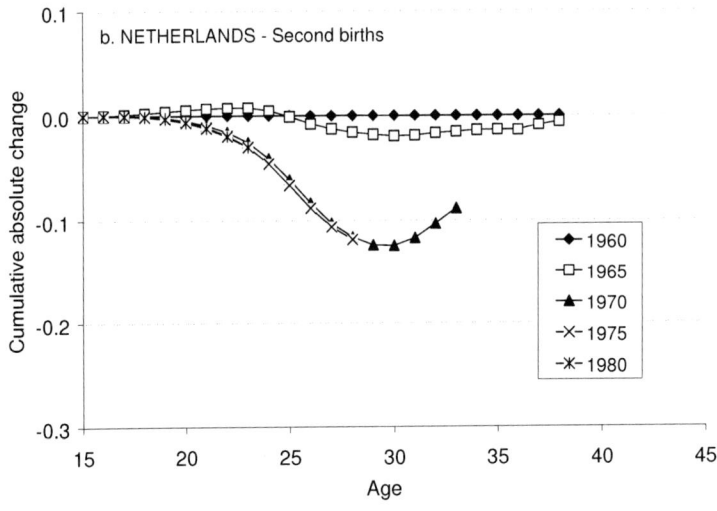

Figure 9:   (Continued)

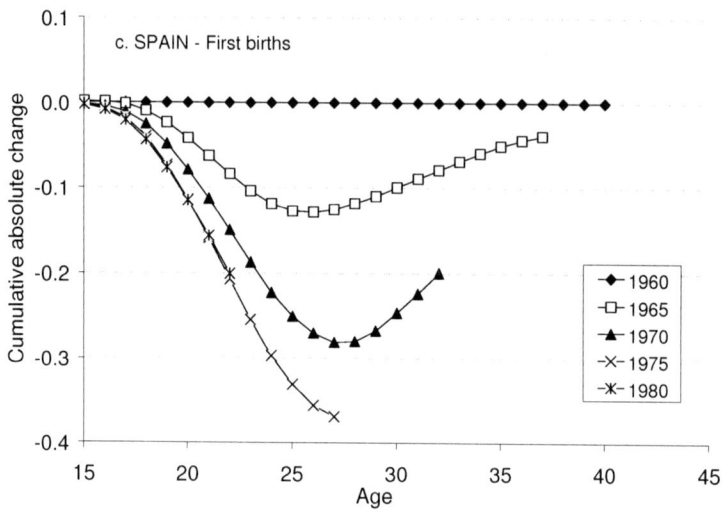

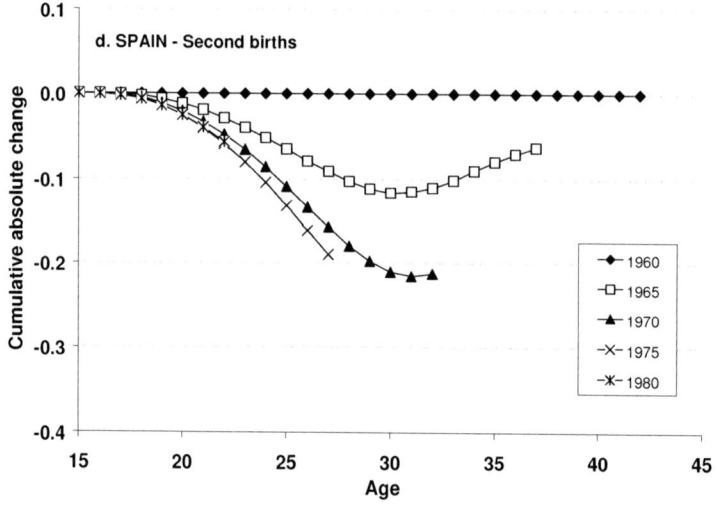

Figure 9:   (Continued)

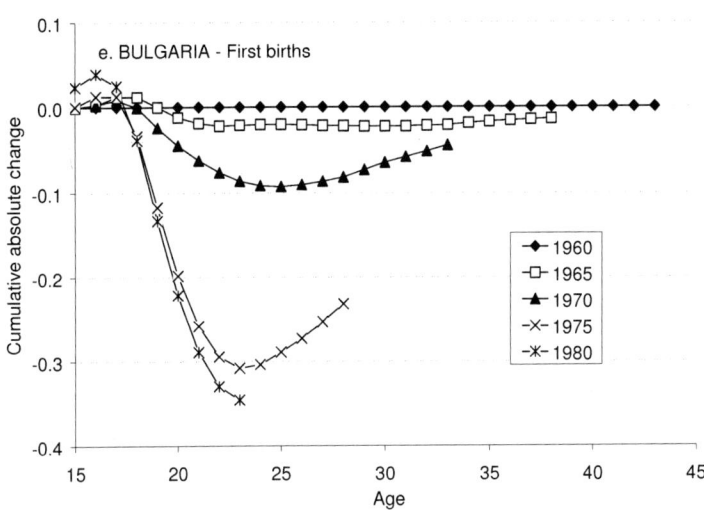

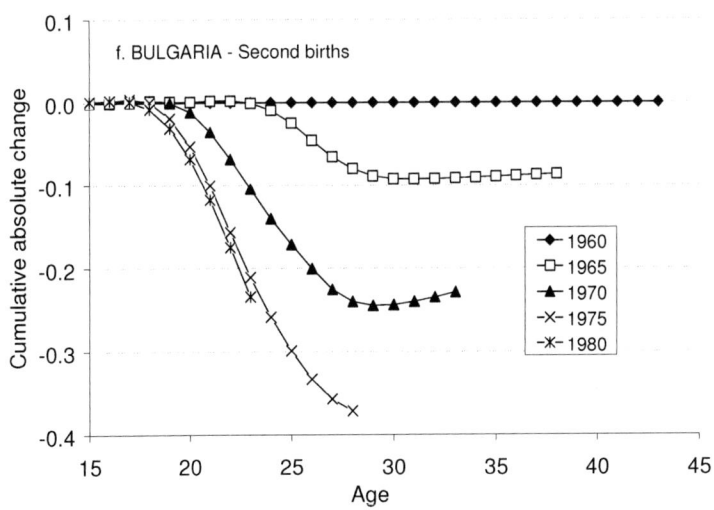

Source: Observatoire Démographique Européen.

In *Spain,* 90 percent of women of the 1960 birth cohort had a first birth by age 42. Each subsequent cohort of the 1960s and 1970s had fewer first births when these women were in their early to mid-twenties (Figures 8c and 9c). For example, by age 27, women of the 1975 cohort had borne 0.37 fewer first births than the 1960 cohort. It appears, nevertheless, that in Spain first birth delay came to a halt among the cohorts of the late 1970s. The curve for the 1980 cohort is equivalent to the 1975 curve, although this is difficult to distinguish in Figure 9c. As women grew older, they had a propensity to recuperate delayed first births; however, so far it cannot be conclusively determined to what extent recuperation has been achieved. Sixty-four percent of Spanish women in the 1960 cohort had a second birth by age 42. Second births were also being delayed when women were young. By the time women of the 1970 cohort were in their early thirties, they had had only about half as many second births as the cohort ten years older. Just as with first births, second births were no longer being delayed among the cohorts of the late 1970s. The propensity to recuperate the delayed second births was also evident, but it was weaker and the eventual outcome yet unknown. Period fertility in Spain had declined to its lowest level by 1999, when the period TFR was at 1.13 births per woman, and it has been gradually rising since then, reaching 1.37 in 2006. This increase was directly related to the fact that childbearing delay was abating.

In *Bulgaria,* 97 percent of women of the 1960 cohort had had a first birth by age 43. Although a moderate delay in first births took place among the 1960s cohorts, it is clear that more than 90 percent of women in these cohorts will eventually become mothers. There was a notable decline of the first birth rate among the 1970s birth cohorts, particularly among young women born early in the 1970s (Figures 8e and 9e). While the 1970s cohorts maintained early childbearing patterns with peak fertility at ages 19 to 20, they also showed a clear propensity to recuperate at least some of the first births delayed at younger ages (Figure 9e). Consequently, their fertility in their late twenties was higher than in previous generations (not shown here). For example, the maximum first-birth deficit of the 1975 cohort compared to the 1960 cohort was –0.31 births, but it later narrowed to –0.23 births by age 28 (Figure 9e). Seventy-six percent of the 1960 cohort had had second births. The proportions having second births declined considerably in subsequent cohorts, especially among those of the late 1960s and the early 1970s. For example, only 28 percent of women in the 1975 cohort had had a second birth by age 28, compared to 57 percent in the 1965 cohort at that age, a difference of 50 percent. Moreover, apparently, the propensity to recuperate second births later in life was weak (Figure 9f). At the same time, the delaying of parenthood slowed down among these cohorts. The fertility age trajectories of the 1975 and the 1980 cohorts became closer to each other than in previous cohorts. The rapid pace of childbearing delay, combined with quantum declines among the cohorts of the late 1960s and early 1970s, was reflected in the period rates. The period TFR declined from

1.82 births per woman in 1990, to its lowest level of 1.09 in 1997. It increased moderately to 1.30 in 2000, and to 1.38 in 2006.

These three examples, together with evidence presented in the country chapters and other literature (Kohler et al. 2002, Sobotka 2004a, Frejka, Sardon 2004, 2006, 2007), illustrate prevailing contemporary patterns of fertility behaviour. The main features are the following:

In the past two to four decades, the postponement of parenthood was an ongoing process in virtually all European countries, and it continues to be so. The almost universal prevalence of childbearing postponement is confirmed in individual chapters and by selected examples in Table 3. Among the cohorts of the 1960s and early 1970s, childbearing by young women declined in virtually all countries. This decline has been more obvious for second than for first births. In general, the rates of decline have been more pronounced in the countries of Southern, Central, and Eastern Europe, and less so in Western and Northern Europe. In the Netherlands, the fertility of young women no longer declined among the 1970s birth cohorts. This means that childbearing postponement has ceased among Dutch women, at least temporarily, if not permanently. Incipient signs of postponement coming to an end can be detected elsewhere, such as among the cohorts of the late 1970s in Spain and Bulgaria (Figures 8 and 9), but also in France, the United Kingdom, and in the Nordic countries.

There is a propensity to recuperate delayed fertility. Recuperation of second births tends to be weaker than that of first births. Recuperation is particularly strong in Northern Europe and in many Western European countries, but is weaker in Southern, Central, and Eastern Europe (cf. country chapters; Frejka and Sardon 2007).

A crucial yet unanswerable question is the extent to which delayed births of the 1970s cohorts will be recuperated as women get older. The experience of the recent past portrayed in the chapters of this book and from other sources indicates higher rates of recuperation in Northern and Western Europe than elsewhere.

Even though it is not known to what degree childbearing will be recuperated, it can be surmised, but not proved conclusively, that quantum declines are a part of the trends of fertility behaviour of women in the midst of their childbearing in a number of European countries, possibly in most of them. For example, the developments in Bulgaria (Figures 8e and 9e; and, even more so, 8f and 9f) illustrate these presumed quantum declines. Especially among second births, the curves for each subsequent cohort are below the preceding ones (Figures 8d and 8f), and data available to date illustrate that propensities to recuperate delayed births appear weak (Figures 9d and 9f). Similar trends occurred in Poland, the Slovak Republic, Slovenia, Romania, Italy, and many other countries.

Table 3: **First and second birth order cumulated cohort fertility rates (CCFRs) up to 27th birthday, selected low fertility countries, birth cohorts 1940, 1950, 1960, 1970, and 1975 (or latest available)**

Country	CCFR up to 27th birthday						Annual change between birth cohorts (percent)				
	1940	1950	1960	1965	1970	1975*	1940-1950	1950-1960	1960-1965	1965-1970	1970-1975*
First births											
Denmark	...	...	0.539	0.451	0.421	0.350	...	...	−3.6	−1.4	−3.7
Sweden	...	...	0.493	0.493	0.427	0.319	...	...	0.0	−2.9	−5.9
England & Wales	0.723	0.630	0.497	0.455	0.433	0.392b	−1.4	−2.4	−1.8	−1.0	−2.5
Netherlands	0.665	0.608	0.395	0.324	0.268	0.268	−0.9	−4.3	−4.0	−3.8	0.1
Austria	...	...	...	0.522	0.471	0.407	...	...	...	−2.1	−2.9
Italy	0.604	0.641	0.514	0.391	0.298	0.298a	0.6	−2.2	−5.5	−5.5	...
Spain	...	...	0.548	0.419	0.278	0.192	...	...	−5.3	−8.2	−7.4
Czech Republic	0.833	0.841	0.842	0.830	0.748	0.536	0.1	0.0	−0.3	−2.1	−6.6
Hungary	0.785	0.797	0.804	0.761	0.661	0.481	0.1	0.1	−1.1	−2.8	−6.4
Bulgaria	0.875	0.893	0.877	0.856	0.787	0.604	0.2	−0.2	−0.5	−1.7	−5.3
Romania	...	...	0.822	0.770	0.712	0.569	...	...	−1.3	−1.6	−4.5
Slovenia	0.753	0.810	0.826	0.726	0.584	0.443	0.7	0.2	−2.6	−4.4	−5.5
Second births											
Denmark	...	0.372	0.213	0.179	0.160	0.140	...	−5.6	−3.5	−2.2	−2.7
Sweden	...	...	0.245	0.247	0.209	0.136	...	...	0.2	−3.3	−8.6
England & Wales	0.465	0.394	0.300	0.257	0.233	0.214b	−1.6	−2.7	−3.1	−1.9	−2.2
Netherlands	0.373	0.331	0.189	0.139	0.106	0.101	−1.2	−5.6	−6.2	−5.4	−1.0
Austria	...	...	...	0.249	0.218	0.181	...	...	...	−2.7	−3.7
Italy	0.290	0.304	0.214	0.143	0.097	0.097a	0.5	−3.5	−8.1	−7.8	...
Spain	...	...	0.215	0.137	0.082	0.054	...	...	−9.1	−10.2	−8.3
Czech Republic	0.491	0.560	0.558	0.504	0.394	0.219	1.3	0.0	−2.0	−4.9	−11.7
Hungary	0.356	0.474	0.460	0.429	0.334	0.200	2.9	−0.3	−1.4	−5.0	−10.2
Bulgaria	0.503	0.568	0.560	0.515	0.360	0.227	1.2	−0.1	−1.7	−7.1	−9.2
Romania	...	0.513	0.504	0.440	0.297	0.224	...	−0.2	−2.7	−7.9	−5.6
Slovenia	0.347	0.400	0.430	0.354	0.252	0.156	1.4	0.7	−3.9	−6.8	−9.6

* or latest available
Source: Frejka and Sardon (2007).
Notes: a=1972, b=1974.

6. Conclusions

Early in the 21st century, about one-quarter of Europe's population live in countries with fertility close to the replacement level. Three-quarters live in countries with fertility considerably below replacement. This general conclusion is arrived at irrespective of whether period or cohort fertility measures are used.

Relative stability of fertility trends has been achieved in most parts of Western and Northern Europe during the 1980s through the early 2000s (cf. Figure 3 and respective country chapters), and among the corresponding cohorts of the late 1940s to the 1960s. Similarly, period fertility was relatively stable in many former state socialist countries during the 1970s and 1980s when corresponding cohort fertility was exceptionally even (corresponding country chapters). In both cases, it remained close to replacement.

It is more difficult to determine accurately the underlying quantum of fertility during periods of changing fertility trends when the respective measures and their adjustments should be considered an approximation. That was the case especially in the former state socialist countries during the 1990s and 2000s. In the early 2000s, total period fertility rates were very low there, around 1.3 to 1.4 births per woman (cf. Figure 3), whereas the adjusted TFRs were around 1.5–1.7 (cf. Table 1). There is no information available yet about fertility of the corresponding birth cohorts of the 1970s and early 1980s. Judging from the trends in cohorts that were in the midst of their childbearing careers by the early 2000s, there are clear indications of an incipient and rather pronounced decline in their completed fertility. Cohort fertility has also been declining in the German-speaking countries and in Southern Europe, although it has not been quite as volatile as in the former state socialist countries. Early in the 21st century, period total fertility in these regions reached low levels of around 1.3-1.4 and the adjusted TFRs were about 1.4-1.5.

In sum, in the mid- 2000s in Western and Northern Europe fertility quantum was moderately below the replacement level, which has been recently reached in the United States; whereas in Southern, Central and Eastern Europe, fertility quantum was considerably below the replacement level. Across Europe, the mean number of births per woman was close to 1.7, but in many countries the period fertility level was considerably lower and stood around 1.4-1.5 births per woman even when the negative tempo distortions are taken into account.

Throughout Europe, a historic transformation of childbearing patterns has been taking place. An early childbearing pattern—typical of the baby boom period of the 1950s and 1960s, and retained in Central and Eastern Europe until the mid-1990s—was being replaced by a late pattern, characterised by a pronounced delay of entry into parenthood. This secular trend towards later childbearing has greatly contributed to the decline and fluctuations in period fertility rates, as they have been negatively affected by changes in the timing of childbearing. Delayed births were eventually being recuperated, especially among childless women, but the extent of recuperation differs by country and region. In Western and Northern Europe, most—at times, all—of the delayed births have been recuperated as women have reached their late twenties and thirties. The extent of recuperation has been notably smaller in the German-speaking countries and in Southern Europe. Thus far, the recuperation of delayed births has been weak in most of the former state socialist countries, especially among second and higher order births.

All in all, despite a recent upward trend in period TFRs, European fertility early in the 21st century was at its lowest point since the Second World War. Surveys of fertility intentions indicate that young adult women in most countries of Europe still prefer to have around two children on average (Testa 2007), but in many countries, a substantial fraction of childbearing desires remains unrealised (e.g. Bongaarts 2001). It is not yet clear whether an increasing number of women currently in their young adult years will desire a very small family size (no children or one child only), but recent evidence for several European countries (Austria, the Czech Republic, the Netherlands, and Spain) shows that young women are increasingly preferring sub-replacement family size (see the respective country chapters). This may lead to a greater cross-country differentiation in family size preferences in Europe, similar to the emerging differentiation in fertility levels. This diversity in fertility is likely to prevail for decades to come, and may eventually lead to a bifurcation in population trends in Europe, bringing long-lasting population decline to the countries with sustained low fertility and low immigration rates.

References

Avdeev, A., and A. Monnier. 1995. A survey of modern Russian fertility, *Population: An English selection* 7: 1–38.

Bolesławski, L. 1993. Polskie tablice dzietności kobiet 1971-1992. Polish fertility tables 1971-1992. Warsaw: Główny urząd statystyczny.

Bongaarts, J. 2002. The end of fertility transition in the developed world, *Population and Development Review* 28(3): 419–443.

Bongaarts, J., and G. Feeney. 1998. On the quantum and tempo of fertility, *Population and Development Review* 24(2): 271–291.

Chesnais, J.-C. 1986. La transition démographique: étapes, formes, implications économiques. Etude de séries temporelles relatives à 67 pays. Cahier n° 113, Paris: INED-PUF.

Council of Europe. 2006. *Recent demographic developments in Europe 2005*. Strasbourg: Council of Europe Publishing.

Demeny, P., and G. McNicoll. 2006. The political demography of the world system, 2000–2050, in P. Demeny and G. McNicoll (Eds.), *Population and Development Review, a supplement to* vol. 32, pp: 254–287.

Dunnell, K. 2007. The changing demographic picture of the UK. National Statisticians annual article on the population, *Population Trends* 130: 9–21.

Eurostat. 2006. Population in Europe 2005. First results. Statistics in Focus, Population and Social Conditions, 16/2006. Luxembourg: European Communities.

Eurostat. 2007. *Population and Social Conditions*. http://epp.eurostat.ec.europa.eu.

Festy, P. 1979. *La fécondité des pays occidentaux de 1870 à 1970*. Travaux et Documents No. 85. Paris: INED – PUF.

Frejka, T. 2004. The 'curiously high' fertility of the USA, *Population Studies* 58(1): 88–92.

Frejka, T., and J.-P. Sardon. 2004. Childbearing Trends and Prospects in Low-Fertility countries: A cohort analysis, Dorbrecht: Kluwer Academic Publishers.

Frejka, T., and J.-P. Sardon. 2005. The direction of contemporary fertility trends in the developed countries: further decline, plateau or upswing? Proceedings of the XXV IUSSP International Conference. Tours: France.

Frejka, T., and J.-P. Sardon. 2006. First birth trends in developed countries: persisting parenthood postponement, *Demographic Research* 15(6): 147–180. www.demographic-research.org.

Frejka, T., and J.-P. Sardon. 2007. Cohort birth order, parity progression ratio and parity distribution trends in developed countries, *Demographic Research* 16(11): 315–374. www.demographic-research.org.

Frejka, T., and J. Ross. 2001. Paths to sub-replacement fertility: the empirical evidence, in R. Bulatao and J. B. Casterline (Eds.), *Global Fertility Transition. Population and Development Review, a supplement to* vol. 27. pp: 213–254.

Gabrielli, G., A. Paterno, and S. Strozza. 2007. *Dynamics, characteristics, and demographic behaviour of immigrants in some south-European countries.* Paper presented at an international conference on "Migration and Development," Moscow: 13–15 September 2007.

Glass, D. 1937. The population problem and the future, *Eugenics Review* 29(1): 39–47. Reprinted in *Population and Development Review* 31(3): 557–572 (2005).

Goldstein, J. 2006. How late can first births be postponed? Some illustrative population-level calculations, *Vienna Yearbook of Population Research* 2006: 153–165.

Hamilton, B. E., J. A. Martin, and S. J. Ventura. 2007. *Births. Preliminary data for 2006.* National Vital Statistics Reports 56(7). December 2007, Atlanta: NCHS and CDC.

Héran, F., and G. Pison. 2007. Two children per woman in France in 2006: are immigrants to blame?, *Population and Societies* 432. http://www.ined.fr/fichier/t_telechargement/ 7659/telechargement_fichier_en_publi_pdf2_pop.and.soc.english.432.pdf.

Kohler, H.-P., and J. A. Ortega. 2002a. Tempo-adjusted period parity progression measures, fertility postponement and completed cohort fertility, *Demographic Research* 6(6): 92–144. www.demographic-research.org.

Kohler, H.-P., F. C. Billari, and J. A. Ortega. 2002. The emergence of lowest-low fertility in Europe during the 1990s, *Population and Development Review* 28(4): 641–680.

Lesthaeghe, R., and L. Neidert. 2006. The second demographic transition in the United States: Exception or textbook example?, *Population and Development Review* 32(4): 669–698.

Lesthaeghe, R., and P. Willems. 1999. Is low fertility a temporary phenomenon in the European Union?, *Population and Development Review* 25(2): 211–228.

Lutz, W., V. Skirbekk, and M. R. Testa. 2006. The low-fertility trap hypothesis: forces that may lead to further postponement and fewer births in Europe, *Vienna Yearbook of Population Research* 2006: 167–192.

McDonald, P. 2000. Gender equity in theories of fertility transition, *Population and Development Review* 26(3): 427–439.

McDonald, P. 2006. An assessment of policies that support having children from the perspectives of equity, efficiency and efficacy, *Vienna Yearbook of Population Research* 2006: 213–234.

Morgan, P. S. 1996. Characteristic features of modern American fertility, in.: J. B. Casterline, R. D. Lee and K. A. Foote (Eds.), *Fertility in the United States. New patterns, new theories.* Supplement to *Population and Development Review 22,* New York: Population Council, pp: 19–63.

Roig Vila, M., and T. Castro Martín. 2007. Childbearing patterns of foreign women in a new immigration country: The case of Spain, *Population-E* 62(3): 351–380.

Sardon, J.-P. 1991. Generation replacement in Europe since 1900, *Population: An English Selection* 3: 15–32.

Schoen, R. 2004. Timing effects and the interpretation of period fertility, *Demography* 41(4): 801–819.

Smallwood, S. 2002. The effect of changes in the timing of childbearing on measuring fertility in England and Wales, *Population Trends* 109: 36–45. www.statistics.gov.uk/ STATBASE/Product.asp?vlnk=6303.

Sobotka, T. 2003. Tempo-quantum and period-cohort interplay in fertility changes in Europe. Evidence from the Czech Republic, Italy, the Netherlands and Sweden, *Demographic Research* 8(6): 151–214. www.demographic-research.org.

Sobotka, T. 2004a. Postponement of childbearing and low fertility in Europe. Amsterdam: Dutch University Press.

Sobotka, T. 2004b. Is lowest-low fertility explained by the postponement of childbearing?, *Population and Development Review* 30(2): 195–220.

Sobotka, T., H.-P. Kohler, and F. C. Billari. 2007. *The increase in late childbearing in Europe, Japan, and the United States.* Paper presented at the 2007 Annual Meeting of the Population Association of America, New York: 29–31 March 2007.

Testa, M. R. 2007. Childbearing preferences and family issues in Europe: evidence from the Eurobarometer 2006 survey, *Vienna Yearbook of Population Research* 2007: 357–379.

Toulemon, L. 2004. Le fécondité est-elle encore naturelle? Application au retard des naissances et à son influence sur la descendance finale, in *Chaire Quetelet 2002*, Academia Bruylant/L'Harmattan, pp: 1–28.

Van Imhoff, E. 2001. On the impossibility of inferring cohort fertility measures from period fertility measures, *Demographic Research* 5(2):23–64. www.demographic-research.org.

VID. 2006. *European demographic data sheet 2006.* Vienna: Vienna Institute of demography, IIASA, Population reference Bureau. http://www.oeaw.ac.at/vid/popeurope/index.html.

Overview Chapter 2:
Parity distribution and completed family size in Europe:
Incipient decline of the two-child family model?[1]

Tomas Frejka[2]

Abstract

By the end of the 20th century the two-child family became the norm throughout Europe. Between 40 and over 50 percent of women in the 1950s and 1960s cohorts had two children. There were some incipient signs that shares of two-child families were declining, especially in Central and Eastern and Southern Europe. An increase in childlessness among recent generations was an almost universal trend. The increase in proportions of one-child families was prominent in CEE and in SE. Wherever shares of childless women and of women with one child continue to grow, the obvious result will be entrenched below replacement fertility. Much depends on progression ratios to first and to second births. In CEE mainly the progression ratios to second births are declining. In the Nordic countries progression ratios to first and to second births were relatively stable and even more so in France. Altogether, most people opt for two children, very few for three or more, the frequency of the one-child family is increasing as are the proportions of people remaining childless. The latter trends were more pronounced in Southern, Central and Eastern Europe and not so much in Northern and Western countries.

---

[1] In this chapter the terms "parity" and "family size" will be used interchangeably. This is not an accurate use of the term "family size," but it has become customary in this context and means the number of children borne by women irrespective of partnership status.

[2] E-mail: Tfrejka@aol.com

1. Introduction

From the middle of the 19th through the second half of the 20th century, the prevailing "large family" model of three or more children was gradually replaced by the two-child family. A diverse set of social, economic, political and cultural developments generated this process. Improved standards of living, advances in public sanitation, and increasing attention to personal hygiene were among the important conditions of declining mortality, particularly due to a drop in infant mortality, which was one reason for the decline in childbearing. Rising costs and declining benefits of children and childrearing were additional reasons for parents of successive generations to have smaller numbers of children. Gender relationships were changing in society and in the family, with increasing proportions of women employed. At the same time, people's economic aspirations and expectations, as well as their growing individualism, materialism, secularism and desire for personal self-fulfillment, were undermining the satisfaction derived from having children. These were among the principal conditions leading to small family size.

This chapter will explore in some detail the demographic developments that generated the two-child family model which prevailed throughout the developed countries by the end of the 20th century (see, for instance, van de Kaa 2001:316-318). A crucial contemporary issue is whether the two-child family norm will last, or whether it will be replaced by societies in which large proportions of parents will decide to have only one child, or no children at all.

The focus will be on actual completed family size distributions and trends. Analyses of desired or ideal family size are not included because these have been dealt with quite extensively in recent literature (for instance, Goldstein et al. 2003; Fokkema and Esveldt 2005; Testa 2006)

2. The data

The analysis of parity distribution in this chapter is conducted with cohort data. Such an approach has the advantage of reflecting quite adequately lifetime developments experienced by families and by women. At the same time, it should be taken into account that statistical information about the contemporary status is outdated. A reliable picture is based on data of cohorts that have completed their childbearing. These data provide an adequate tool for analyzing trends, but the end point provides information about generations that were in their prime childbearing years one, two, or even three decades ago.

Data used in the overview analysis are from the country chapters complemented by those of the *Observatoire Démographique Européen*. The pathways of constructing parity distributions depend on the data available in the respective country. They are derived from population censuses or from vital statistics. A combination of both sources can also be applied, and at times these sources can be supplemented by informed professional estimates. Population census-based parity distributions utilize data on women of individual ages who have completed childbearing by number of children ever born. Vital statistics-based parity distributions use single-year, age-specific cohort fertility rates by single-year cohorts and by individual birth order to compute birth order total cohort fertility rates. In the analysis four family-size categories were used: childless women, women with one child, women with two children, and women with three or more children.

Data were not available for all European countries; therefore only three groups were used. Criteria for creating these were geographic and substantive. In very general terms, the countries in the respective groups experienced common socioeconomic and political developments during the 20th century. The groups are:

Northern and Western Europe: Denmark, Norway, Sweden, France, England & Wales, Netherlands, Austria and West Germany (included only in Panel A of Figure 1).

Southern Europe: Greece, Italy, Spain, and Portugal

Central and Eastern Europe (formerly socialist countries): Czech Republic, Slovak Republic, Slovenia, Poland, Lithuania, Bulgaria, Romania, and Russian Federation

3. Family size trends

3.1 Northern and Western Europe

In the four family-size categories, several developments common to a number, often a majority, of countries stand out (Figure 1):

In the long run, the proportion of childless women experienced an extended decline that reached a low plateau among the 1930s cohorts; a subsequent reversal occurred, and shares of childless women reached 15 to nearly 30 percent in the 1960s cohorts.

Among the cohorts born early in the 20th century, the shares of childless women were between 20 and 30 percent in the countries for which data were available (Figure 1, Panel A). From thereon, a gradual decline took place involving at least 30 cohorts. Among the 1930s and early 1940s cohorts, the central cohorts that generated the "baby boom," the proportions of childless women were clustered in a narrow range of 9 - 12 percent. In subsequent cohorts, a renewed increase in childless women is taking place. Among cohorts completing their childbearing early in the 21st century, i.e., the birth cohorts of the early 1960s, the share of childless women in several countries, such as Austria, the Netherlands, England & Wales, and Sweden, was between 15 and 20 percent. In contrast, shares of childless women in Denmark and France were low, close to 10 percent.

In Western Germany, the precise proportion of childless women is not known, but there is no doubt that it was rising steeply among the 1960s cohorts (Figure 1, Panel A). Some authors estimated the childlessness share to be as high as 30 percent in the mid-1960s cohorts (Germany chapter; Dorbritz, Ruckdeschel 2007). To a significant degree, childlessness had become a matter of deliberate choice (Höpflinger 1991). Among young people in Western Germany, there are two main groups: "those who live with children and as a rule are also married, as opposed to those who have chosen not to have children, the vast majority of whom do not marry" (Germany chapter). Low fertility has become a matter of considerable concern to the German government, which has started to implement policy measures aimed at creating incentives and conditions that encourage childbearing (Auth 2006; Prskawetz et al. 2006).

The principal reasons for the relatively high levels of childlessness among the cohorts born around 1900, and among those of the 1960s, were very different. Quite large proportions of women born in the late 19th and early 20th centuries remained single, and almost all of these did not have children. In part this was due to the large number of young men killed during the First World War (Germany chapter). Also, the unusually severe consequences of the Great Depression of the 1930s were reflected in generally low levels of fertility and high rates of childlessness. Relatively frequent childlessness in recent decades is related to the complex changes that have taken place as young women spend more time acquiring advanced education as well as building up their careers, and thus having to cope with the tensions between working and childrearing. The above reasoning often applies equally to other countries, and these developments are discussed in greater detail in the country chapters and in overview chapters 4, 5, and 6.

The two-child family became the norm following a steady long-term increase that reached a saturation point approximately with the birth cohorts born around 1950 (Figure 1, Panel C).

The proportion of women with two children was around 20 percent in the cohorts born early in the 20th century; smaller than the shares of childless women, as well as the shares of one-child families and large families with three or more children (Figure 1, Panel C). The prevalence of the two-child family gradually grew from one generation to the next, and reached a peak among the cohorts of the late 1940s and early 1950s. As discussed in most country chapters, the two-child family became the norm, both in reality and in the general perception of the public. In almost all populations of Northern and Western Europe, a slight decline followed, and the shares of women with two children were clustered to a remarkable extent around 40 percent in the 1960s birth cohorts.

A less pronounced, and shorter-lived, increase in the shares of large families with three or more children occurred up to the prime baby boom cohorts of the 1930s; this was followed by a decline and stabilization (Figure 1, Panel D).

A more detailed analysis of large families indicates that the decline in the shares of families with four and more children was much faster than the decline in families with three children (not shown here). In Austria, for instance, large families decreased by 75 percent between the 1935 and the 1965 cohorts, and constituted about five percent of all families in the mid-1960s birth cohort. The share of the three-child family had declined by a mere 22 percent, with an almost stable 15 percent share of all families in the mid-1960s cohorts (Austria chapter).

Contrary to general perception, proportions of one-child families hardly changed over time, with quite a wide variation between countries (Figure 1, Panel B).

For the time being, the one-child family is not a very common choice in most Northern and Western European countries. In the Sweden chapter it is noted that "having only one child is a rarely chosen family pattern."

3.2 Southern Europe

The time series for Southern European populations are shorter than for the other countries, but commonalities in parity distribution trends can be detected nevertheless (Figure 2).

Among the cohorts of the late 1940s and 1950s, the proportions of childless women were low, around 10 percent. These have been increasing among the cohorts of the 1960s (Figure 2, Panel A), although the absolute values of the percentages for the youngest cohorts in the available time series are probably higher than in reality[3] (Sobotka 2004, chapter 5). But the trend of growth is the important aspect. The increase in childlessness has been the steepest in Italy, where, among the youngest cohorts, close to a fifth of all women apparently remain without children.

Indisputably, shares of one-child families have been on the increase starting with the cohorts born in the 1940s (Figure 2, Panel B). In the 1960s birth cohorts, about one-

---

[3] This is caused by imperfect estimation methods, which tend to underestimate the numbers of first births and thus overestimate women remaining childless among the youngest cohorts.

Figure 1:   **Proportions of women, childless, or with one, two or three and more children, selected Northern and Western European countries, birth cohorts 1900-1965**

Panel A

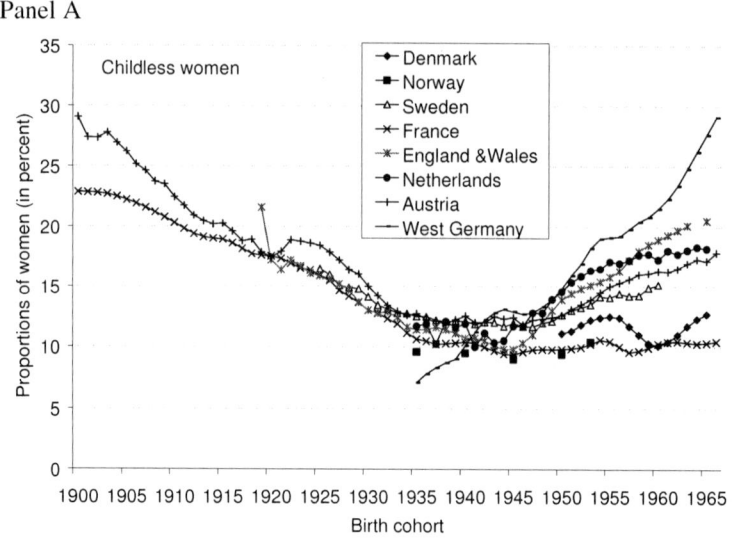

Panel B

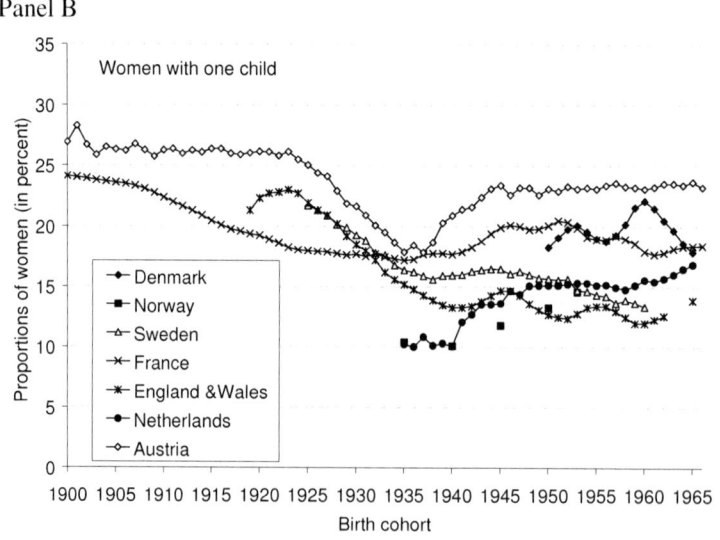

Figure 1: (continued)

Panel C

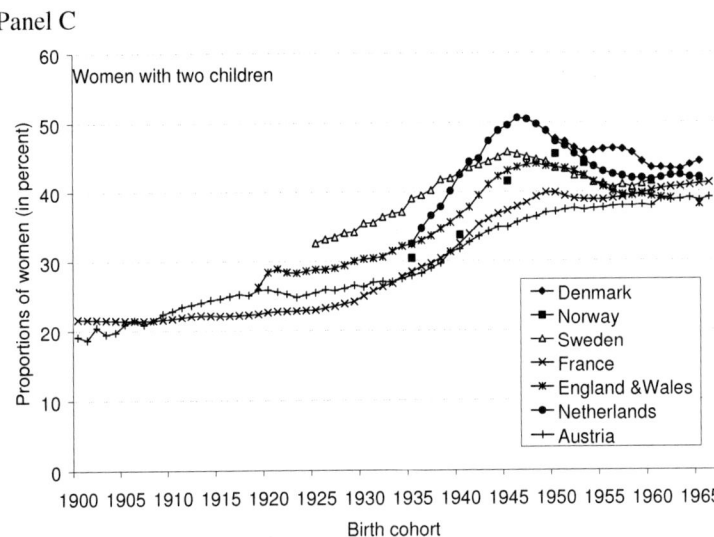

Panel D

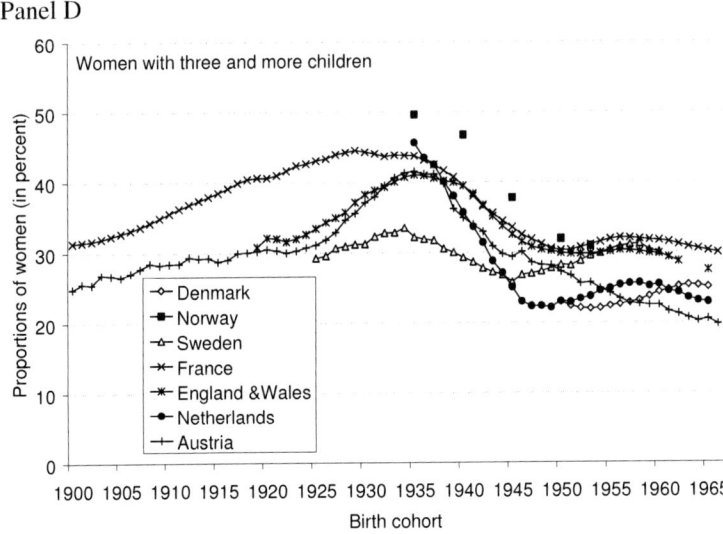

Source: Country chapters and *Observatoire Démographique Européen.*

Figure 2: **Proportions of women, childless, or with one, two or three and more children, selected Southern European countries, birth cohorts 1920-1965**

Panel A

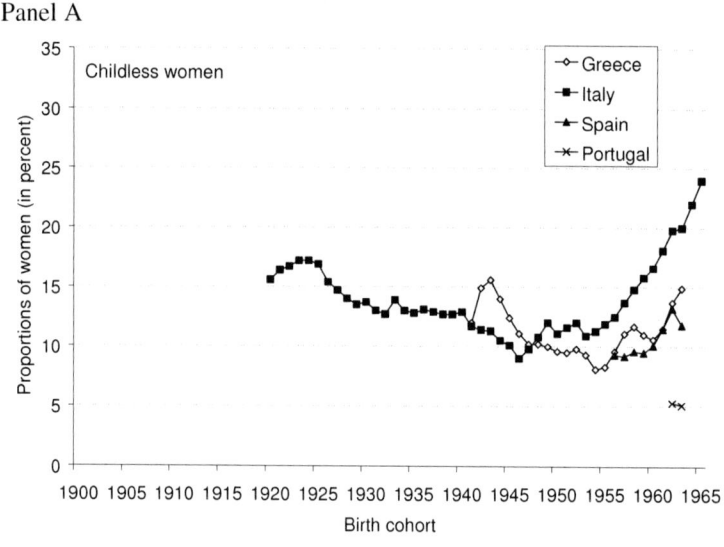

Panel B

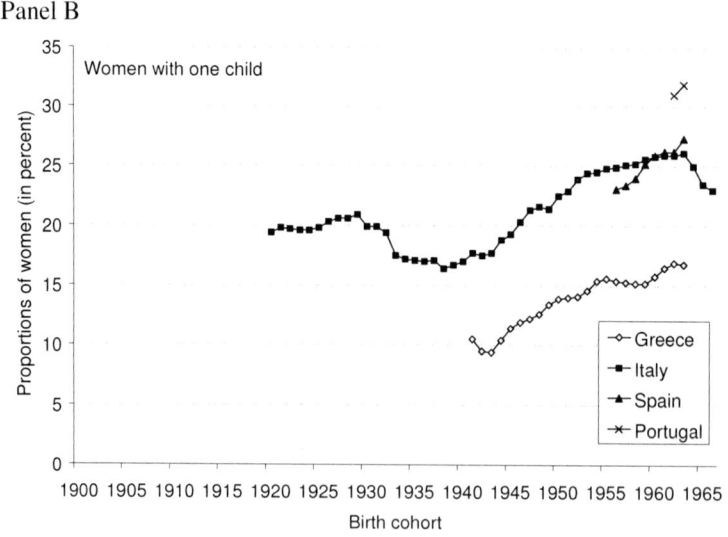

Figure 2: **(continued)**

Panel C

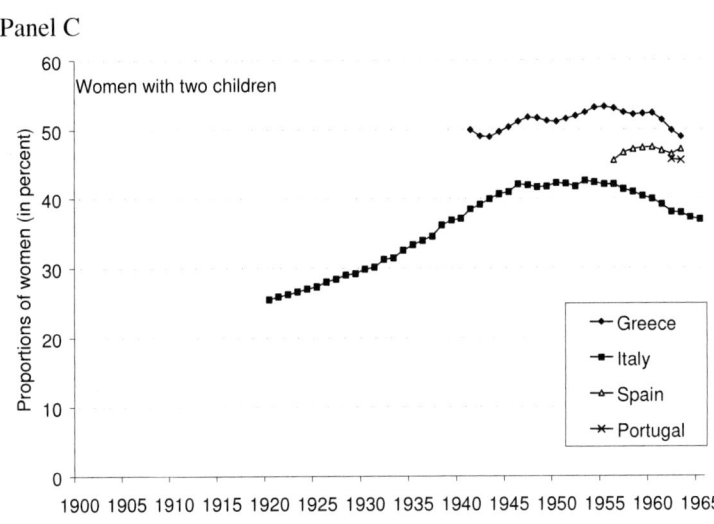

Panel D

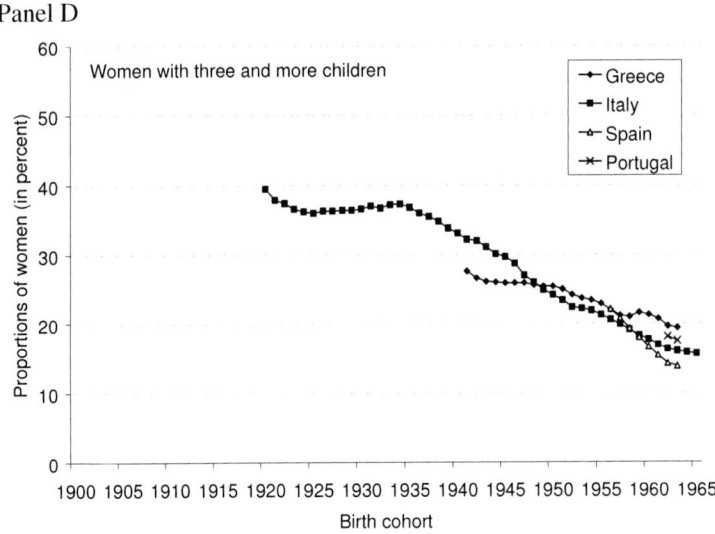

Source: Country chapters and *Observatoire Démographique Européen.*

quarter of women in Italy and Spain had only one child. In Portugal, the proportion of one-child families was even higher; in Greece, lower.

The overwhelming majorities of women in the birth cohorts of the 1940s and 1950s had two children (Figure 2, Panel C). The two-child family was firmly established as the norm. An incipient decline in the percentages can be detected among the 1960s cohorts; in Italy, even among the cohorts of the late 1950s. The authors of the Italy chapter point out that, in the 1960 cohort, women with two children are outnumbered by the sum of mothers of an only child and of childless women.

The decline in the proportions of large families of three and more children was consistent in its direction, as were values for all the Southern European countries (Figure 2, Panel D). In Italy, the only country with a long time series, large families were still the norm among the 1920s cohorts, with almost a 40 percent share. The gradual decline started in the 1930s birth cohorts. Among the cohorts of the 1960s, less than 20 percent of women had large families. The trend direction indicates that this decline was still in progress among younger women.

3.3 Central and Eastern Europe

The countries for which data are available undoubtedly display common trends, yet at the same time there is a notably greater heterogeneity than in the other two regions (Figure 3).

Shares of childless women were apparently quite high in most of these countries among the cohorts born early in the 20th century (Figure 3, Panel A). These gradually declined to a level of around 10 percent and less. The low levels of childlessness were typical among the cohorts of the 1930s, and even more so among the 1940s and 1950s cohorts, essentially during the period of stable authoritarian rule. The childless shares started to increase among the cohorts of the 1960s. The rise in the shares of childless women is a recent phenomenon. The analyses in practically all the country chapters indicate that this growth is likely to continue in the foreseeable future.

While shares of the one-child family underwent some fluctuations in the majority of Central and Eastern European countries, levels in these countries were relatively stable except among the youngest birth cohorts (Figure 3, Panel B). The Russian population did not comply with this pattern of long-term stability. The revolutionary changes of the political system and the subsequent unsettled conditions during the first half of the 20th century are reflected in the changes of the parity distribution in Russia (Figure 3 and Russia chapter). In the late 19th and early 20th centuries, the proportion of Russian families with one child was low; its share was only eight percent among the generations born around 1900. But the share of one-child families in Russia increased rapidly thereafter, reaching three times that level among the 1920s cohorts. Starting with the cohorts of the mid-1930s, the proportion of one-child families has been notably higher in Russia than in any of the other countries. A considerable increase in one-child families occurred in the youngest cohorts, those born in the late 1950s and 1960s. Similar rates of growth of one-child families took place in all these countries among the youngest generations, but at lower levels (Figure 3, Panel B).

The two-child family experienced steady growth almost throughout the entire period of observation. The proportions were apparently between 10 and 30 percent among the cohorts born early in the 20th century, and increased to about 40 to 60 percent among the 1950s birth cohorts (Figure 3, Panel C). In most countries, the peak share was reached with the cohorts born around 1960. Among the cohorts of the 1960s, this proportion stabilized or experienced an incipient minor decline. The two-child family was firmly established as the norm. On average, it was as prevalent as the other three groups combined. In the Czech Republic, Slovenia and Bulgaria, the share of the two-child family was unusually high among the cohorts of the 1950s and early 1960s, 55 percent and higher.

In most countries of this region, shares of women with three or more children were slowly and steadily declining throughout almost the whole period of observation (Figure 3, Panel D). There were a few exceptions. In Bulgaria, a lower proportion of large families was already observable among cohorts of the 1930s. On the other hand, in Romania shares of large families increased, and were relatively high among the cohorts of the 1930s and 1940s as a result of the forceful pro-natalist policies of the Ceauşescu regime. In Poland, the relatively high proportion of women with large families remained unchanged for the cohorts of the late 1940s and the 1950s. In many countries, declines in shares of the large family were still continuing among the 1960s birth cohorts.

3.4 The entire continent and the overall picture

Based on the above exploration, answers to two crucial questions can be outlined:

What were the principal trends characterizing family size during the 20th century?
Which changes in family size were important in shaping fertility trends?

In the interest of averting any confusion that might otherwise arise, a reminder is warranted: namely, that this analysis and its findings deal with developments up to and including the late 1980s only. Completed cohort fertility data were used for this

Figure 3:   Proportions of women, childless, with one, two or three and more children, selected Central and Eastern European countries, birth cohorts 1900-1965

Panel A

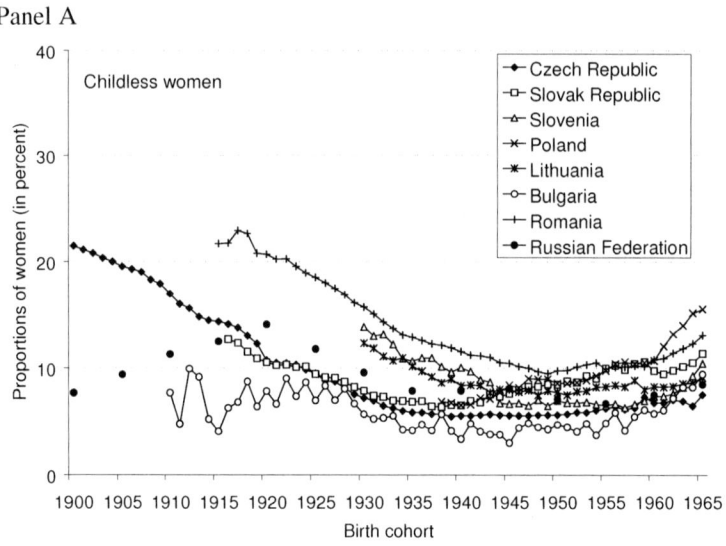

Panel B

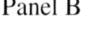

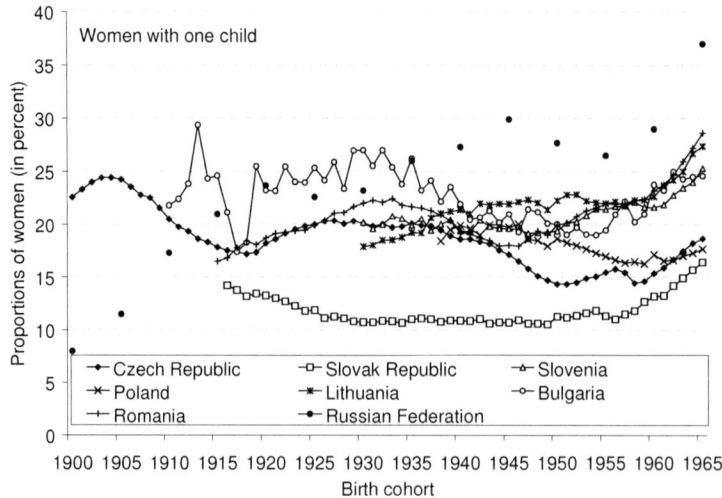

Figure 3:   (Continued)

Panel C

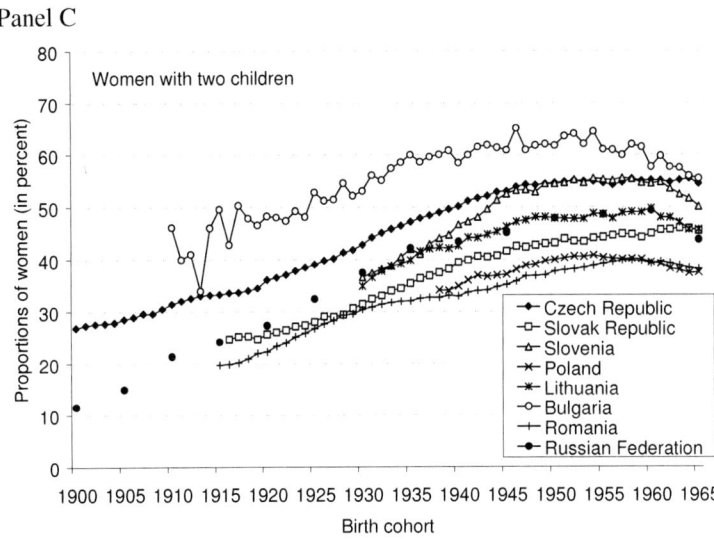

Panel D

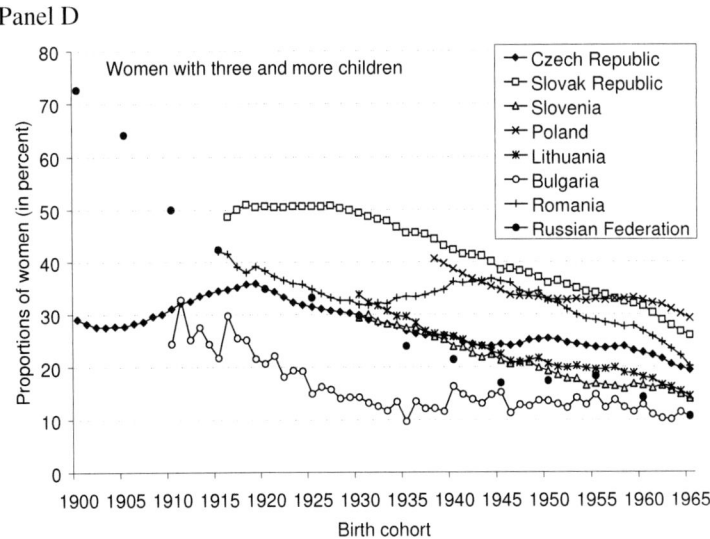

Source: Country chapters and *Observatoire Démographique Européen.*

analysis, which precludes the possibility of learning about changes in family size during the most recent 10 to 15 years. It should also be noted that, while not all European countries were part of the analysis thus far, a sufficiently large number were included that these countries can be considered representative of the entire continent.

The most prominent feature in the development of parity distributions during the second half of the 20th century was the gradual ascension of the two-child family model, which established its undisputed reign notably among the cohorts of the 1950s. In virtually every country, the share of women with two children reached the 40 percent mark (Panels C, Figures 1, 2 and 3). In some populations, women with two children comprised the absolute majority of all families, i.e., over 50 percent constituted two-child families.

Among the 1950s, and more so among the 1960s, birth cohorts, signs of an incipient erosion of the two-child family model can be detected. In over half of the Central and Eastern European countries, and in the Southern European countries, there was a decline in the proportion of two-child families among these cohorts. We will return to this development below.

The decline in the shares of large families was another prevailing trend (panels D, Figures 1, 2 and 3). Detailed analyses show that it was mainly the proportions of really large families of four and more children that were declining (Country chapters; Frejka, Sardon 2004 and 2007). The shares of three-child families were decreasing at a moderate pace, and their proportions were stabilizing in some countries. There were also differing regional variants of the large family trends. In the Northern and Western European countries, there was an increase of large families in the middle of the 20th century, culminating among the baby boom cohorts born in the 1920s and 1930s. A rapid decline in large families followed, which ended among the 1950s cohorts. In the Southern, Central and Eastern European countries, the decline of large families was moderate and continuous.

An increase in childlessness among recent generations was an almost universal trend. The timing of this trend differs between countries and regions. In Northern and Western Europe, this increase started with the birth cohorts of the late 1940s; in Southern Europe, among the 1950s cohorts; and in Central and Eastern Europe, it started with the 1960s cohorts. There were a number of exceptions to this trend. The proportions of childless women in France did not grow, and childlessness fluctuated in Denmark. The increases in childlessness were moderate among the 1960s cohorts in some of the Central and Eastern European countries, such as the Czech and Slovak Republics. The socioeconomic analyses in the country chapters support the notion that increases in childlessness are likely to continue. In a comprehensive investigation of childlessness in cohorts that have already entered the reproductive ages, Sobotka (2005) arrived at the conclusion "that childlessness will increase gradually in almost all industrialized countries, although the timing and the magnitude of this change varies across countries. … In the high-childlessness regions--especially West Germany and England & Wales--final childlessness among women born after 1970 is likely to come close to 25 percent and will almost certainly remain under 30 percent, while the more common levels will range between 15 and 22 percent."

The prevalence of the one-child family was relatively large and growing in Central and Eastern European countries, as well as in Southern Europe. In most Northern and Western European countries, trends in the shares of the one-child family were flat and relatively low.

As indicated above, there were incipient signs of erosion of the two-child family norm. This could be observed mainly in the Central and Eastern European countries, whereas the two-child family norm appeared to hold steady in Northern and Western Europe. Among the birth cohorts of the late 1950s and the 1960s, the proportions of childless women, as well as those of women with one child, experienced considerable relative increases (Table 1). The increments were at the expense of large and of two-child families. In some countries, the proportions of childless women were increasing faster than the shares of one-child families, especially in countries where two-child families were losing ground, such as Slovenia, Poland and Bulgaria. While the relative increase of childless women was considerable, the growth in the proportions of one-child families was also important.

Table 1: **Changes in proportions of family size between 1955 and 1965 birth cohorts, Central and Eastern European countries**

Country	Percent change in proportion of family size between 1955 and 1965 birth cohorts (1955=100)			
	Three and more children	Two child	One child	Childless
Czech Republic	82	100	121	120
Slovak Republic	76	103	145	114
Slovenia	83	91	118	160
Poland	89	93	104	159
Lithuania	74	94	124	111
Bulgaria	72	91	127	194
Romania	70	97	130	131
Russian Federation	59	90	140	127

Source: Country chapters and *Observatoire Démographique Européen.*

3.5 Cohorts completing childbearing early in the 21st century

The average family size of the cohorts completing their childbearing around the year 2000 is, at best, at the replacement level: it ranges from 1.50 to 2.05, or, in lay language, from one and a half to two children (Table 2).

It cannot be stressed enough that a great deal of variety in the parity composition prevails as the principal feature.

In comparing the three regions, some might consider it counterintuitive that the smallest shares of large families were in Southern European (SE) countries, while the largest shares of these families were in Northern and Western Europe (NWE). The two-child family dominates throughout the continent, but especially in Central and Eastern Europe (CEE). The largest shares of the one-child family can also be found in CEE countries; the smallest, in NWE. The smallest proportions of childless women tend to be in CEE and the largest in NWE.

When looking at individual countries, various extremes emerge. The Russian Federation had the largest share of one-child families, combined with small proportions of childless women and a small share of large families. The country with the largest share of two-child families was Bulgaria, which also had numerous one-child families, but few large families and childless women. Norway, Sweden and France had the largest shares of families of more than three children. The largest shares of childless women were in Italy, followed by England & Wales, the Netherlands and Austria[4].

---

[4] The proportion of childless women was estimated to have been even larger in West Germany, but data were not available for the whole parity distribution (see Figure 1, Panel A).

Table 2: **Parity distribution in percent, selected European countries, 1965 or latest available birth cohort**

Country, Region	Cohort	Parity (in percent)				Total cohort fertility rate
		0	1	2	3+	
Northern & Western Europe						
Denmark	1965	12.7	17.9	44.3	25.1	1.93
Norway	1953	10.4	14.6	44.1	30.9	2.05
Sweden	1960	15.1	13.4	41.5	30.0	2.04
France	1965	10.3	18.4	41.2	30.2	2.03
England & Wales	1960	18.9	12.0	39.3	29.8	1.89
Netherlands	1965	18.2	16.9	42.0	22.9	1.78
Austria	1965	17.2	23.7	38.6	20.5	1.65
Southern Europe						
Greece	1963	14.9	16.8	48.9	19.4	1.79
Italy	1965	24.0	23.5	36.9	15.6	1.51
Spain	1963	11.8	27.3	47.1	13.8	1.67
Portugal	1963	5.1	31.9	45.5	17.5	1.84
Central & Eastern Europe						
Czech Republic	1965	7.5	18.7	54.4	19.4	1.93
Slovak Republic	1965	11.4	16.4	45.5	26.7	2.04
Slovenia	1965	10.5	25.3	50.1	13.9	1.77
Poland	1965	15.5	17.7	37.5	29.3	2.00
Lithuania	1965	9.5	28.3	47.3	14.9	1.73
Bulgaria	1965	9.4	24.6	55.4	10.6	1.83
Romania	1965	13.1	28.6	38.2	20.1	1.91
Russian Federation	1965	8.5	37.0	43.8	10.7	1.65

4. Parity progression ratios (PPRs)

Statistics on the propensity to progress from one parity to the next provide an additional perspective, namely, these illuminate various paths of family formation. Parity progression ratios portray changes in patterns of family formation that occurred during the 20th century, and enable the comparison between countries during this period. As only a smaller number of countries with such data were available, just two groups were formed for this analysis. The Northern, Western and Southern European countries are in one group (Figure 4), and the available Central and Eastern European countries are in a second group (Figure 5). The relatively small number of countries implies that generalizations have their limitations. Nevertheless, the following analyses provide a reasonably adequate idea of what has transpired.

4.1 Northern, Western and Southern Europe (in short, the "West")

The propensity to have a first child moved along similar paths in all these populations among the cohorts of the 1930s and early 1940s (Figure 4, Panel A). This trend even increased somewhat, with close to 90 percent of women in the baby boom cohorts having a first birth. Beginning with the cohorts of the mid 1940s, the PPRs 0→1 began to decline in a number of countries, and remained stable in others. In France the propensity to have a first child remained at the 90 percent level through the cohorts of the 1960s, with Denmark not far behind. A moderate yet steady decline in the PPRs 0→1 started among the cohorts of the late 1940s in the Netherlands, England & Wales, and Austria. In the cohorts of the early 1960s, the propensity to have a first child was between 80 and 82 percent in the latter three countries. In Italy the decline of the PPR 0→1 started with the cohorts of the mid 1950s, and was steep so that, among the 1960s cohorts, only 75 to 80 percent of women had a first birth.

There was a considerable variety in the PPRs 1→2 in the West (Figure 4, Panel B). England & Wales, Sweden, the Netherlands, France and Greece had ratios at or above 0.80. In contrast, Austria and especially Italy experienced declines in the PPRs 1→2, and among the cohorts of the 1960s only about 70 percent of women with one child went on to have a second birth.

The retreat from the baby boom is especially visible in the declines of the progression ratios from second to third births, and even more so in a prolonged decline of the PPRs 3→4 (Figure 4, Panels C and D). The declines of the PPRs 2→3 occurred in most countries among the cohorts of the late 1930s and the early 1940s. Among the cohorts of the 1950s and 1960s, these ratios settled at levels over 0.35; in Italy and Austria, the decline continued even among the cohorts of the 1950s, with only around 30 to 35 percent of women with two children going on to have a third birth.

What is important for the overall level of fertility in individual countries is the combined result of trends and levels of all parity progression ratios. In contemporary low-fertility populations, it is mainly the progression to first, second and third births. To illustrate this point, two cases will be compared. Italy experienced a rapid decline of PPRs 0→1 with levels below 0.80 in the 1960s cohorts. The pathway for the PPRs 1→2, as well as the PPRs 2→3, was also one of decline and eventual low levels (Figure 4, Panels A, B and C). In contrast, the French population had high and steady PPRs 0→1 at the 0.90 level; it did not experience any decline of the fairly high PPRs 1→2; and although there was an initial decline in the progression to third births, these PPRs settled at the highest level for all countries among the youngest cohorts (Figure 4, Panels A, B and C). Consequently, the total cohort fertility rates among the mid 1960s cohorts were about 1.5 in Italy, and 2.0 in France (Council of Europe 2006).

4.2 Central and Eastern Europe (in short, the "East")

The progression ratios to first births were consistently high during the socialist era in all the Central and Eastern European countries, between 0.90 and 0.95 (Figure 5, Panel A). Signs of declines show up among the cohorts of the 1960s, most notably in Poland.

The levels of the PPRs 1→2 differed greatly between countries, but the trends were not too varied (Figure 5, Panel B). By far the lowest level of PPRs 1→2 was in the Russian Federation. Interestingly, progression to second births increased up to the 1950s cohorts in the Czech Republic, and some increase could also be detected in Poland. A common feature for all these populations was a notable subsequent decline in the PPRs 1→2, which usually started with the cohorts born around 1960. In the Russian Federation, this decline was the fastest.

The progression ratios to third births were declining among most cohorts in question (Figure 5, Panel C). The levels were distinctly higher in Poland and the Slovak Republic, which were the countries with higher fertility at that time.

A gradual decline occurred in the PPRs 3→4 up to the 1950s cohorts (Figure 5, Panel D), after which the percentage of women with three children who continued on to have a fourth child consolidated at between 20 and 40 percent. This may seem high, but it is actually of minor consequence because the intensity of third birth fertility rates was already extremely low in these countries (Frejka, Sardon 2007).

Overall, the trends of changes in the parity progression ratios in the East were in analogous directions. There was a considerable spread in the variety of levels between countries, except for the PPRs 0→1. The persistently lowest PPRs 1→2 in the Russian Federation constituted a serious deviation consistent with the prominence of the one-child family in that country since the 1940 cohorts (Figure 3, Panel B). The common decline in the PPRs 1→2 among the cohorts of the late 1950s and early 1960s constitutes an important element among the indications suggesting a possible start of an erosion of the two-child family model.

Figure 4:   Parity progression ratios, Northern, Western and Southern Europe, birth cohorts 1930-1966

Panel A

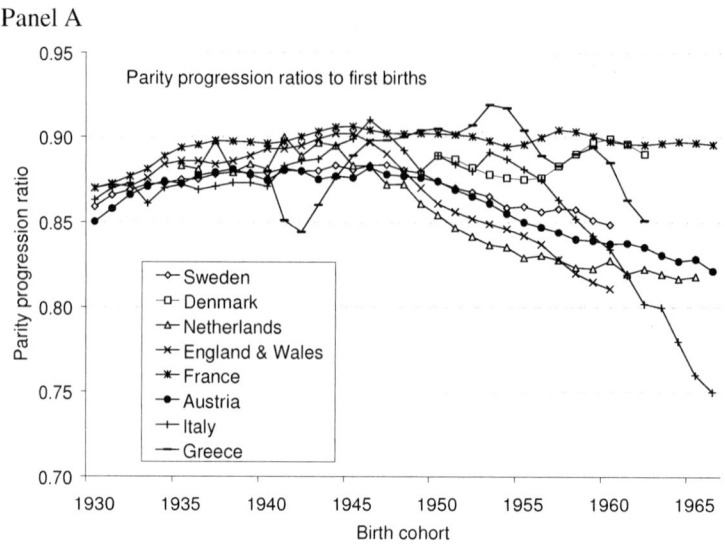

Panel B

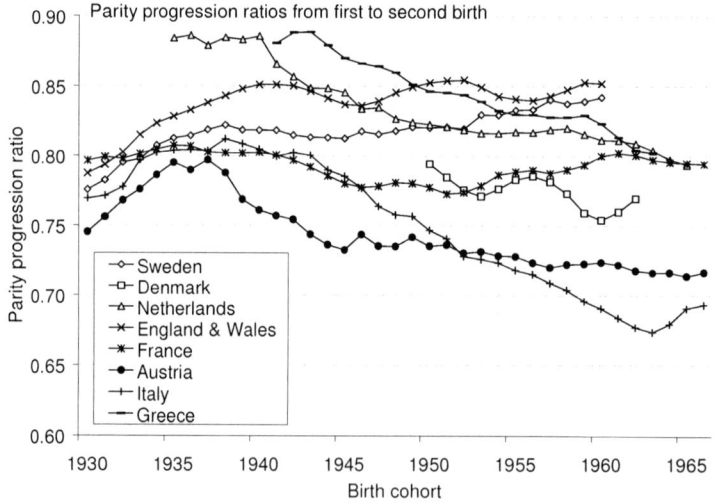

Figure 4:   (Continued)

Panel C

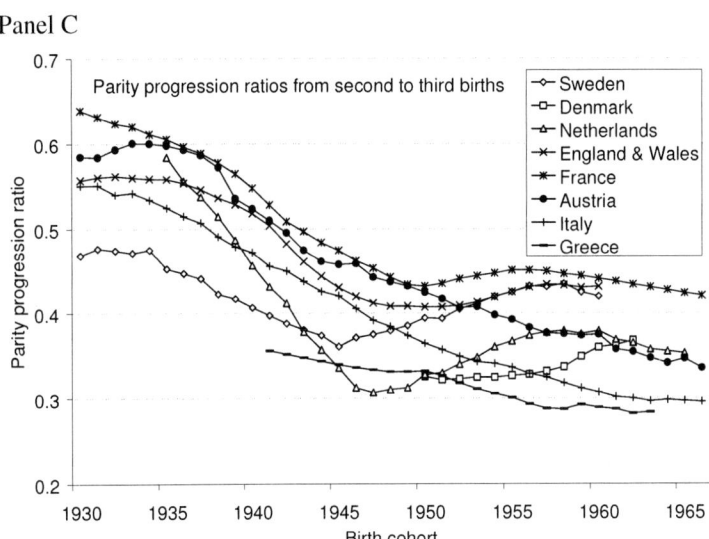

Panel D

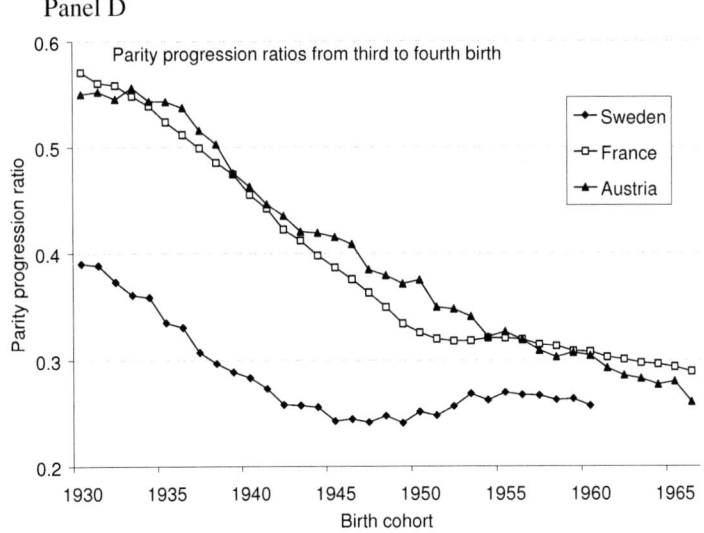

Source: Country chapters and *Observatoire Démographique Européen.*
Note: Data for Denmark, Netherlands, England & Wales, Italy and Greece not available.

Figure 5:   Parity progression ratios, Central and Eastern Europe, birth cohorts 1930-1966

Panel A

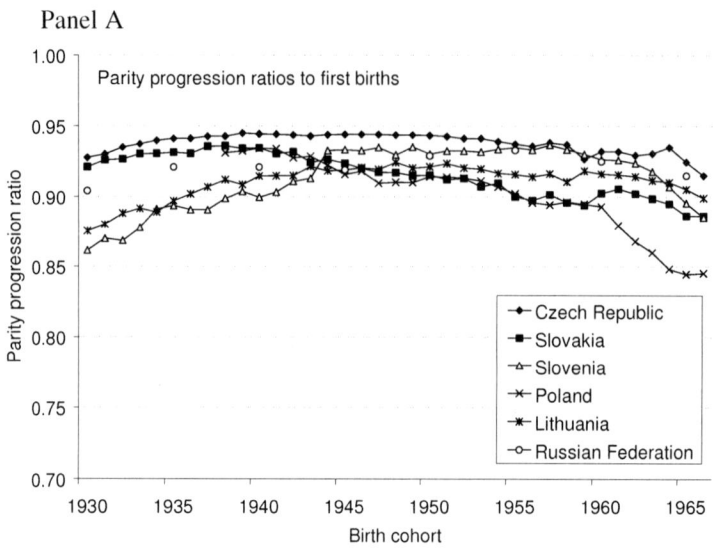

Panel B

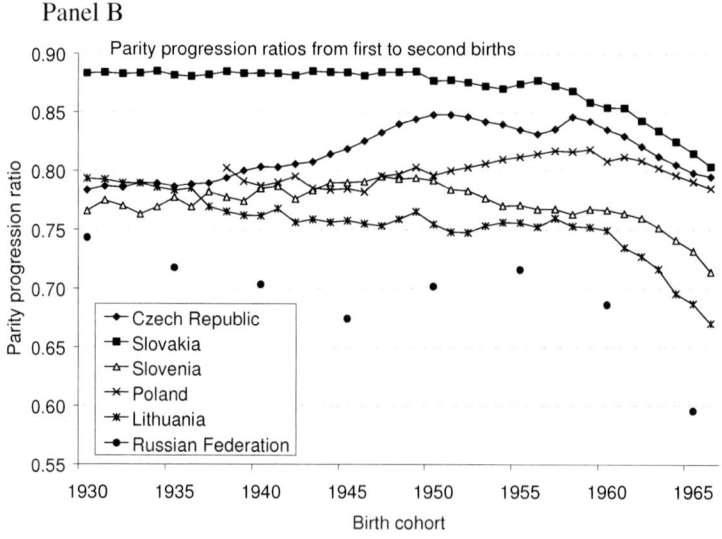

Figure 5:   (Continued)

Panel C

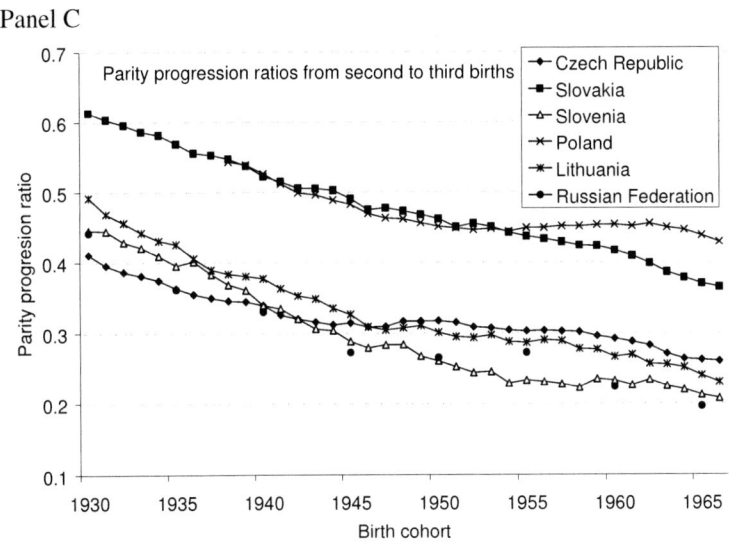

Panel D

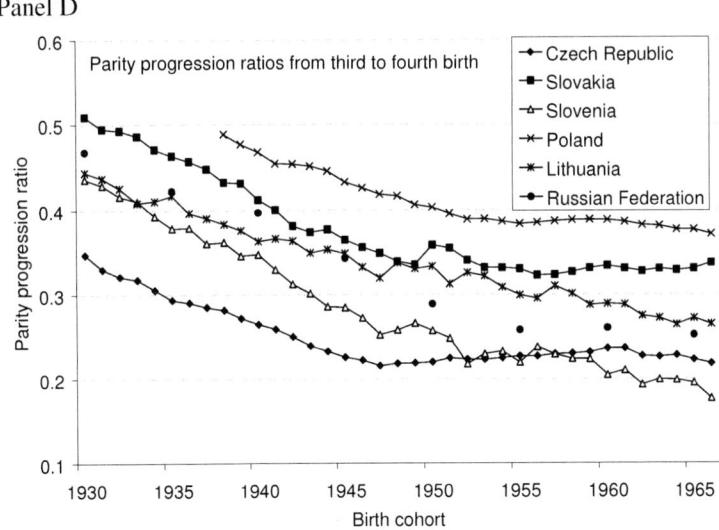

Source: Country chapters and *Observatoire Démographique Européen.*

5. Conclusions

The two-child family was well established in almost all European countries towards the end of the 20th century. But how long is this dominance of the two-child family going to last? Shares of childless women were growing among cohorts of the 1950s and 1960s, yet it is too early to tell when, and at what level, these shares might stabilize. Proportions of one-child families were stable in Northern and Western Europe, and were increasing in Southern Europe and the Central and Eastern European countries. So far it appears that proportions of childless women are growing faster than shares of women with one child. In some countries, however, shares of the one-child family were growing rapidly, and their proportions were becoming close to equal to those of the two-child family, notably in Romania and the Russian Federation. Shares of large families were continuing to decline in Southern, Central and Eastern Europe, and were quite stable in Western and Northern Europe. The overall analyses in the country chapters and in other overview chapters indicate that a comeback of the large family is not a realistic prospect.

There were some incipient signs that the two-child family might be starting to lose its prominent position. Will it be replaced mostly by childless women, or by the one-child family? Neither of these alternatives appears likely in the near future. But in a few countries, shares of the small family (defined as a combination of childless and one-child families) were close to matching the two-child family shares among the early to mid-1960s cohorts. Considering that fertility continued to decline in most countries during the 1990s and early 2000s (cf. overview chapter 1), and keeping in mind that shares of large families are not likely to increase, it is only reasonable to conclude that the weight of "small families" is increasing at the expense of the two-child family among the cohorts of the 1970s, and possibly also among the cohorts of the early 1980s. We will know for sure when these cohorts approach the end of their childbearing years.

References

Auth, D., and B. Holland-Cruz. (Eds.) 2006. Grenzen der Bevölkerungspolitik. Strategien und Diskurse demographischer Steuerung. Opladen: Verlag Barbara Budrich.

Council of Europe. 2006. *Recent demographic developments in Europe 2005.* Strasbourg: Council of Europe Publishing.

Dorbritz, J., and K. Ruckdeschel. 2007. Kinderlosigkeit in Deutschland – Ein europäischer Sonderweg? Daten, Trends und Gründe, in D. Konietzka and M. Kreyenfeld (Eds.), *Ein Leben ohne Kinder.* Wiesbaden: Verlag für Sozialwissenschaften,.

Frejka, T., and J.-P. Sardon. 2004. *Childbearing Trends and Prospects in Low-Fertility countries: A cohort analysis.* Dorbrecht: Kluwer Academic Publishers.

Frejka, T., and J.-P. Sardon. 2007. Cohort birth order, parity progression ratio and parity distribution trends in developed countries, *Demographic Research* 16(11): 315–374. www.demographicresearch.org.

Goldstein, J., W. Lutz, and M. R. Testa. 2003. The emergence of sub-replacement family size ideals in Europe, *Population Research and Policy Review* 22: 479–496.

Fokkema T., and I. Esveldt. 2005. Family size – wishes and limitations, *Studia Demograficzne* 2(2005): 35–53.

Höpflinger, F. 1991. Neue Kinderlosigkeit. Demographische Trends und gesellschaftliche Spekulationen. *Acta Demographica.* 1:81-100, Physica Verlag, Heidelberg.

Prskawetz, A., I. Buber, T. Sobotka, and H. Engelhardt. 2006. Recent changes in family policies in Austria and Germany: a response to very low fertility, *Entre Nous* 63:27–29.

Sobotka, T. 2004. *Postponement of childbearing and low fertility in Europe.* Amsterdam: Dutch University Press.

Sobotka, T. 2005. *Childless societies? Trends and projections of childlessness in Europe and the United States.* Unpublished manuscript.

Testa, M. R. 2006. *Childbearing preferences and family issues in Europe.* Special Eurobarometer 253/Wave 65.1 – TNS Opinion & Social, European Commission.

Van de Kaa, Dirk J. 2001. Postmodern fertility preferences: from changing value orientation to new behavior, in Bulatao, A. Rodolfo and J. B. Casterline (Eds.), *Global Fertility Transition. Supplement to Population and Development Review.* 27: 290-331.

Demographic Research: Volume 19, Article 5
research article

Overview Chapter 3:
Birth regulation in Europe:
Completing the contraceptive revolution

Tomas Frejka[1]

Abstract

Early in the 21st century modern contraception -- primarily hormonal methods, advanced IUDs, sterilization and condoms -- has become the main instrument of birth regulation in Northern and Western Europe and gaining ground in Southern Europe and the formerly state socialist countries of Central and Eastern Europe. Legal induced abortion use, which was highly prevalent in Central and Eastern Europe, has been declining since the demise of authoritarian regimes around 1990. Nonetheless, abortions are still used in countries of the former Soviet Union and the Balkans, where the "abortion culture" had been deeply ingrained. Liberal abortion legislation, modern induced abortion technology, and modern contraceptives, have enhanced women's health, been instrumental in childbearing postponement, have been a factor in changing partnership relations, and in the evolution of values regarding sexuality, reproduction, and childbearing, but they have not been a principal cause of contemporary low fertility. Assisted reproductive technology (ART) is emerging and having a slight positive impact on fertility in some countries.

---

[1] E-mail: Tfrejka@aol.com

1. Introduction

Contraception and induced abortions were the principal means of regulating fertility in Europe in recent decades. Both were known already in the ancient cultures of Egypt, Greece, Rome and other countries (Himes 1936; van de Walle 1999), but were not widely practiced prior to the 19th century.

In addition to abstinence, the most widespread contraceptive method of the 19th and early 20th centuries was *coitus interruptus* – withdrawal (Santow 1993). The practice of induced abortion was also widespread. With time, other contraceptive methods were increasingly used, namely the douche, the rhythm method (also known as the *calendar method* or *periodic abstinence*) and condoms. The first intrauterine devices (IUDs) were introduced in the 1920s, but were not in general use before the 1960s. The U.S. Food and Drug Administration approved oral hormonal contraception, the "pill," in 1960; this marks the initiation of the era of truly modern contraception. The generally accepted contemporary classification of modern contraceptives includes sterilization, condoms and barrier methods in addition to IUDs, and various forms of hormonal contraception, such as the pill, injectables and implants. (We will use this terminology even though the characterization "modern" is historically inaccurate.) Rhythm, withdrawal, prolonged abstinence and douching are considered traditional methods. One reason for distinguishing between modern and traditional methods is the difference in their effectiveness in preventing conception. Modern methods are very effective when properly administered, whereas traditional methods tend to have high failure rates. When a modern contraceptive method is used consistently for 12 months, fewer than one pregnancy per 100 women-years will materialize, compared to 14 – 26 pregnancies when traditional methods are used[2] (United Nations 2000).

In the second half of the 20th century, several European countries had legal restrictions on the use of contraceptive methods, reflecting the position and influence of religious institutions, notably Christian churches. In the Netherlands, for example, "it was forbidden to sell or advertise contraceptives" in the 1960s, but "in 1969 the [Dutch] government removed the statutory prohibition on contraceptives" (Netherlands chapter). In principle, none of these restrictions are any longer in force early in the 21st century.

Abortion laws can be classified into five broad categories, reflecting various degrees of restrictiveness: (1) strict prohibition, or abortion only allowed to protect the woman's life; (2) abortion also permitted to protect a woman's physical health; (3) abortion permitted to protect a woman's physical and mental health; (4) abortion permitted on socioeconomic grounds; and (5) abortion permitted on demand during a

---

[2] Although the male condom is considered a modern method its effectiveness is low: the probability of failure is 14 pregnancies per 100 women-years during 12 months of use.

prescribed period of the pregnancy without restriction as to reason. Induced abortions were almost universally illegal in the first half of the 20th century. After 1950, laws were liberalized in most European countries, first in the formerly state-socialist countries of Central and Eastern Europe in the mid-1950s, and gradually elsewhere. As of the early 21st century, induced abortions are permitted without any restriction as to reason in almost all European countries (Rahman et al. 1998), although a few countries have some legal constraints, and there are two significant exceptions. The most restrictive laws are still in force in Ireland. In Poland, abortion was permitted on socioeconomic grounds in 1956, but the law was revised in 1993 to permit abortion only when a pregnancy threatens the woman's life or health, when a pregnancy is the result of a crime, or if the foetus appears to be severely and incurably damaged (Kulczycki 1995).

The legal status of abortion may entail various consequences, such as increased health risks or the need to travel to other countries to obtain an abortion. Where restrictive laws are in force, the health risks can be considerable because induced abortions may not be performed in optimal hygienic conditions with advanced medical procedures. Following the imposition of extensive restrictions in eligibility for an induced abortion in Romania in October 1966, the abortion-related maternal mortality rate increased from 16.9 per 100,000 live births in 1965, to 151.3 in 1982, a nine-fold increase. Throughout the 1980s, 85 to 90 percent of maternal deaths in Romania were due to abortions (Baban 1999). The response to restrictive legislation in some countries is that women with a strong motivation to interrupt an unwanted pregnancy will travel to another country to obtain an abortion. "In Ireland … an increasing number of women have been travelling to England for abortion services" (Henshaw et al. 1999). The health risks to these women are negligible because of the good quality of the services in England. Nonetheless, even with liberal legislation the quality of abortion services may differ from one country to another, with differential effects on women's reproductive health.

The principal contemporary medical methods of pregnancy termination are vacuum aspiration and Mifepristone (RU-486) for early abortions, as well as dilatation and curettage (D&C). Up until the second half of the 20th century, the health risks associated with induced abortions were considerable. It was with the development of antisepsis that D&C became a relatively safe procedure when performed by qualified medical personnel. The introduction of vacuum aspiration roughly coincided with the widespread legalization of abortion (van de Walle 2003). RU-486 was invented in France in 1980, and has become a widely used method in a number of European countries. This method was used, for example, in 57 percent of induced abortions in 2005 in Sweden (Socialstyrelsen 2006)

Customarily, only the means to prevent conception and births -- contraception and induced abortion -- have been subsumed under the concept of birth regulation. In recent decades, however, various methods of assisted reproduction have been increasingly used by couples facing infertility, and these methods have become relevant for fertility trends (e.g., Stephen 2000). Assisted reproductive technology (ART) has led to a rise in the frequency of multiple births (Czech Republic chapter), and arguably has also had a slight positive impact on fertility rates, especially at higher reproductive ages (Hoorens et al. 2007, Sobotka et al. 2007). Leridon's (2004) study shows that assisted reproduction can partly offset the negative effects of fertility postponement on the ability to conceive. These findings justify the inclusion of such activities in the "birth regulation" concept.

The first human conceived by in vitro fertilization (IVF) was born in 1978 in England (Steptoe and Edwards 1978). A few other methods of ART have been developed since then, of which the most prominent is the intracytoplasmatic sperm injection (ICSI), which is commonly used in the case of male-factor infertility. The use of ART differs greatly between countries. These variations can be attributed to a number of factors, including differences in the provision of ART by the various national health care systems, differences in the legislative regulation of ART, and varying levels of access to ART treatments (Schenker 1997). In most European countries with available statistics on assisted reproduction, the proportion of children born after an ART treatment ranges between one and three percent, with Macedonia recording a very low volume of 0.2 percent, and Denmark reporting the highest success rate of 3.9 percent in 2003 (Anderson et al. 2007, these data exclude intrauterine inseminations).

2. Contraception

It is possible to get a general idea of levels and trends in contraceptive use in the four main regions of Europe in the past two decades from Table 1[3].

---

[3] The United Nations Population Division periodically provides an overview of contraceptive use around the world. Nationally representative sample surveys of women of reproductive age (usually restricted to women who are married or in a union) conducted by governments and international organizations are compiled and regional averages are estimated. The two most recent global overviews refer to 1998 and 2005 (United Nations 2001 and 2006), but reflect developments preceding those years because national surveys are conducted irregularly.

Table 1: **Contraceptive use and use of modern methods, by regions in Europe, as reported in 1998 and 2005, reflecting years prior to these dates**

| Region | Year reported | Percentage of couples using | | Percentage of users employing modern methods |
		any method	modern method	
Eastern Europe[a]	1998	69	31	44
	2005	62	36	58
Northern Europe	1998	78	77	98
	2005	79	75	95
Southern Europe	1998	69	31	46
	2005	69	49	71
Western Europe	1998	75	71	94
	2005	74	70	95

Sources: United Nations 2001, 2006.
Note: [a]The formerly state-socialist countries of Central and Eastern Europe.

The main observations that can be drawn from these data are as follows:

Contraceptive prevalence was higher in Northern and Western Europe than in Eastern and Southern Europe;

The use of modern contraceptives was almost universal in Northern and Western Europe;

Although relatively low, the use of modern contraceptives increased substantially in Eastern Europe and especially in Southern Europe during recent years.

The transition to the dominant use of modern contraceptives by the majority of populations, habitually referred to as "the contraceptive revolution" (Westoff & Ryder 1977), took place in Northern and Western Europe during the 1960s and 1970s. In Southern Europe, this occurred mostly during the 1980s and 1990s, and is still ongoing in the 2000s (see country chapters). In the formerly socialist countries of Central and Eastern Europe, major changes in contraceptive behaviour got under way with the collapse of the authoritarian regimes (For examples see Table 2 and the chapters on the Czech Republic, Poland, Russia, and Slovakia).

Table 2: **Percentage currently using contraception, married women of reproductive age[a], selected European countries, 1971-1999**

Country	Year	Any method	Prevalence of modern methods						Percentage of users employing modern methods
			Total	Sterilization	Pill	IUD	Condom	Withdrawal	
Czech	1991	78	53	2	7	17	27	25[b]	68
Republic	1993	69	45	3	8	15	19	22	65
	1997	72	63	12	23	14	13	7	88
Romania	1978	58	5	..	1	0	3	26	9
	1993	57	15	1	5	11	4	34	26
	1999	64	30	3	8	7	9	29	47
Finland	1971	77	54	0	20	3	31	16	70
	1977	80	78	4	11	29	32	2	98
	1989	77	75	16	11	26	20	1	97
Spain	1977	51	20	0	13	1	5	22	39
	1985	59	38	5	16	6	12	16	64
	1995	81	67	20	15	8	24	11	83
France	1972	64	21	0	11	1	8	33	33
	1978	79	48	5	27	10	6	22	61
	1988	81	67	7	30	26	4	7	83
	1994	75	69	8	36	20	5	3	92

Sources: United Nations 2001, 2006.
Notes: a – Women currently married or in consensual unions, usually ages 15-44 or 15-49; b - includes rhythm.

There was considerable variation between countries in the composition of contraceptive methods used, and in their trends of use over time. Taking into account that contraceptive methods tend to be used differentially depending on age (mainly, on the age of women), an almost universal increase in the use of the more effective methods, sterilization and the pill can be observed (Table 2). Conversely, the use of traditional methods has declined across the board, as exemplified by the trends in the use of withdrawal.

One specific development is worth pointing out. The overall use of sterilisation has generally been increasing. Nonetheless, the delay of childbearing, with a growing number of women "catching up" towards the end of their reproductive period, has led to some decline in the use of sterilisation at those ages. In Great Britain, for example, "since the 1980s, particularly among couples in their 30s and early 40s, the popularity of sterilisation as a method of contraception seems to have decreased, whilst among women aged 45–49 it appears to have increased" (Botting and Dunnell 2000). This phenomenon is apparently occurring in several Western countries (see, for example, Figure 19 and its discussion in Netherlands chapter).

When looking at the mix of contraceptives being used and the trends of use of specific contraceptives, a clear distinction can be made between those countries where the contraceptive revolution has run its course, and those countries where change is still in progress. In those countries where the contraceptive revolution is complete, the use of traditional methods is now almost zero. In a number of countries, such as the Czech Republic and Spain, change in the use of contraceptives was progressing rapidly during the 1990s, and the patterns of use are coming close to those of countries with a completed transformation. Romania is an example of a country where changes in contraceptive use still have a long way to go. Despite a significant ongoing metamorphosis, fewer than half of all couples in Romania were using modern contraceptives in 1999, but the transformation no doubt continued during the 2000s (Romania chapter).

3. Induced abortions

"Abortion culture" is the term succinctly characterizing the nature of birth regulating behaviour in the formerly socialist countries of Central and Eastern Europe for the four decades of the 1950s through the 1980s (Stloukal 1999). Liberal abortion legislation, coupled with health systems advancing curative, rather than preventive, medicine, made induced abortions easy to obtain and socially acceptable. With the exception of Hungary, the GDR, and parts of the former Yugoslavia, modern contraceptives, especially the pill, were difficult to obtain, and most couples were using traditional ineffective contraception (Stloukal 1995; Sobotka 2003). Withdrawal, and, to a lesser extent, the rhythm method and condoms, were being employed by a majority of users (Frejka 1983; David 1999).

There were major differences between these countries in the incidence of induced abortions. For the most part, women had an average of one to two lifetime abortions. But in the Soviet Union and Romania, the total induced abortion rate around 1960 was on the order of five to almost eight lifetime abortions per woman (Frejka 1983).

Birth prevention behaviour changed significantly during the 1990s and early 2000s following the collapse of the totalitarian regimes in the formerly socialist countries, although some reshaping was seeping in prior to that. The incidence of induced abortion decreased in all these Central and Eastern European countries (Table 3) together with a major shift to modern contraceptives (Tables 1 and 2). The real decline of induced abortions might not have been quite as impressive as official data depict due to likely incomplete registration. By the early 2000s, countries of Central Europe with reliable abortion registration experienced levels close to those prevalent in Western Europe, but there were a number of countries where a considerable proportion of women were still resorting to induced abortion. This was particularly true in the countries of the former Soviet Union and in the Balkans (Sobotka 2003), where the "abortion culture" had been deeply ingrained, living conditions for diverse socio-economic strata of the population were improving unevenly and gradually, and it was taking time for birth preventing behaviour to modernize.

Table 3: **Legal induced abortions, rates (per 1000 women of reproductive age) and total abortion rates, selected countries, 1980–2003**

Country	Rates of legal induced abortion				Total induced abortion rate[c]			
	1980	1990	1996	2003	1980	1990	1996	2003
Croatia[a]	50.3	40.1	12.9	6.5	1.5	1.2	0.4	0.2
Czech Republic	32.3	47.7	20.7	12.6	1.0	1.4	0.6	0.4
Hungary	36.3	41.2	34.7	25.8	1.1	1.2	1.0	0.7
Romania[a]	u	181.7	78.0	34.8	u	5.5	2.3	1.0
Russian Federation[a]	[123.1]	[109.3]	68.4[e]	44.5	3.7	3.3	2.0[e]	1.3
Russian Federation (see chapter)						3.4[d]	2.5	1.6
Finland	20.4	11.1	10.0	10.8	0.6	0.3	0.3	0.3
Sweden	20.7	21.3	18.7	20.2	0.6	0.6	0.6	0.6
Spain[a]	u	4.3	5.7	8.5	u	0.1	0.1	0.2
Germany	u	8.5	7.6	7.7	u	0.3	0.2	0.2
France	21.6	16.4	16.6	16.5	0.6	0.5	0.5	0.5
France (see chapter)	19.0[f]	14.0[d]	14.2	14.1	0.6[f]	0.5[d]	0.5	0.5
Netherlands[b]	6.7	5.2	6.5	8.6	0.2	0.2	0.2	0.3

Sources: Henshaw et al. 1999 (for columns 1980, 1990, and 1996); Sedgh et al. 2007 (for column 2003); Rossier and Pirus (2007) for France; papers in this volume.

Notes: a – Incomplete or of unknown completeness; b – Residents only; c – The total induced abortion rate is the average number of induced abortions per woman during her lifetime if present levels were to prevail. It is commonly estimated by multiplying rates per 1000 women of reproductive age by 30 (the number of years between age 15 and age 45). Data in the table are either such estimates or those cited in papers of this volume; d – 1991; e – 1995; f – 1981; u – Unknown.

Throughout Western Europe, especially following the introduction of modern contraceptives in the 1960s and 1970s, levels of induced abortions were low, and abortion was apparently employed to a large extent as a backup measure. The total induced abortion rates (TIARs) were generally below 0.6 abortions per woman (Table 3), with no major fluctuations over time. A relatively high level of induced abortions by Western European standards is not necessarily taken as problematic in a particular country. The fact that France has one of the highest TIARs in the West (at the level of 0.5 to 0.6) appears to be accepted as normal (France chapter). In Sweden, TIARs are equally high, which can be attributed to about 20 percent of couples using traditional methods of contraception; this proportion has remained stable for several decades (Sweden chapter). Even though there are efforts to increase the use of modern contraceptives in Sweden, these have not been very successful. Yet apparently authorities are not much concerned, possibly because "currently more than half of the induced abortions are performed before the 7th week of pregnancy" (Sweden chapter). In Spain, on the other hand, the TIAR has been much lower than in France and Sweden. However, as the numbers of induced abortions, and thus their incidence, have been increasing in Spain since decriminalization in 1985, the level of induced abortions is perceived as high, especially among young people, and "may be regarded to be a consequence of shortcomings in sex education, for these subjects are not included in school curricula" (Spain chapter).

4. Effects

The significant advancements in contraceptive and induced abortion technologies, and their relatively easy and widespread availability, are phenomena of the second half of the 20th century. Presumably this could imply that they have had a profound impact on fertility levels and trends. Was that the case? What would the course of fertility have been towards the end of the 20th century without modern contraceptive technology, and without liberal abortion legislation? If the absence of the latter features had been the only societal development that was different over the past half century, fertility trends might not have been much different than they were in reality. Remember that over half of Europe's population was reproducing at below the replacement level in the 1920s (Kirk 1946), and that this was brought about by employing mainly withdrawal, condoms and illegal abortions. Restricted childbearing motivation was the critical factor. For a more modern example, let us note that developments in Poland in the 1990s suggest that legislative changes may have only negligible visible fertility consequences. The rescinding of liberal abortion legislation in 1993 apparently had only a marginal effect on declining fertility, although without the ban fertility might have declined faster. On the other hand, under certain circumstances the legal curtailment of induced abortion, combined with limited access to contraception, can affect fertility markedly, as was the case in Romania after 1966. There fertility was retained at a relatively high level compared to most other formerly state-socialist countries through the late 1980s.

According to this line of reasoning, liberal abortion legislation and modern induced abortion technology, as well as the availability of new contraceptives, may have facilitated a behaviour that people found preferable in any case, and this may have been its main effect. Even without the liberal abortion legislation, without vacuum aspiration and RU-486, and without the improved contraceptive technology, childbearing trends of the past several decades would most likely have been similar to what actually occurred. It is the motivations shaped by living conditions, as well as by values, norms and attitudes, that modify childbearing behaviour. People would have used whatever contraception was available, backed up by some illegal abortions, to achieve their goals. The changed abortion legislation, together with modern abortion and contraceptive technologies, made it easier for people to have the number of children they desired.

Several additional, overlapping, crucial effects surface when childbearing developments of the past 50 years are examined in greater detail.

Modern contraceptives have reduced the incidence of unwanted and mistimed pregnancies and births, which, in turn, has reduced the incidence of legal and illegal induced abortions. The latter is a significant contribution to improved reproductive health.

Modern contraceptives have contributed to a decline in unwanted and mistimed pregnancies and births at all ages. In most countries, this decline has been more pronounced among young women, especially teenagers.

Modern contraception and liberal abortion legislation have been instrumental in enabling women and couples to postpone childbearing to higher ages. Postponed fertility generates period fertility that is lower than what would otherwise be the case, and can be a factor in declining lifetime childbearing.

The use of modern contraceptives, complemented by relatively easy access to legal induced abortions, provides women (couples) with tools that allow them to time pregnancies more effectively than was previously possible, and thus to have greater control over life-cycle events, such as education, employment, career development and marriage (Presser 2001; Sobotka 2004).

The use of modern contraceptives, complemented by relatively easy access to legal induced abortions, constitutes one out of a number of basic components/phases of the second demographic transition (van de Kaa 2001). At the same time, the application of modern contraceptives and liberal abortion legislation are instrumental in generating other characteristics of the SDT, namely postponement of marriages and births, and the separation of sex and procreation. These characteristics are, in turn, preconditions for new forms of partnership and family behaviour, as well as changes in values and norms on sexuality, reproduction and childbearing.

These developments can be seen as evidence that modern contraception and liberal induced abortion legislation have had unmistakable and highly significant fertility effects, as well as broader social effects. These family planning tools have improved people's lives, enhanced women's health, and been instrumental in childbearing timing and postponement. In addition, enhanced control over fertility has been a factor in changing partnership relations, and in the evolution of values and norms on sexuality, reproduction and childbearing.

References

Anderson, N. A., A. V. Goossens, L. Gianaroli, R. Felberbaum, J. de Mouzon, and K. G. Nygren. 2007. Assisted reproductive technology in Europe, 2003. Results generated from European registers by ESHRE. *Human Reproduction* 22(6): 1513–25.

Baban, A. 1999. Romania, in H. P. David (Ed.), From Abortion to Contraception: A Resource to Public Policies and Reproductive Behavior in Central and Eastern Europe from 1917 to the Present. Westport, Connecticut: Greenwood Press, pp: 191-221.

Botting, B., and K. Dunnell. 2000. Trends in fertility and contraception in the last quarter of the 20th century. *Population Trends 100, UK National Statistics* http://www.statistics. gov.uk/articles/population_trends/fertconttrends_pt100.pdf.

David, H. P. (Ed.) 1999. From abortion to contraception. A resource to public policies and reproductive behavior in Central and Eastern Europe from 1917 to the present. Westport, Connecticut: Greenwood Press.

Frejka, T. 1983. Induced Abortion and Fertility: a Quarter Century of Experience in Eastern Europe, *Population and Development Review* 9(3): 494–520.

Henshaw, S. K., S. Singh, and T. Haas. 1999. Recent trends in abortion rates worldwide, *International Family Planning Perspectives* 25(1): 44–48.

Himes, N. E. 1936 (reprinted 1963). *Medical History of Contraception.* New York: Gamut Press.

Hoorens, S., F. Gallo, J. A. K. Cave, and J. C. Grant. 2007. Can assisted reproductive technologies help to offset population ageing? An assessment of the demographic and economic impact of ART in Denmark and UK, *Human Reproduction* 22(9): 2471–2475.

Kirk, D. 1946. *Europe's Population in the Interwar Years.* Princeton, NJ: League of Nations and Princeton University Press

Kulczycki, A. 1995. Abortion policy in post-communist Europe. The conflict in Poland, *Population and Development Review* 21(3): 471–505.

Leridon, H. 2004. Can assisted reproduction technology compensate for the natural decline in fertility with age? A model assessment, *Human Reproduction* 19(7): 1549–1554.

Presser, H. B. 2001. Comment: A gender perspective for understanding low fertility in post-transitional societies, in R. A. Bulatao and J. B. Casterline (Eds.), *Global fertility transition. Supplement to Population and Development Review* 27: 177–183.

Rahman, A., L. Katzive, and S. K. Henshaw. 1998. A global review of laws on induced abortion, 1985–1997, *International Family Planning Perspectives* 24(2): 56–64.

Rossier C., and C. Pirus. 2007. Estimating the number of abortions in France, 1976–2002, *Populatio E* 62(1): 57–88.

Santow, G. 1993. Coitus interruptus in the twentieth century, *Population and Development Review* 19(4): 767–792.

Schenker, J. G. 1997. Assisted reproduction practice in Europe: legal and ethical aspects, *Human Reproduction Update* 3(2): 173–184.

Sedgh G., S. K. Henshaw, S. Singh, A. Bankole, and J. Drescher. 2007. Incidence and recent trends in legal abortion worldwide, *International Family Planning Perspectives* Forthcoming September 2007.

Sobotka, T. 2003. Re-emerging diversity: rapid fertility changes in Central and Eastern Europe after the collapse of the communist regimes, *Population-E* 58(4–5): 451–486.

Sobotka, T. 2004. *Postponement of childbearing and low fertility in Europe*. Doctoral thesis, University of Groningen, Amsterdam: Dutch University Press.

Sobotka, T., M. Hansen, T. Jensen, and N. E. Skakkebaek. 2007. Will fertility among Danish women remain stable due to assisted reproduction? Assessing the role of in vitro fertilization in sustaining cohort fertility rates. PAA Annual Meeting, New York.

Socialstyrelsen (The National Board of Health and Welfare, Centre For Epidemiology, Sweden), 2006. *Aborter 2005*. www.socialstyrelsen.se.

Steptoe, P. C., and R. G. Edwards. 1978. Birth after the reimplantation of a human embryo, *Lancet* 2(8085): 366.

Stephen, E. H. 2000. Demographic implications of assisted reproductive technologies, *Population Research and Policy Review* 19(4): 301–315.

Stloukal, L. 1995. Demographic aspects of abortion in Eastern Europe: A study with special reference to the Czech Republic and Slovakia. PhD Thesis, Canberra: Australian National University.

Stloukal, L. 1999. Understanding the 'abortion culture' in Central and Eastern Europe, in H. P. David (Ed.), From Abortion to Contraception: A Resource to Public Policies and Reproductive Behavior in Central and Eastern Europe from 1917 to the Present. Westport, Connecticut: Greenwood Press, pp 23-37.

United Nations. 2001. *Levels and Trends of Contraceptive Use as Assessed in 1998*. ST/ESA/SER.A/190. New York: United Nations

United Nations. 2006. *World Contraceptive Use 2005*. New York: United Nations.

Van de Kaa, D. J. 2001. Postmodern fertility preferences: from changing value orientation to new behavior, in R. A. Bulatao and J. B. Casterline (Eds.), *Global fertility transition. Supplement to Population and Development Review* 27: 290–331.

Van de Walle, E. 1999. Towards a demographic history of abortion, *Population. An English Selection* 11: 115–132.

Van de Walle, E. 2003. Induced abortion: history, in P. Demeny and G. McNicoll (Eds.), *Encyclopedia of Population*, New York: MacMillan Reference USA, pp: 527–529.

Westoff, C. F., and N. B. Ryder. 1977. *The Contraceptive Revolution*. Princeton: Princeton University Press.

Demographic Research: Volume 19, Article 6
research article

Overview Chapter 4:
Changing family and partnership behaviour:
Common trends and persistent diversity across Europe

Tomáš Sobotka [1]

Laurent Toulemon [2]

Abstract

Following the era of the 'golden age of marriage' and the baby boom in the 1950s and 1960s, marriage has declined in importance, and its role as the main institution on which family relations are built has been eroded across Europe. Union formation most often takes place without a marriage. Family and living arrangements are currently heterogeneous across Europe, but all countries seem to be making the same shifts: towards fewer people living together as a couple, especially in marriage; an increased number of unmarried couples; more children born outside marriage; and fewer children living with their two parents. The relationship between these changing living arrangements, especially the decline of marriage, on the one hand, and the overall level of fertility, on the other, is not straightforward. In most countries, marriage rates and fertility declined simultaneously. However, the aggregate relationship between marriage and fertility indices has moved from negative (fewer marriages imply fewer births) to positive (fewer marriages imply more births). Thus, the decline of marriage, which is a part of the second demographic transition (see Overview Chapter 6), cannot be considered an important cause of the current low fertility level in many European countries. On the contrary, in European countries where the decline of marriage has been less pronounced, fertility levels are currently lower than in countries where new living arrangements have become most common.

[1] Vienna Institute of Demography (VID). E-mail: tomas.sobotka@oeaw.ac.at
[2] Institut national d'études démographiques (INED). E-mail: toulemon@ined.fr

1. Introduction

Families and living arrangements in developed countries have changed dramatically since the 1960s. The major features of this change, such as the gradual decline of marriage and the growth of cohabitation, the postponement of union formation and childbearing, the rise in union instability, and the disconnection between marriage, sex, and reproduction, have been observed in all regions of Europe, and have been analysed in detail in dozens of publications and research articles (e.g., Kuijsten 1996, Lesthaeghe and Moors 2002, Billari 2005, Prioux 2006). These developments also constitute major behavioural landmarks of the second demographic transition, discussed in depth in Overview Chapter 6, and they are widely reflected in different country chapters in this volume.[*] Family life and the meaning of family have undergone a profound change. Intimate partnerships and sexuality, but also the relationships between parents and their children, have moved away from the realm of normative control and institutional regulation, giving rise to the new ideal of reflexive 'pure relationships' based on mutual consent and the recognition of individual autonomy (Giddens 1992). As noted in the France chapter, family has become "less of a place to reproduce generational and gender hierarchies, and more of a special space where individuals forge their identity" (Toulemon et al. 2008:524).

The ongoing transformation of the family is evidenced by the spread of family forms and living arrangements other than the nuclear families of (married) couples with children. Cohabiting unions, 'living apart together' partnerships, same-sex partnerships, one-parent families, and single living have increased in prominence. The boundaries between family and non-family life have become less clear-cut; Ahlburg and de Vita (1992: 2) observed that family patterns in the United States are so fluid that "the U.S. Census Bureau has difficulty measuring family trends." Legislative changes are also beginning to reflect the new family landscape. New laws and regulations on registered partnerships (of both homosexual and heterosexual couples), same-sex marriages, and, in the case of the Netherlands, the option of a 'flash annulment' of marriage without a prior divorce procedure (see the Netherlands chapter), further contribute to the diversity in family patterns. Arguably, the perception of what constitutes a family has changed as well. Kiernan's (2004) analysis of 1998 Eurobarometer data shows that children, rather than partnership status, appear to be more salient in defining families: according to the survey results, 59 percent of respondents consider a cohabiting couple with children to be a family, whereas 48 percent consider a married couple without children as a family.

---

[*] All overview and country chapters referred to herein are part of Special Collection 7: Childbearing Trends and Policies in Europe and can be found online at: http://www.demographic-research.org/special/7/.

On the other hand, just 27 percent of respondents consider a childless cohabiting couple to be a family. In line with this distinction, research on family change in Germany often focuses on the issue of 'polarisation' between family life and other forms of private life (Schulze and Tyrell 2002), whereby family is usually defined on the basis of the presence of children in the household (see Germany chapter).

The pace of change in family life and living arrangements varies across countries, cohorts, and social groups. Thus, the catchphrase 'convergence to diversity' best characterises the situation in which most countries follow a similar trajectory of family changes, but at the same time retain many distinct patterns of family behaviour (Kuijsten 1996). The increase in diversity is also manifested in the timing and sequencing of early life transitions. Events like home leaving, marrying, and becoming a parent often do not conform to the norms regarding the 'proper' sequence of events, and take place outside the previously accepted boundaries between youth and adulthood (Rindfuss 1991, Corijn and Klijzing 2001, Heinz and Krüger 2001).[3]

This contribution reviews trends and cross-country diversity in family, partnership behaviour, and living arrangements in contemporary Europe. Given the wide scope of this topic, we paint this picture with a broad brush, referring the reader to country-specific chapters and other studies for more details. Discussion of the roots of the observed changes in family behaviour is kept to a minimum; some of these factors are mentioned in Overview Chapter 6, which examines the concept of the second demographic transition and reviews changes in family-related values and attitudes in Europe. This study first outlines trends and regional differences in home-leaving patterns. Section 3 examines the evidence on the gradual retreat of marriage, especially from the lives of young adults. Section 4 discusses the rising importance of unmarried cohabitation, its diverse forms, and legislative responses to it. Section 5 summarises the evidence on the rise of other living arrangements, especially single living and 'living apart together' relationships, and discusses the increase in age at union formation. Section 6 analyses the rising rates of divorce and union dissolution, while Section 7 outlines the declining role of marriage for childbearing, highlights the broad diversity in non-marital childbearing in Europe, and notes the surprisingly widespread incidence of single motherhood. In conclusion, Section 8 discusses the relevance of family changes to fertility rates.

---

[3] Several studies emphasise a need for a more precise definition and measurement of different processes that supposedly lead to an increasing heterogeneity of individual life course experiences. Using different measures of 'de-standardisation,' Brückner and Mayer (2005) provide evidence of such a process in the domain of family formation in West Germany in the second half of the 20th century (they find, however, an increased homogeneity in cohort experiences of education and labour market participation). Similarly, Elzinga and Liefbroer (2007: 246) find "strong support to the idea that the family life trajectories of young adult women all across Western world are becoming more destandardised" (see also footnote 9).

Tables and graphs in our study draw from a number of different data sources, including official statistics and published expert estimates and analyses. We focus especially on the countries covered in this collection, but selected figures and tables also show data for other countries and for broader European regions. This selection, as well as the choice of countries, was in part determined by the limited data availability, especially with respect to long-term time series and specific topics that are not commonly reported in the official vital statistics, such as living arrangements, cohabitation, and leaving the parental home. The Fertility and Family Surveys, FFS (see http://www.unece.org/pau/ffs/; Macura and Beets 2002), constitute a unique source of comparable data on living arrangements of adults and children, and on fertility, in Europe. The major drawback of using the FFS lies in their age: Most of the surveys were conducted in 1992-1997, and the collected data thus typically provide a picture of family change and living arrangements up to the late 1980s and the early 1990s. The Gender and Generation Surveys currently being conducted (http://www.unece.org/pau/ggp/) will provide more comparable and updated figures (Vikat et al. 2007). The results presented in this chapter, which are based on the FFS, illustrate well the ongoing family transformations, but they may not fully reflect the actual patterns of living arrangements. Specifically for Central and Eastern Europe, the Fertility and Family Surveys often reflect the household and family patterns prevailing in the late stages of state socialism, i.e., before 1990, and do not capture the rapid transformation in living arrangements in the 1990s.

2. North-South contrasts in home-leaving patterns

Departure from the parental home is a key event in the life of a young adult, and is commonly seen as a precondition to living with a partner and becoming a parent. Two studies based on the FFS (Corijn and Klijzing 2001, Billari, Philipov, and Baizán 2001) provide a comparative analysis of the timing and patterns of home leaving in Europe. They depict wide differences in home-leaving behaviour of the cohorts born around 1960, with the two most contrasting patterns prevailing in Southern Europe and in the Nordic countries (See Table 1 based on Billari, Philipov, and Baizán 2001; see also Billari 2004). In Southern Europe, the 'latest-late' pattern (Billari 2004) dominates: home leaving takes place late, especially for men who often reside with their parents even after reaching the age of 30, and it has been delayed among the cohorts born in the 1950s (Corijn and Klijzing 2001: Table 13.1) and 1960s (Italy chapter). In Northern Europe, both women and men leave home at a young age (median age for Swedish women is under 19), there is little diversity in the age at home leaving between individuals, and almost everyone leaves before the age of 30. Most of the post-communist countries did not display a particularly early or late home-leaving pattern at the time of the FFS, but ages at leaving home were more diverse in these countries, as many men and women continued to reside with their parents until their early thirties (Corijn and Klijzing 2001).

Table 1:   Home-leaving patterns among cohorts born around 1960; selected countries of Europe

Country	Median age			Never left home by age 30 (%)		Percentage leaving home after first union	
	Men	Women	Difference	Men	Women	Men	Women
Northern Europe							
Sweden	20.2	18.6	1.6	2	1	6	6
Western Europe (incl. German-speaking countries)							
Austria	21.8	19.9	1.9	16	6	28	20
France	21.5	19.8	1.7	9	5	5	3
Germany (East)	22.4	20.6	1.8	8	4	19	28
Germany (West)	22.4	20.8	1.6	11	4	11	11
The Netherlands	22.5	20.5	2.0	5	2	NA	NA
United Kingdom	22.4	20.3	2.1	11	5	NA	NA
Southern Europe							
Italy	26.7	23.6	3.1	32	20	8	9
Spain	25.7	22.9	2.8	25	14	11	11
Central and Eastern Europe							
Czech Republic	23.8	21.2	2.6	18	16	31	34
Hungary	24.8	21.3	3.5	27	17	32	35
Lithuania	20.3	19.8	0.5	20	22	28	32
Poland	25.8	22.5	3.3	37	23	27	29
Slovenia	20.9	20.5	0.4	15	13	23	27

Source: Billari, Philipov, and Baizán 2001 (based on the FFS data).

In Central and Eastern Europe, this long co-residence of children with their parents is mostly involuntary. In the past, it was attributable to a lack of housing coupled with a rigid, centrally organised system of distribution, which meant that housing was often available only to families with children. The housing shortage, now more in terms of cost than availability, is still an important obstacle to home leaving in this region (Czech Republic and Slovenia chapters). Combined with a rapid expansion of higher education, the persistent housing shortage explains the observed trend towards delayed home leaving in these countries (see also Section 5.1). It also helps to explain another interesting feature of the Central-Eastern European home-leaving pattern; namely, a high proportion of first unions that start before leaving the parental home. Around one-third of women in the Czech Republic, East Germany, Lithuania, Poland, and Slovenia entered a union while still living with their parents. With the exception of Austria, this proportion fell below 12 percent for other countries shown in Table 1 (especially in France and Sweden, where this pattern was an exception, experienced by three and six percent of women, respectively).[4]

Differences in welfare regimes, combined with long-term cultural differences between the East and the West (Hajnal 1965), and between the North and the South of Europe (Reher 1998), also explain many cross-country differences in European home-leaving patterns (Billari 2004). Besides the availability of housing, specific institutional and economic factors, such as employment, income, and spatial distribution of tertiary education, are often identified as important determinants of home leaving (e.g., Holdsworth 2000; Billari, Philipov, and Baizán 2001; Aassve et al. 2002; Mulder, Clark, and Wagner 2002). Dense regional networks of universities in Italy and Spain enable many young people to pursue studies while remaining with their parents, whereas in the Netherlands, a generous student loan system, combined with relatively long distances to higher educational institutions, mean that many young people leave the parental home at a younger age in order to attend university (the Netherlands chapter). Interestingly, employment and earnings are particularly important in the late-leaving and weak welfare state countries of Southern Europe, where young adults who have a job and a higher income leave the nest earlier. These factors do not play any significant role for home leaving in the early-leaving and 'Social Democratic' welfare countries of Northern Europe, where young adults leave home irrespective of their employment status and personal income. In Northern Europe, young people thus often experience poverty, even if only for a short period, after leaving home (Aassve et al. 2002).

In addition to these factors, young adults ('mama's boys') in Italy and Spain often prefer to stay in the parental home, even when they have gained economic independence (Italy chapter, Dalla Zuanna 2001), and this prolonged 'cohabitation' is willingly accepted by their parents (Manacorda and Moretti 2006). The Spain chapter notes that "…the greater freedom of movement enjoyed by adult children (…) and growing household welfare, along with the social differentiation between sexuality and procreation, have weakened the pressures for leaving the parental home at an early age" (Delgado et al. 2008:1086). The progressively postponed departure of children from the parental home in Mediterranean countries has been often interpreted as an outcome of economic insecurity, prolonged education, and limited availability of affordable housing, combined with the persistence of strong family ties between generations; but also as a problematic manifestation of a general 'delay syndrome,' and an unwillingness

---

[4] We expect that these general patterns of home leaving were retained for younger cohorts in most parts of Europe. The available data indicate, however, that home-leaving among younger cohorts has occurred at much later ages in Central and Eastern Europe (see also different country chapters and Section 5.1).

of young adults to assume adult roles and responsibilities (Dalla Zuanna 2001). Delayed home leaving in these countries is intrinsically linked to delayed union formation and delayed parenthood (e.g., Billari 2004), which may eventually have a negative effect on completed fertility rates (Kohler, Billari, and Ortega 2002).

Countries also differ greatly in the extent to which home leaving is coupled with union formation. For the cohorts born around 1960, these two events were most closely related in Belgium (Flanders) and Southern Europe (especially for women; 76 percent of Spanish and Italian women left home at the time they married). In Norway and Sweden, but also in the Baltic countries (data available for Latvia and Lithuania), the timing of leaving home and union formation did not overlap for a large majority of young adults (Billari, Philipov, and Baizán 2001). In the Nordic countries, but also in the Netherlands and the United Kingdom, leaving the parental home remains a mark of independence and signifies the transition to adulthood (e.g., Holdsworth 2000). Consequently, many young people leave home early simply to achieve independence through residential autonomy (the Netherlands chapter, Sweden chapter). It is also important to note that in many countries where late home leaving is common the patterns of departure of young adults from the parental home are more fuzzy and less easily measurable, as many young men and women experience spells of living independently and returning to their parents. These moves are often related to migration for employment or education, but also to changes in income or partnership status.

3. The gradual retreat of marriage

The evidence of the gradual retreat of marriage in all parts of Europe is overwhelming. Marriage rates have declined—to very low levels in some places—and couples are marrying at later ages. Growing numbers of marriages are ending in divorce or separation, and consensual unions have increasingly replaced marriage among younger people. Especially in Northern and Western Europe, marriage has been historically far from a universal institution, and many people married at relatively late ages (Hajnal 1965). But the rapid decline in the centrality of marriage in the lives of individual men and women after the 'golden age of marriage' in the 1950s and the 1960s, when marriage was very common and took place early in life (Festy 1980), is remarkable. As Thornton, Axinn, and Xie (2007: 4-5) observe for the United States, "marriage has become less central in organizing economic production, consumption, and the transfer of property across generations. It has become less influential in delineating the relationships between men and women, the transition to adulthood, and the identity for men and women. It has also become less relevant as a context of sexual expression, living arrangements, and the bearing and rearing of children. In addition, marriage has become less sacred, being increasingly viewed as a secular rather than religious institution." Clearly, the character and the meaning of marriage have undergone a remarkable transformation. Most people still perceive marriage as an ideal and as the most desirable living arrangement (see Overview Chapter 6), but they marry for different reasons, and at different points in their lives, than in the past. This is well illustrated by changes in the sequencing of early life course events, and the changing relationship between cohabitation, pregnancy, marriage, and childbearing, which is briefly analysed in Section 7. As in the case of home-leaving patterns and other living arrangements, the diversity in Europe is enormous, and our overview only scratches the surface of some region-specific peculiarities. Our main focus is on the decline in marriage rates, the rapid trend towards postponement of marriages, and the diminishing prevalence of marriage among young adults.

3.1 The end of universal marriage

The near-universal decline in first marriage rates in Europe, and the increase in the proportion of people who never marry, can be documented by diverse indicators. We focus on the period indicator of the total first marriage rate, and the cohort indicator of the proportion of women who have never married by the age of 50. The former indicator is based on period age-specific first marriage rates ('incidence rates'), which are computed for all women, irrespective of their current family status. It is not an accurate indicator of the intensity of first marriages, as it is distorted by the changes in the age-specific composition of population by marital status (see also Appendix). However, as a simple measure readily available for most countries in Europe, it provides a rough evaluation of marriage trends over time.

Figure 1 depicts trends in the total first marriage rates (TFMR) in different regions of Europe since 1950. The substantial decline in the TFMR first began in the mid-1960s in Sweden and, more gradually, in other Nordic countries. Other regions followed suit: Western European countries experienced a steep fall in first marriage rates during the 1970s; Southern European countries in the late 1970s and the 1980s; and the post-communist countries of Central and Eastern Europe during the 1990s. Thus, between 1960 and 2000, all European regions shifted from being characterised by high first marriage rates, with the TFMR values typically around 1, to low total first marriage rates around 0.6 (somewhat higher in South-eastern Europe). In Central and Eastern Europe, the TFMR remained very high until 1990, and the decline in marriage rates after the fall of the Iron Curtain was particularly steep and rapid. Consequently, the lowest TFMRs in the early 2000s were recorded in the former communist countries. In this region, Slovenia was the main exception, where the steep decline in TFMR had already begun in 1980, a few years after long-lasting cohabiting unions were made *de facto* equalised with marriage (the change took place in 1976, see Slovenia chapter). A more gradual decline also took place in Hungary and East Germany. A recent slight rise in first marriage rates, observed in many countries, is not necessarily linked to the underlying increase in first marriage intensity, but may rather be a consequence of a slowdown in the pace of first marriage postponement.

Figure 1:   Period total first marriage rates in different regions of Europe, 1950-2005

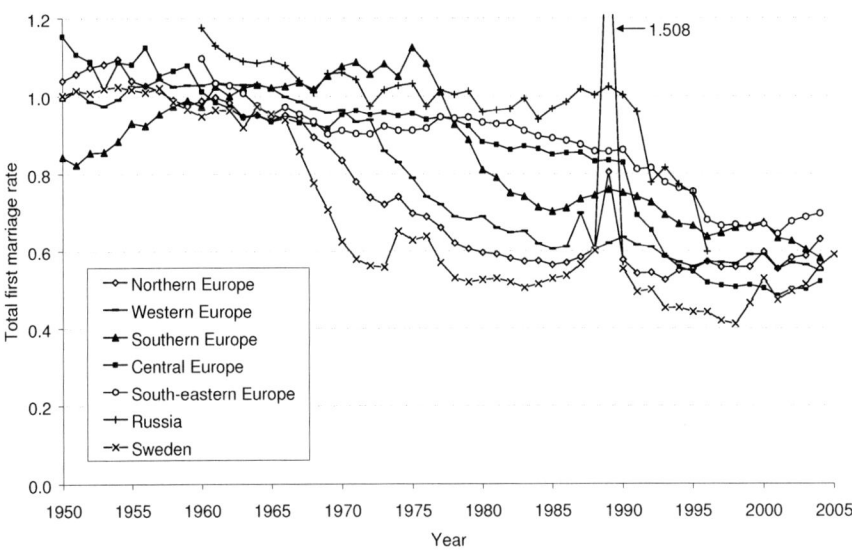

Source: Council of Europe (2006), Sardon (1991 and 1993), Eurostat 2008.
Notes: Data are not weighted by the population size of given countries and regions.
The 'marriage-boom' in Sweden in 1989 is related to changes in public pensions for widows, effective from 1990 (see Sweden chapter, Andersson 1998).
Countries are grouped into regions as follows:
Western Europe: Austria, France, Western Germany, the Netherlands, Switzerland, and the United Kingdom;
Northern Europe: Denmark (data available from 1955), Finland (from 1955), Norway, and Sweden;
Southern Europe: Italy, Portugal, and Spain;
Central Europe: Croatia (from 1960), Czech Republic, Eastern Germany (from 1960), Estonia (from 1970), Hungary, Latvia (from 1970), Lithuania (from 1970), Poland, Slovakia (from 1960), and Slovenia (from 1970)
South-eastern Europe: Bulgaria and Romania.

This recent convergence in period total first marriage rates is not yet visible in the cohort proportion of women ever married by age 50. However, with the exception of several post-communist societies, there was a steep increase in the proportion of never-married women among the late 1950s and the early 1960s cohorts (see Figure 2 for the trend in the proportion of ever married in the countries included in this collection). Thus, the near universality of marriage, typical for the 1930s and 1940s cohorts, has been replaced by a more diverse pattern, whereby a large and gradually increasing fraction of women remain unmarried throughout their reproductive lives. For those born in 1945, between 89 and 96 percent of women have been married at least once in most countries shown in Figure 2 (Sweden has the lowest proportion of ever married, 87 percent). For those born in 1965, the estimated proportion of ever married by age 50 exceeds 90 percent only in Bulgaria and the Czech Republic, whereas it falls below 75 percent for France, Slovenia, and Sweden (see also Prioux 2006). Sweden displays the most pronounced rise in the proportion of never married at age 50, estimated at 37 percent among women born in 1965.

Figure 2:   Cohort proportion of ever-married women by age 50 in selected countries of Europe; birth cohorts 1930-1966

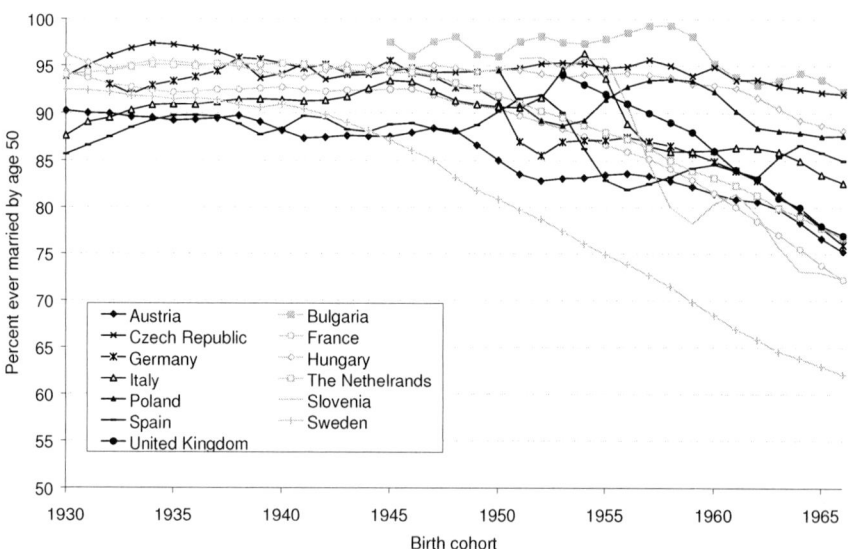

Source: Council of Europe (2006).
Note: The proportion of ever married has been partly estimated for the cohorts born in the mid-1950s and later.

3.2 Long-lasting postponement of marriages

The trend in the mean age at first marriage evolved in parallel with the trend in period first marriage rates. Marriage postponement started shortly after the onset of the decline in first marriage rates; countries that experienced this decline first were also the first to experience delayed marriages. The rapid increase in the mean age at first marriage is a clear marker of a disconnection between sex, marriage, and reproduction (see also Section 7.2 below). Sweden, where first marriage postponement started in the late 1960s, can again be considered a 'forerunner' of new family behaviour. In contrast to the TFMR, the mean age at first marriage still remains widely differentiated in Europe, especially along the 'East-West divide'. Most post-communist countries, which were characterised by an early marriage pattern until the 1980s, experienced an intensive postponement of marriages only after 1990. Consequently, they still have a younger age at marriage (typically between age 23 and 26 for women) than the countries of Western and Southern Europe (typically, at age 27 to 29 years) and the Nordic countries (mean age 29 to 31 years). However, Central and Eastern Europe has also become heterogeneous in this respect, with the countries of the former Soviet Union (except the Baltic countries) retaining the lowest mean age of women at first marriage, at around 23 years in 2004 (see also Ukraine chapter); and several countries of Central Europe (Czech Republic, Hungary and Slovenia) exceeding age 26, with Slovenia reaching 27.8 in 2004. In some parts of Eastern Europe, prevailing social norms still encourage early marriage. In the Ukraine, participants of focus group discussions "felt pressure from parents and peers to marry and have at least one child early rather than risk becoming an 'old maid'" (Perelli-Harris 2008:1151).

Due to a combination of marriage decline and marriage postponement, the proportion of married people has declined rapidly, especially among men and women under age 30. This shift was particularly pronounced in the post-communist countries of Central and Eastern Europe, where early marriages remained common until the early 1990s (e.g., the Czech Republic and Slovakia chapters). At present, marriage has almost disappeared from the lives of young adults in many parts of Europe. In fact, Figure 4 shows that there has been a remarkable convergence in the proportion of people married at young ages, especially for men. For instance, the proportion of men married at age 22 fell to six percent in Romania, and to one to three percent in six other countries analysed in Figure 4 (the Czech Republic, France, Hungary, Italy, the Netherlands, and Sweden)[5]. Similarly, the proportion of women married by age 20 fell to 16 percent in Romania, and to two to four percent in the latter six countries, while in 1980 it was as

---

[5] Due to shortage of space and limited data availability, we do not present the corresponding figures for all the countries included in this collection.

high as 49 percent in Hungary and Romania. Except in Romania, relatively few men (less than 15 percent) and women (13-31 percent) were married by age 25; again, a clear convergence occurs across countries. A marked decline in the proportion married is also observed at age 30, although considerable cross-country differences prevail: only 21 percent of Swedish men and 32 percent of Swedish women were married at that age, compared with 60 percent of Romanian men and 72 percent of Romanian women.

As the universality of marriage declines, marriage becomes more a manifestation of individual values and preferences, but is also subject to pragmatic decision-making, as unmarried people react more sensitively to macro-level policies and other factors that can facilitate or hinder marriage. This 'instrumentalization of marriage' (Salles 2006) can lead to distinct marriage booms and busts that occur in reaction to the actual or expected changes in public pensions, taxation, or marriage allowances. Such distinct marriage booms took place in Sweden in 1989 (Figure 1, see Sweden chapter and Andersson 1998), and in Austria in 1972, 1983, and 1987 (Austria chapter, Prioux 1993) In addition, short-term marriage booms may also be caused by such factors as 'lucky' dates in the calendar, like, for example, July 7, 2007 (07-07-07).

Figure 3:   Period mean age at first marriage for women, 1960-2004

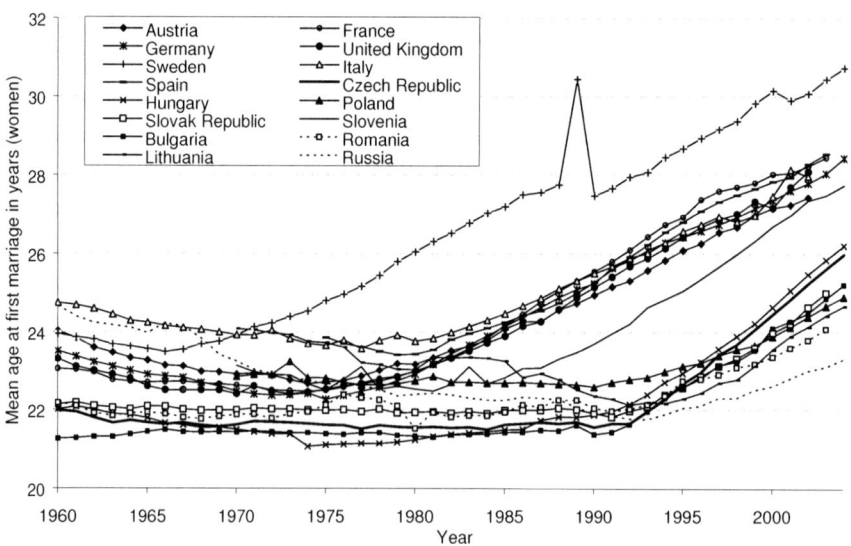

Source: Council of Europe 2006, Russian Federation chapter.

4. The rise of cohabitation and the diversity of cohabiting unions

The substantial rise in unmarried cohabitation, noted in most country chapters, constitutes a hallmark of the ongoing changes in family life in most developed countries. The unexpected spread of cohabitation and its diversity were initially neglected in sociological literature (Smock 2000). In recent decades these issues have been the subject of extensive demographic research in Europe (e.g., Trost 1979 and 1981, Hoem and Rennermalm 1985, Hoem 1986, Leridon and Villeneuve-Gokalp 1989, Liefbroer 1991, Blom 1994, Manting 1994, Blossfeld 1995, Prinz 1995, Toulemon 1997, Kiernan 1999 and 2004, Haskey 1999, Mills 2000, Murphy 2000, Nazio and Blossfeld 2003, Kasearu 2007) as well as in the United States (e.g., Bachrach 1987, Bumpass and Sweet 1989, Rindfuss and VandenHeuvel 1990, Smock 2000, Bumpass and Lu 2000, Heuveline and Timberlake 2004, Thornton, Axinn, and Xie 2007). Contemporary research shows that the character and stability of cohabitation vary greatly between individuals, between countries, and over time. In this section, we provide a rough outline of cohabitation in contemporary Europe, and refer the reader for more detail to the more specific literature listed above.

Unmarried cohabitation is not a new phenomenon. It has been historically practiced in many countries of Central, Western, and Northern Europe among people who could not afford to marry, or who were not legally entitled to marry (e.g., separated individuals who could not dissolve their marriages); and, in the case of Sweden, also among some intellectuals opposed to church marriages (Villeneuve-Gokalp 1991, Kiernan 2004, Probert 2004). The reasons behind the contemporary spread of cohabitation tend to vary, however. Rindfuss and VandenHeuvel (1990: 704) argue that the rise in cohabitation is "the result of historical changes in the dating and sexual relationships among unmarried individuals (…) which in turn are grounded in the rise of individual in Western ideology." There are different typologies of cohabitation (e.g., Prinz 1995, Heuveline and Timberlake 2004, Kasearu 2007), but the most frequent distinction is that drawn between cohabitation as a stage in the marriage process, and cohabitation as an alternative to marriage (Rindfuss and VandenHeuvel 1990). It is apparent that cohabiting unions are very heterogeneous, and include individuals with different social characteristics and very different expectations about the nature of their relationship (Murphy 2000). Although cohabiting unions are frequently compared to marriage, Rindfuss and VandenHeuvel (1990) suggest that they also have some attributes typical of single living.

Figure 4:   Proportion of women and men married at ages 20 (22), 25, and 30 in selected countries of Europe

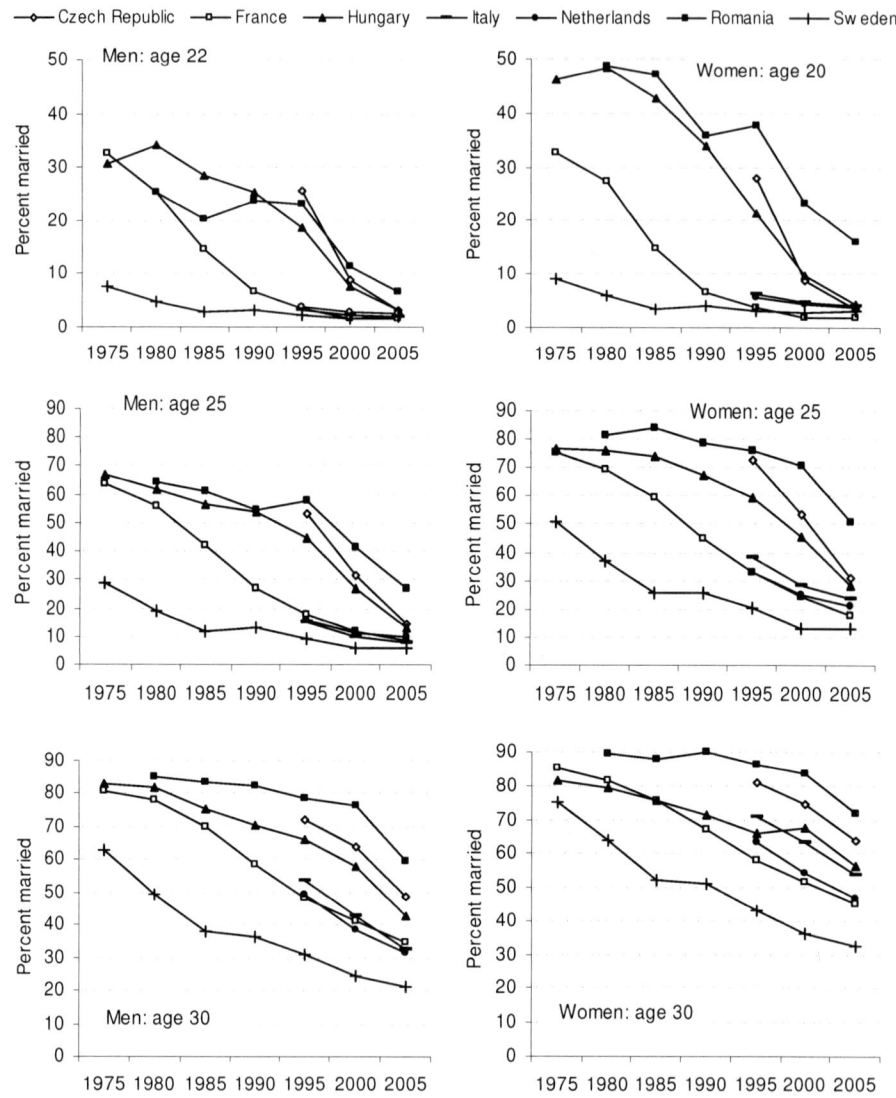

Source: Authors' computations based on Eurostat (2007).

Usually, cohabitation first spreads as a rather marginal phenomenon of relatively short duration, either among divorced and separated people, or as a short pre-marital experience—a sort of a 'trial marriage,' or as a part of the courtship process. During that first phase, marriage intensity may increase due to shotgun marriages (Munoz-Pérez and Prioux 2005). In this stage, cohabitation is not 'competing' with marriage, and is usually not seen as an appropriate arrangement for childbearing. Over time, cohabitation becomes increasingly popular and accepted by the society. It becomes a habitual or even a 'normative' form of entry into union for those who eventually plan to get married, but it also serves as a substitute for marriage: it lasts longer, becomes widely adopted among young adults (e.g., Toulemon 1997, Nazio and Blossfeld 2003) and "enters the arena of reproduction" (Smock 2000). Although unmarried cohabitation may eventually become a 'marriage-like' relationship, it is still not a complete substitute for marriage. First, unmarried partnerships remain more fragile than marriages (Prinz 1995, Smock 2000), even when children are born (Toulemon 1995, Andersson 2002 and 2003); and, second, the degree of legal recognition of cohabiting couples and their children differs widely across countries: as the registration of fathers is not compulsory in all countries, some children born to cohabiting mothers do not have a 'legal father.' Furthermore, in most societies, long-term cohabitation is more typical of economically disadvantaged couples, as individuals in an economically secure position are more likely to convert their cohabitation into marriage (Kravdal 1999, Oppenheimer 2003, Kiernan 2004).

Many European countries partly deviate from the general picture sketched above. But trends over time comprise three main stages, which are widely shared across countries (e.g., Blossfeld 1995, Toulemon 1997, Haskey 1999, Bumpass and Lu 2000, Mills 2000, Murphy 2000, Nazio and Blossfeld 2003, Steele et al. 2006, see also Russia chapter):

1) *Diffusion*: An increasing proportion of young adults enter a consensual union at the beginning of a partnership, and this eventually becomes a majority practice;
2) *Permanency*: Cohabitation lasts longer and is less frequently converted into marriage;
3) *Cohabitation as a family arrangement*: Pregnancy gradually ceases to be a very strong 'determinant' of marriage among cohabiting couples, and, as a result, childbearing among cohabiting couples becomes common.

Moreover, with the further spread of cohabitation, unmarried couples with children may become similar to married ones. The study of British women by Steele et al. (2006) found that, among younger cohorts of women born in 1970, childbearing reduced the couples' risk of separation, suggesting that the presence of children 'cements' cohabiting partnerships. On the other hand, when cohabitation is widespread, couples married without prior cohabitation become more selected, and their risk of dissolution is smaller (Liefbroer and Dourleijn 2006).

In many countries, in the space of a few decades, cohabitation has almost completely replaced marriage as a normative choice of a first union (e.g., Sweden chapter). In France, a massive rise in cohabitation occurred between 1965 and 1995, when the proportion of couples starting their union by cohabitation soared from 10 to 90 percent (Toulemon 1997). In Austria and the Netherlands, the rule, 'cohabitation first, marriage later or never,' was widely embraced by the cohorts born in the 1960s and later (Austria and the Netherlands chapters). In Russia, the rise of cohabitation was dramatic among the cohorts born after 1960 (Russian Federation chapter), whereas in Hungary, a similar change occurred among the cohorts born between 1965 and 1975 and in the Czech Republic among the 1970s cohorts that reached adulthood after the political regime change in 1989 (Hungary and the Czech Republic chapters). Until recently it appeared that some countries, especially in Southern Europe, but also Poland or Romania, were relatively 'immune' to the erosion of marriage and the spread of cohabitation. Recent evidence, however, indicates that cohabitation is now spreading in these societies as well. For instance, Rosina and Fraboni (2004) found evidence of a "progressive diffusion" of cohabitation among younger generations of Italians, especially those living in Central and Northern Italy, and with higher levels of education. Cohabitation also spread rapidly in the 1990s in Spain, although the incidence of cohabitation remains limited there (Spain chapter). The Bulgaria chapter points out that the rise in cohabitation became particularly pronounced after the mid-1990s, i.e., some years after the start of the political transition. In Slovakia, where cohabitation remains less common among young adults, there was a marked rise during the 1990s in the proportion of women cohabiting in their twenties (Slovakia chapter). In some other post-communist countries, including Poland, Romania and Ukraine, cohabitation remains rather limited, and its prevalence is increasing only gradually (Poland, Romania, and Ukraine chapters). Albania, where the new living arrangements have not gained any significance yet, constitutes a notable exception: according to the 2005 data, only 0.2 percent of people aged 15-29 cohabited there (Gjonca et al. 2008:278).

Heuveline and Timberlake's (2004) study based on the FFS data provides the most thorough analysis of the diversity of cohabitation in Europe. It presents life table estimates of adulthood premarital cohabitation and childhood exposure to premarital cohabitation during the three-year reference period prior to the FFS survey, i.e., in the late 1980s and the early 1990s. The study distinguishes countries where cohabitation remained a *marginal phenomenon*, and those where it was a *prelude to marriage* (i.e., of a relatively short duration, and with a low frequency of childbearing), a *stage in the marriage process* (i.e., usually leading to marriage, but often after a birth of a child or children), an *alternative to being single* (i.e., of relatively short duration and frequently ending in a separation rather than marriage), an *alternative to marriage* (i.e., of longer duration and frequently involving childbearing), and a status *indistinguishable from marriage*. Such a categorisation ignores the huge diversity of cohabiting couples in each country, and neglects rapid changes over time. Despite these limitations, cross-country contrasts remain large enough to justify this crude differentiation. Table 2 reproduces selected life table indicators estimated from another study based on the FFS (Andersson and Philipov 2002) for women in thirteen European countries and the United States, using the typology of countries proposed by Heuveline and Timberlake. Southern European countries (Italy and Spain), together with Poland, appear on the 'marginal' side of the cohabitation spectrum, with rather traditional Poland showing the highest resistance to cohabitation: only four percent of women were experiencing cohabitation as a first union by age 28, and only two percent of children were born to cohabiting couples (see also Poland chapter).

Sweden is the only society where cohabitation as a family-building institution evolves to be indistinguishable from marriage, and where children are born to cohabiting parents almost as frequently as to married parents (Heuveline and Timberlake 2004, see also Thomson 2005). Almost nine out of 10 Swedish women entered cohabitation as a first union by age 28, and 45 percent of all children were born to cohabiting couples. However, even in Sweden, childbearing intensities are still higher in marriage than in cohabitation, cohabiting unions are of a shorter duration, and many cohabiting unions are typically transformed into marriages, especially after the birth of the first or the second child (Sweden chapter). Cohabitation as an *alternative to marriage* was typical for France, and, outside of Europe, for Canada; whereas cohabitation as an *alternative to single living* was typical only for two non-European societies: New Zealand and the United States (Heuveline and Timberlake 2004). All the remaining European countries analysed by Heuveline and Timberlake belonged to the two categories in which cohabitation typically leads to marriage (*prelude to marriage* and *stage in marriage process*).

With a growing pressure to provide legal recognition of same-sex partnerships, but also with the rise of cohabitation, unmarried couples in an increasing number of European countries can either achieve a specific legal status by registering their partnership, or may be automatically granted some of the advantages and obligations conferred upon married couples. The legal approach to cohabiting couples varies widely across countries (Barlow 2004, Waaldijk 2005). In some countries, a functional approach is adopted, giving cohabiting couples some of the privileges of marriages

Table 2: **Selected life table estimates of cohabitation experience among women, based on the FFS analysis and the typology of cohabitation developed by Heuveline and Timberlake (in percent)**

Role of cohabitation	Country	Period of estimation	Incidence by age 28	Ending in marriage within 5 years	Ending in separation within 5 years	Children born to cohabiting parents
Marginal	Poland	1986-91	4	46	5	2
	Italy	1990-95	8	43	32	4
	Spain	1989-95	17	31	40	4
Prelude to marriage	Belgium (Flanders)	1985-92	28	53	17	4
	Czech Republic	1992-97	46	59	20	7
	Hungary	1988-93	27	47	32	6
Stage in marriage process	Austria	1990-96	67	43	24	19
	Finland	1979-92	76	48	25	13
	West Germany	1986-92	48	46	29	11
	Latvia	1989-95	51	48	34	11
	Slovenia	1989-95	50	52	14	16
Alternative to single	United States	1989-95	52	46	45	11
Alternative to marriage	France	1988-94	71	38	28	23
Indistinguishable from marriage	Sweden	1978-93	87	31	34	45

Sources: Data estimated by Andersson and Philipov (2002: Tables 4, 20, 21, and 30) on the basis of the FFS surveys. The typology of cohabitation was developed by Heuveline and Timberlake (2004: Table 4).

Notes: Most of the life table estimates of the incidence of cohabitation, conversion of cohabitation to marriage and the percentage of children born to cohabiting couples by Andersson and Philipov come very close to similar estimates provided by Heuveline and Timberlake (2004: Table 4). Data by Andersson and Philipov shown in this table are computed with the competing-risks life table method.

without requiring them to register their union (i.e, Australia, Canada, and to some extent, the United Kingdom, see Barlow 2004). This is also the case in Slovenia, where, since the adoption of the Marriage and Family Relations Act in 1976, long-lasting cohabitation has "practically the same legal consequences for the couple and their children as marriage" (Stropnik and Šircelj 2008:1031). In Sweden, this functional approach is applied to opposite-sex cohabiting couples, while same-sex cohabiting couples may register their partnerships (this is also possible in other Nordic countries, following the pioneering example of Denmark from 1989, see Festy 2006). In many other European countries, cohabiting couples of the opposite sex are treated as unrelated persons, and are not granted any other rights or privileges; whereas same-sex couples, who are not entitled to marriage, can achieve legal recognition by registering their partnership. In Spain, same-sex couples are allowed to marry and partnership registration is possible in some regions as well (Barlow 2004). Countries allowing partnership registration also widely differ in the number of rights and benefits, including parental rights, granted to registered couples (Waaldijk 2005, Festy 2006). Belgium and the Netherlands grant access to marriage, as well as to partnership registration, to both same-sex and opposite-sex couples; whereas France does not authorize gay marriage, but provides access to 'civil registration' to all couples. According to Barlow (2004: 65-66), French and Belgian civil partnerships come closest to recognising cohabitation as a specific family life arrangement that is distinct from marriage, and that endows couples with increased family-style rights and obligations.

In countries where opposite-sex couples were also allowed to register their partnerships, such as France and the Netherlands, they soon outnumbered same-sex couples seeking registration. In France, the new form of civil union, called *Pacte civil de solidarité* (PACS), became relatively popular soon after it was introduced in 1999 (France chapter). In 2005, a record number of 59,800 PACS were registered, compared with 271,600 marriages (see Prioux 2006 and France chapter). This evidence suggests that there is a substantial demand among cohabiting couples to obtain legal recognition of their partnership without getting married. The new forms of registered partnerships and their variety across countries also blur some of the boundaries between marriage and cohabiting union, and constitute a challenge for demographic research on union formation.

5. Changes in living arrangements of young adults and the delayed entry into first union

5.1 Living arrangements of young adults

In addition to unmarried cohabitation, other living arrangements have become more widespread. This section, dealing with living arrangements of young adults, is further complemented with an analysis of living arrangements of 'younger' parents (under age 45) in Section 7.3. There is lack of coherent data that would allow us to easily analyse and compare recent changes in the importance of various living arrangements for young adults across Europe. To provide at least a broad snapshot, we employ two different data sources for a number of countries grouped into broader regions: census data showing household arrangements of men and women in 2000 or 2001 (Eurostat 2008, see Table 3);[6] and the period life tables, estimated by Andersson and Philipov (2002) on

---

[6] We excluded countries with incomplete records on the selected living arrangements, namely France, Latvia, and Lithuania.

the basis of the FFS data, and pertaining to the 1980s and the early 1990s (Appendix Table A1). Census data, presented in Table 3, distinguish between the three main types of living arrangements of young adults (living with parents, living single, living with a partner). For those who live with a partner, we also show the percentage cohabiting and the percentage with children.

Regional contrasts in the fraction of young adults still living in the parental home are broadly consistent with the analysis of home-leaving patterns in Section 2, although the percentages are higher than would correspond to the median age at home leaving for the 1960 cohort, reported in Table 1. This indicates that the 'nest-leaving' has been generally postponed in most countries during the last two decades. Northern Europe, especially Denmark, and parts of Western Europe (especially for women) continue to display a rather low percentage of young adults living with parents. Particularly for men, living in the parental home often becomes a permanent living arrangement throughout their young adult years. In Southern Europe, between 48 percent (Portugal) and 60 percent (Italy) of men aged 20-34 still live with their parents. This finding is consistent with the FFS life table analysis, according to which young adult men in Italy and Spain spend around a half of their time between ages 15 and 39 living with their parents. A high percentage of young adults, especially men, in Central and Eastern Europe also co-resided with their parents around 2000; this proportion equals that observed in Southern Europe for men in the Czech Republic, Poland, Slovakia, and Slovenia; and for women in Slovenia.

In countries with an early home-leaving pattern and larger availability of affordable housing, especially in Northern and Western Europe, many young adults who have left the parental home live alone or share a household with their friends or age-mates for longer periods of time (the Netherlands chapter). In all analysed countries, living single is more common among young men than among women, which is also shown in the FFS data: in Nordic countries, men spend between 12 and 15 percent of time between ages 15 and 39 living single, and as much as 19 percent in West Germany (Table 3; see also Germany chapter). In Southern Europe, Ireland, and most of Central and Eastern Europe, living single is still a rather marginal experience, especially for women. There are, however, signs that more young adults now live single in some Central European countries than was common in the past (the Czech Republic, Estonia, and Slovakia in Table 3, see also the Czech Republic chapter). Low affordability of housing remains a paramount factor, limiting a faster spread of this living arrangement (the Czech Republic and Slovenia chapters).

Living in union constitutes the most common living arrangement for the group of women aged 20-34 as a whole (except Italy, Slovenia, and Spain), but for young men in Austria, Ireland, post-communist Central Europe, and Southern Europe, it is more common to live with parents than to live with a partner. Only around a quarter of young adult men live in union in Greece, Italy, Slovenia, and Spain. Central and Eastern European countries are characterised by a high percentage of unions with children, suggesting that many couples still have children soon after they start living together. This region is also most diverse with respect to the percentage of couples who cohabit (see also Overview Chapter 6), although a word of caution is warranted here: Many young adults do not register changes in their address when they move out of the parental home to live single or to cohabit, and they also tend to report their official place of residence in the census, especially if they come back to the parental nest from time to time. This leads to a potential over-reporting of living in the parental home, and underreporting of living single and of unmarried cohabitation in the census data.[7]

Many young adults who live with their parents or as singles have a steady partner living at a different address. This arrangement, frequently called 'living apart together' (LAT), has in part substituted postponed union formation. It is commonly perceived as an intermittent relationship, which is "monogamous in nature and an arrangement that is more than a temporary, fleeting, or casual relationship." (Haskey 2005:36; see also Villeneuve-Gokalp 1997). LAT often comes close to 'steady dating,' which was also commonly practised in the past, but LAT is usually considered as a more stable and lasting situation, in which partners perceive themselves as living as a couple, although not in the same dwelling. It may also involve shorter spells of co-residence ('semi-cohabitation,' 'weekend couples'). Because of their unclear definition and diverse character, LAT relationships have not been extensively studied to date (Haskey 2005 lists studies conducted in different developed countries). Haskey's estimates for the United Kingdom show that LAT is particularly common among men and women in their early twenties. Of those who are unmarried, four out of ten people aged 20-24 are in an LAT relationship, as are one-quarter of those aged 25-34. Pinnelli's (2001: 61-62) analysis of the FFS data shows that, in a typical European country, 12-13 percent of women aged 20-39 are in an LAT relationship, with Poland having the lowest proportion, 2.8 percent; and Italy having the highest proportion, 20.5 percent. Different definitions, however, may yield different estimates of the prevalence of this phenomenon (Haskey 2005).

For many couples, a LAT arrangement was chosen as a (temporary) solution dictated by their current circumstances, most frequently housing constraints (Villeneuve-Gokalp 1997, Pinnelli 2001). Nevertheless, in some countries living apart together is seen as a desirable way to live by an increasing share of the population (the

---

[7] We do not know how large is the bias in the census data attributable to this 'failure' to report the actual residence (and thus the actual living arrangement). In the Czech Republic, for instance, the level of cohabitation reported in the census data is well below that reported in the surveys (Zeman 2003, the Czech Republic chapter).

Netherlands chapter). Sobotka and Testa (2008) have found that LAT was most frequently preferred as a living arrangement by younger men and women in Germany: in Western Germany, 12 percent of childless women and 14 percent of childless men aged 18-39 expressed preference for an LAT relationship. It is plausible that LAT arrangements are on the rise, especially in Southern Europe and Central and Eastern Europe, owing to the expansion of higher education and the low affordability of housing. In the case of Southern Europe, where more young adults co-reside with their parents, cultural preferences may also play a role. LAT provides young adults with some advantages of cohabitation, especially of having a sexual relationship, without a need to establish their own household. In countries with progressively delayed home leaving patterns, parents have increasingly accommodated the rising demand for privacy on the part of their adult children, and commonly allow their children to pursue a sexual relationship with their partners in the parental home (see Dalla Zuanna 2001: 146 for Italy; the increased freedom and autonomy of adult children living with parents is also noted in the Spain chapter).

Table 3:   Living arrangements among women and men aged 20-34, in percent (2000-2001)

WOMEN	In parental home	Single, no children	In union	Other	Of those in union	
					Cohabiting	With children
Northern Europe						
Denmark	5.2	26.9	61.3	6.6	50.3	60.4
Finland	11.0	17.8	58.3	12.8	48.8	57.1
Norway	19.8	15.5	53.6	11.1	45.4	72.8
Western Europe						
Ireland	31.9	3.7	38.6	25.8	31.0	59.4
The Netherlands	14.6	17.4	61.3	6.7	39.3	52.7
United Kingdom	15.9	8.0	52.4	23.7	38.5	58.6
German-speaking countries						
Austria	23.3	12.7	51.2	12.8	27.5	72.4
Germany	18.1	17.2	56.6	8.1	26.6	63.3
Switzerland	15.5	17.4	53.0	14.1	23.8	57.8
Southern Europe						
Greece	34.3	5.2	47.3	13.3	6.7	74.6
Italy	45.6	4.8	42.7	6.9	8.5	68.6
Portugal	34.1	4.0	54.6	7.3	12.3	74.6
Spain	45.9	4.4	37.7	12.0	15.6	62.3
Central and Eastern Europe						
Czech Republic	28.7	8.3	47.5	15.5	9.2	85.6
Estonia	16.0	10.6	52.9	20.5	40.8	81.7
Hungary	25.8	5.6	55.1	13.6	21.2	78.1
Poland	32.7	6.5	46.8	14.1	4.3	85.1
Romania	22.2	2.6	64.2	10.9	12.0	80.7
Slovak Republic	33.5	8.0	47.2	11.3	3.8	90.1
Slovenia	43.4	2.7	42.0	12.0	23.0	86.8

Table 3: **(Continued) Living arrangements among women and men aged 20-34, in percent (2000-2001)**

MEN	In parental home	Single, no children	In union	Other	Of those in union	
					Cohabiting	With children
Northern Europe						
Denmark	10.1	41.2	48.4	0.4	56.3	54.1
Finland	22.3	21.6	47.0	9.1	54.0	51.1
Norway	31.7	25.1	39.3	3.9	50.6	68.0
Western Europe						
Ireland	44.2	5.5	30.5	19.9	34.8	55.2
The Netherlands	26.7	23.0	46.7	3.6	46.1	45.0
United Kingdom	28.0	12.1	43.7	16.1	43.8	53.9
German-speaking countries						
Austria	38.4	16.4	37.1	8.1	32.6	68.0
Germany	31.0	24.6	41.2	3.2	31.8	57.9
Switzerland	25.2	22.2	38.1	14.4	28.7	51.5
Southern Europe						
Greece	49.5	6.0	26.4	18.1	9.5	64.9
Italy	60.0	7.1	26.9	5.9	9.9	61.8
Portugal	47.6	4.7	42.8	5.0	13.2	69.5
Spain	56.1	6.2	26.9	10.8	18.2	55.6
Central and Eastern Europe						
Czech Republic	46.5	14.0	34.2	5.4	10.5	82.5
Estonia	32.3	14.1	44.6	8.9	44.5	78.6
Hungary	41.9	6.8	41.4	9.9	24.4	73.8
Poland	50.7	8.8	35.3	5.2	4.5	82.4
Romania	40.5	3.5	48.5	7.5	14.6	75.5
Slovak Republic	49.1	12.8	34.6	3.5	4.2	88.1
Slovenia	62.8	4.5	26.5	6.2	26.3	82.7

Source: Own computations based on the 2000-2001 Census data provided by Eurostat (2008).

Complex households including more than one nuclear family are still present in Southern Europe, as well as in Central and Eastern Europe, in part because a significant share of cohabiting or married young adults live with their parents (see Section 2), but also because many lone mothers and fathers reside with their parents or other relatives. For instance, in Southern Europe—specifically, in Greece, Italy, and Spain—25 to 40 percent of lone parents live with other relatives (Chambaz 2000). These arrangements belong, together with single parents and people living in institutions and student houses, to the last category ('Other') in Table 3.

5.2 Delayed entry into first union

The decline of marriage has not been fully offset by an increase in unmarried cohabitation. Consequently, the proportion of adults living in union has decreased, mostly because of the delay of entry into a first union, but also because of more union disruptions that are not rapidly followed by a second union (Philipov 2006). The age at entering first co-residential union has increased most rapidly in Southern Europe, and only gradually in Northern and Western Europe. In France, the median age of women at first union has increased in conjunction with prolonged education and rising unemployment (Prioux 2003). For both women and men born in the early 1970s, the age has risen by more than two years, from a low of 21.5 (women) and 23.8 years (men) among the late 1950s cohorts (see Figure 5). In countries with a late home leaving age and relatively low prevalence of cohabitation, the median age at first union for women has increased with much higher intensity, leading to greater cross-country diversity (Figure 5). For instance, the mean age at entering first union among Italian women increased from 22.5 among the 1951-55 cohorts to 26.5 among the 1966-70 cohorts. The increase has been even more intensive for Italian men, among whom only a quarter had started living with a partner by age 27 in the youngest cohort observed (1966-70, see Ongaro 2001: Table 8.1).

Figure 5:   Cohort median age at entering first union for women and men in selected countries of Europe

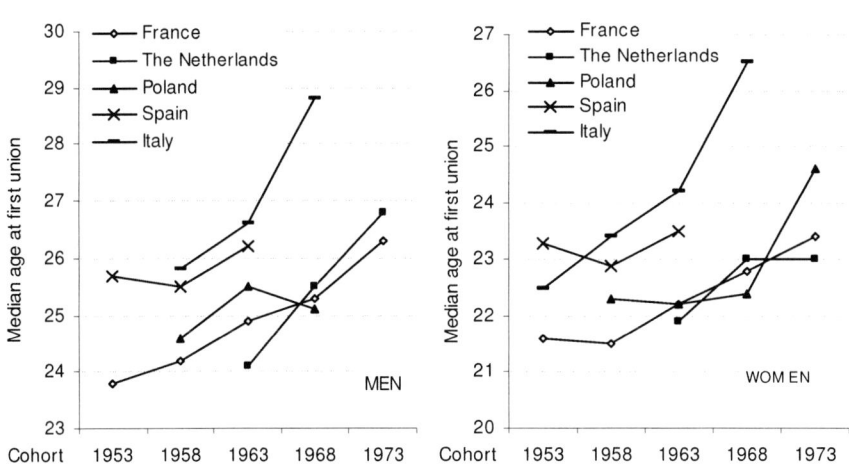

Source: Prioux 2003 for France (pp. 574-575, Table B in Appendix II) and data tables in country studies in Corijn and Klijzing 2001.
Notes: For all countries except France data were computed for 5-year cohort groups and do not refer to the one particular cohort
          shown in the graphs: e.g., 1953 holds for 1951-55. Data for Poland show median age at first marriage for the cohorts displayed
          in the figure, as cohabitation was very rare.

6. Rising divorce rates: Large differences in Central and Eastern Europe

At the beginning of the 21st century, most European countries are experiencing high divorce rates, typically two to five times higher than in the 1960s. In a number of countries, including all the Nordic countries, Belgium, United Kingdom, the Czech Republic, Estonia, and Russia, the period total divorce rate (TDR) has reached around 0.5, indicating that under a long-term continuation of current divorce rates, around one-half of all marriages will end up in divorce. In addition, cohabiting unions, which are increasingly common, have higher levels of dissolution than marriage, implying that union dissolution has become a common experience for contemporary Europeans, especially those born after 1960. Consequently, living arrangements and family forms have also become more diverse due to the rising numbers of divorced and separated individuals living alone, with their children, or with their new partners (an arrangement aptly termed 're-partnering'). Experiencing family disruption and living with a single mother or with a stepparent have become increasingly common experiences for children (Heuveline, Timberlake, and Furstenberg 2003, see also Section 7.3).

There has been a universal trend of increasing divorce rates since the 1970s in all parts of Europe (Figure 6). The range of the total divorce rate (TDR) in Europe is currently very wide, from fewer than 10 divorces per 100 initial marriages, to more than 50. However, in contrast to some other indicators of family behaviour, there is no consistent East-West differentiation in divorce rates. Some countries of Central and Eastern Europe exhibit very high divorce rates typical of Northern Europe and parts of Western Europe (e.g., the Czech Republic, Hungary, and almost all the countries of the former Soviet Union), while a number of more traditional or socially conservative countries (e.g., Macedonia, Poland, and Romania) exhibit divorce rates that are well below the European average (e.g., Romania chapter). In Southern Europe, divorce rates also remain relatively low, although they increased markedly after 1990, when the TDR was still at or below 0.1. Some countries of the former Soviet Union can be considered 'forerunners' of the trend towards high divorce rates, experiencing the highest divorce levels in Europe during the 1950s and the 1960s (e.g., Estonia, Latvia, Russia, and Ukraine), with Latvia already registering a total divorce rate of 0.5 in the late 1960s. The Russian Federation chapter suggests that high divorce rates in Russia were in part linked to the high frequency of 'shotgun marriages' that led to high intra-family tension, and to conflicts with relatives.

Time trend data on dissolution rates of unmarried unions are generally not available, with the exception of the dissolutions of registered partnerships in countries where this form of un-married union is legally recognised and recorded in vital statistics. Life table analysis of the FFS data by Andersson and Philipov (2002: Table 20) shows that, in most European countries, between one-fifth and one-third of cohabiting unions dissolve within five years, with Spain reaching the highest dissolution rate of 40 percent (and, outside of Europe, the United States reaching an even higher rate of 45 percent; see Table 2 above). As in the case of marriage, the rates of dissolution of unmarried couples may become increasingly linked to the presence of children (Steele et al. 2006).

Figure 6: **Total divorce rates in selected countries of Europe, 1960-2004**

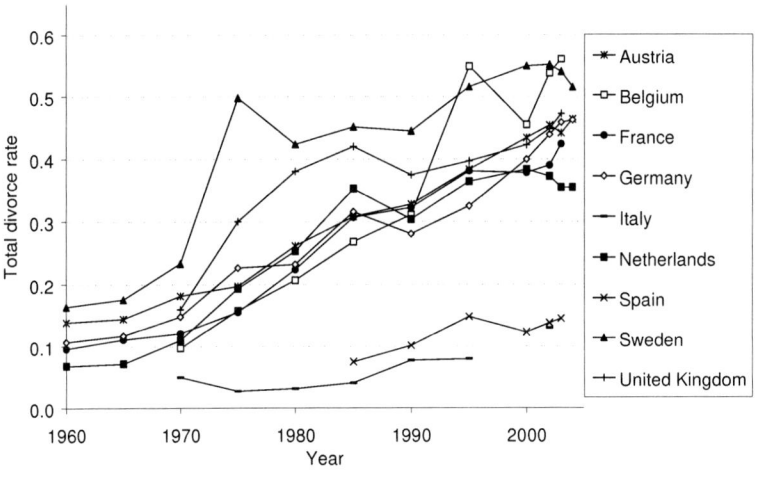

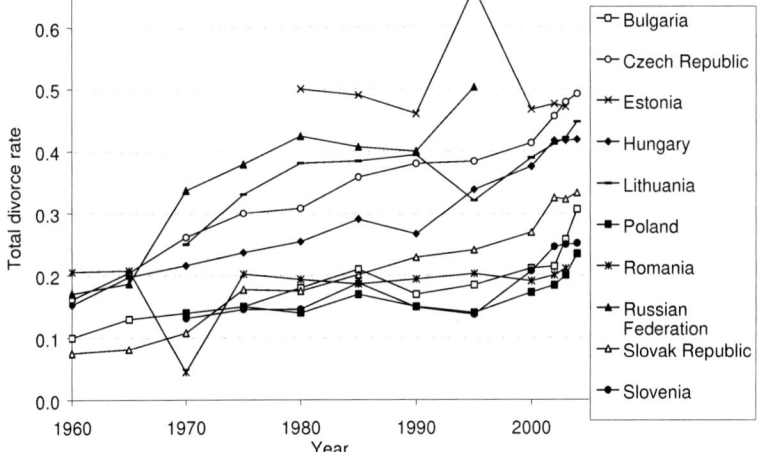

Source: Council of Europe, 2006.

The increasing economic independence of women, which is closely linked to their participation in the labour force, made divorce increasingly possible,[8] as did the introduction of welfare provisions for women who are not economically active (the Netherlands chapter; see also Kalmijn 2007). Despite the continued negative perception of divorce in some countries (e.g., Romania chapter), divorce rates are unlikely to remain low in societies where divorce is still rare, and the current cross-country heterogeneity will probably diminish in the future. The frequency of divorce is partly influenced by legislation (Stevenson and Wolfers 2007). In some countries, permissive legislation contributes to the 'normalisation' of divorce (e.g., the Netherlands chapter), whereas in other countries it makes divorce rather difficult to obtain, for example, by not allowing an easy divorce by mutual consent. Moreover, legislation in a number of countries, including Ireland, Italy, and Spain, stipulates legal separation as a precondition or an alternative to full-fledge divorce. In 2001, a new form of marriage dissolution, termed 'flash annulment' or 'lightning divorce,' opened up in the Netherlands. It came about as an unexpected consequence of the legislation authorizing registered partnerships (Barlow 2004). Under this procedure, a couple mutually downgrades their marriage into a registered partnership, which can subsequently be easily dissolved without being recorded as a divorce (the Netherlands chapter).

7. The declining importance of marriage for childbearing and childrearing

7.1 Marriage is no longer a precondition to childbearing and the key step in the transition to adulthood

The increase in mean age at marriage is a consequence of the postponement of almost all transitions to adulthood (completion of education, union formation, starting a first job, and, in many countries, leaving the parental home), and of an increasing propensity among young adults to enter a union without marriage, and to delay or even forego marriage when they live as a couple. These changes have been extensively analysed with the FFS data (Billari, Philipov and Baizán 2001, Corijn and Klijzing 2001, Macura and Beets 2002, Prioux 2006). The declining importance of marriage is further illustrated by the data on the rise of cohabitation (see also Section 4) and by the rising

---

[8] In addition to providing economic independence, labour force participation of women may contribute to partnership instability by expanding their as well as men's opportunities to meet a new partner (Stevenson and Wolfers 2007).

diversity of sequences in the early life course transitions, and in the ages when these transitions are commonly experienced.

For younger cohorts, marriage does not seem to have any relevance as a setting for sexual expression: in many countries, the mean age at first marriage is now more than ten years higher than the median age at sexual debut, which is typically around 17-18 in most countries of Europe (Bozon 2003, Kontula 2003, these figures refer to the early 1970s cohorts) and very few couples experience first sex after marriage (see also Overview Chapter 6). The general trend is also characterised by a weakening of the relationship between first union, first birth, and marriage. In a growing number of countries, marriage has become rather unusual as a form of first union, whereas periods of cohabitation, both pre-marital and serving as an alternative to marriage, are increasing in duration (see Section 4). In Western and Northern Europe, as well as in Estonia, only a minority of women born in the 1960s married 'directly,' without previous cohabitation (Prioux 2006).

Furthermore, marriage is no longer seen as the only appropriate arrangement for childbearing. Many people who intend to have a child do not feel any rush to marry, and pregnancy is not a very strong determinant of marriage either. This is in contrast to the situation in the early 1970s, when unmarried cohabitation did not last long, and the probability of marrying was very high among cohabiting couples. Many first marriages took place during the woman's pregnancy, probably due to the social pressure to give birth within marriage (see chapters on Austria, England and Wales, the Netherlands, and France; Toulemon 1995). With the increasing use of more efficient contraception, especially the pill, couples could delay first marriage, as well as the birth of their first child. In the view of van de Kaa (1994), the spread of modern contraception facilitated changes in values and attitudes related to sexuality and reproduction which, in turn, have led to the disconnection of marriage from procreation, and to the rise of new living arrangements. Thus, contraceptive technology, which had the potential to strengthen the link between marriage and reproduction by reducing unwanted pre-marital and extramarital pregnancies, also made it possible to have almost risk-free sexual intercourse without being married. Contraception thus opened the way to a new model of reproduction, which is only loosely linked to marriage. As a result, there are fewer conceptions followed by a 'shotgun marriage,' more long-lasting unions which are not converted to marriages, and fewer births conceived during the first years of marriage. These changes have taken place since the 1970s in Austria, France, the Netherlands, the United Kingdom, and in many other countries of Western and Northern Europe; but only since the early 1990s in the Czech Republic, and even more recently in Poland, Bulgaria, Romania, Slovakia, and the Ukraine (see the respective chapters).

As a result, there is no longer a dominant standard biography of family formation (Rindfuss 1991; Germany chapter). The once 'normative' pathway of 'direct' marriage (without previous cohabitation) followed by childbearing has been increasingly replaced by a number of alternative pathways: in some societies, the sequence of cohabitation – marriage – childbearing has become most common, while in other countries, the sequence of 'cohabitation–first or second birth–marriage' is now the most prevalent pattern, and many couples with children do not marry at all.[9] The increasing frequency of marriages involving the 'legitimisation' of children can be illustrated by the example of France, where the proportion of marriages of couples with child(ren) increased rapidly during the 1980s and the 1990s, from five to seven percent in the 1950s through the 1970s, to 29 percent in 2000 (Munoz-Pérez and Prioux 2005: 354, Annex 4). The phenomenon of shotgun marriages (i.e., the sequence of 'pregnancy, within or outside cohabiting union–marriage–first birth') initially increased in prevalence as a result of an early decline in the relevance of marriage for sexual activity, and the associated rise in unplanned ('accidental') conceptions. As marriage was still considered important for childbearing, many couples decided to 'legalise' their union before childbirth, while other couples conceived a child once they had finalised their plans to marry. The frequency of shotgun weddings later declined as a result of a loosening tie between marriage and childbearing, and pregnant women are now more likely to start cohabiting or remain in a cohabiting relationship instead of marrying in response to a pregnancy (Smock 2000, Steele et al. 2006, Toulemon 1995). In Western and Northern Europe, the share of first marriages that were preceded by a premarital conception peaked between 1965 and 1975, and subsequently declined between the mid-1970s and the late 1990s (Austria chapter; see Figure 7 for trends in shotgun marriages in selected countries). A similar development took place about a decade later in Southern Europe. Meanwhile, in Central and Eastern Europe, marriages 'under the pressure of pregnancy' remained very common, at least until the 1990s, and a large majority of children conceived outside marriage were eventually born within marriage (the Czech Republic and Slovakia chapters; see also Munoz-Pérez 1991, Castiglioni and Dalla Zuanna 1994).

---

[9] Elzinga and Liefbroer (2007: 247) note that the evidence in the Netherlands and Sweden, where almost all young people enter their first union through cohabitation, suggests that new standards of behaviour may be emerging over time, leading eventually to a 're-standardisation' of family behaviour and living arrangements.

Figure 7: **Percentage of first marriages following a conception in Austria, the Czech Republic, England and Wales, and France, 1950-2006**

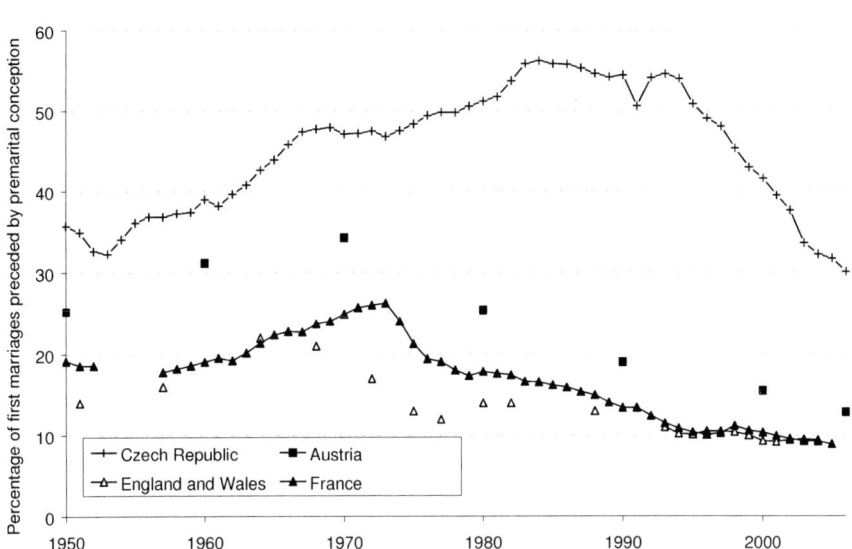

Source: Austria the Czech Republic, and England and Wales chapters; own calculations from Beaumel et al. 2007, Hobcraft 1996, and ONS 2007.
Note: Percentage of pre-marital conceptions refers to the fraction of all marital first births in a given year that took place within eight months following the marriage (Czech Republic and Austria) or the percentage of marriages with pre-maritally conceived birth (England and Wales and France).

As marriages have been postponed more intensively than births, and the share of extramarital births has remained highest at younger ages, first marriages now take place in most countries at higher ages than first births. This pattern is most pronounced in Sweden, where first marriage takes place on average almost three years later than the birth of a first child, suggesting that marriages have become more frequent among parents than among childless couples. Among the countries analysed in Table 4, only Italy and several countries of Central and Eastern Europe (the Czech Republic, Poland, and Russia) recorded a higher mean age of mothers at first birth than the mean age of women at first marriage in 2005.

Table 4: **Mean age at first birth and at first marriage among women in selected European countries, 1970 and 2005[1]**

	Mean age at first birth			Mean age at first marriage			Age at first birth - Age at first marriage [2]	
	1970	2005	Change	1970	2005	Change	1970	2005
Austria	24.1	27.2	3.1	22.9	28.6	5.7	0.3	-1.4
	(1984)						(1984)	
Bulgaria	22.1	24.7	2.6	21.4	25.8	4.4	0.7	-1.1
Czech Republic	22.5	26.6	4.1	21.6	26.4	4.8	0.9	0.2
France	24.0	27.7	3.7	22.6	29.4	6.8	1.4	-1.7
Hungary	22.8	26.7	3.9	21.5	26.7	5.2	1.3	0.0
Italy	25.1	28.7	3.6	23.9	28.5	4.6	1.2	1.5
	(1997)			(2003)				(1997)
Lithuania	24.0	24.9	0.9	23.2	25.0	1.8	0.8	-0.2
	(1978)			(1978)	(2004)		(1978)	(2004)
The Netherlands	24.8	28.9	4.1	22.9	29.1	6.2	1.9	-0.2
Poland	23.4			22.8				
	(1971)	25.8	2.4	(1971)	25.4	2.6	0.6	0.4
Romania	22.6	24.8	2.2	21.9	25.4	3.5	0.7	-0.6
Russian Federation	23.1	24.1	0.9	22.5	23.3	0.8	0.6	0.7
	(1978)			(1978)	(2004)			(2004)
Slovenia	23.7	27.7	4.0	23.1	28.5	5.4	0.6	-0.8
Spain	25.1	29.3	4.2	23.9	29.3	5.4	1.2	0.0
	(1975)			(1975)				
Sweden	24.2	28.7	4.5	23.9	31.5	7.6	-0.3	-2.8
	(1974)			(1974)				
England and Wales	23.7	27.3	3.6	22.4	27.2	4.8	1.3	-0.8
					(2000)			(2000)

Source: Eurostat 2007, Council of Europe 2006, Russian Federation chapter, and national statistical offices.

Notes: (1) To make the data on the mean age at first birth comparable, this table includes only countries that collect data on biological ('true') birth order of children or countries for which expert estimates for the biological birth order are available. Thus, we do not include data for Germany and we use the following estimates on the mean age at first birth: France (France chapter, Toulemon and Mazuy 2001), Russian Federation (Russian Federation chapter), and England and Wales (Smallwood 2002 and ONS 2007).

(2) For countries where data on both mean age at first birth and at first marriage in 1970 and 2005 are not available, the computation of the difference between these ages is shown for another year (as indicated in brackets). This year does not always correspond to the years shown in the previous columns of the table (also indicated in brackets when different from the default years).

7.2 More children born outside marriage, to an unmarried couple or to a single mother

The disconnection of childbearing from marriage is most clearly illustrated by a steep rise in the proportion of non-marital births over the last three decades that began in many countries in the early 1970s (earlier in Northern Europe, see Figure 8). This does not imply a similar increase in the frequency of single motherhood, as extramarital births are, with increasing frequency, taking place in the context of stable cohabiting partnerships (see below). In total, one-third of all births in the EU-25 occurred outside marriage in 2005, up from five percent during the 1960s, and 18 percent in 1990 (Eurostat 2006a). This change accelerated in Central and Eastern Europe after the breakdown of state socialism in 1989, and in Italy and Spain after 1995. The recent rise in extramarital childbearing in the latter two countries might seem surprising, given the persistent importance of marriage and traditional family bonds in these societies (Reher 1998; Dalla Zuanna 2001). It is linked to the rise in cohabitation (see Rosina and Fraboni 2004 for Italy), but also to an influx of immigrants from the countries where extramarital childbearing is common (see Spain chapter). In most societies where childbearing outside wedlock had remained rare until recently, such as Belgium, Italy, or Poland, it is a common phenomenon now. Only in Albania, Cyprus, and Greece do extramarital births remain marginal, accounting for less than six percent of all births in 2005. Albania, where only 0.5 percent of births in 2003 were non-marital, is the most extreme outlier (Albania chapter). A growing number of countries and regions register a majority of births outside marriage. In 2005, Estonia, Iceland, Norway, Sweden, and the former GDR (East Germany) were in this group, and it is likely that Bulgaria, France, and Slovenia will follow suit. Interestingly, in the Nordic countries that experienced an early and dramatic rise in extramarital childbearing, the proportion has stabilized since the late 1990s, after reaching a level of about half of all births. First births, in particular, frequently occur outside marriage (Austria, the Czech Republic, Hungary, and the Netherlands chapters). For instance, almost one-half (49.6 percent) of first births in Austria were outside marriage in 2005, compared with 36.5 percent of all births (Austria chapter).

Despite common trends, contemporary Europe is characterised by considerable diversity in non-marital childbearing. As in the case of divorce, this division does not follow simple geographical boundaries or old geo-political lines. The countries of Central and Eastern Europe, in particular, remain very diverse in this respect, comprising countries with both very low and very high percentages of non-marital births. Differences within countries also remain pronounced, following long-established religious and cultural divisions, as well as different historical patterns (e.g., the Czech Republic chapter). Germany constitutes a specific case of persistent regional differentiation in non-marital childbearing: the already high percentage of non-marital births in Eastern Germany shot up further after unification in 1990, whereas the percentage of non-marital births in Western Germany increased gradually, remaining below the EU average (Figure 8; see Germany chapter for an overview of various hypotheses for this divergence; see also Konietzka and Kreyenfeld 2002 and Salles 2006). Differences between ethnic groups can also be large. For example, the Bulgaria chapter notes a very steep rise in the ratio of extramarital births among the Roma population—to around 55 percent in 2001—which can be explained by a rise in *de facto* marriages that are not legally registered, and that are recognised only within the Roma community.

Childbearing outside marriage covers various family forms, which have different implications for the economic position and well-being of parents and their children (Heuveline, Timberlake and Furstenberg 2003; Kiernan 2004). It is essential to make a distinction between children born within consensual unions, and those born outside a stable partnership union. For the latter group, it is often difficult to differentiate between mothers who bring up their children without a father, and couples who do not live together, but have some relationship and act as a 'parental couple.' Some mothers who do not live with a partner, and who are thus identified as 'lone mothers,' may in

Figure 8:   Percentage of children born outside marriage in selected countries and regions of Europe (1950-2005)

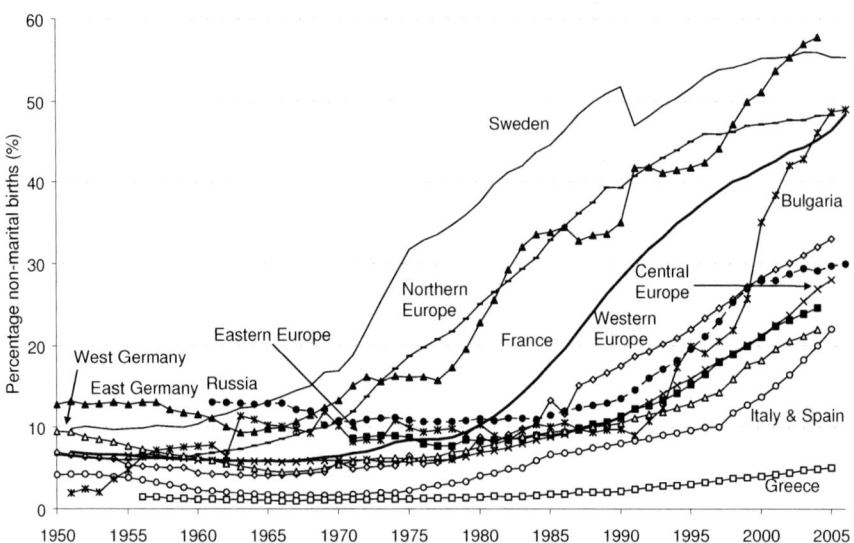

Source: Council of Europe 2006, Eurostat 2006a and 2006b, Grünheid 2006.
Notes: Regional data are not weighted by the population size of given countries.
Countries are grouped into regions as follows:
Western Europe: Austria, Belgium, France, Germany, Ireland, Luxembourg, the Netherlands, Switzerland, United Kingdom;
Northern Europe: Denmark, Finland, Iceland, Norway, Sweden;
Central Europe: Croatia, Czech Republic, Hungary, Poland, Slovakia, Slovenia;
Eastern Europe: Belarus, Moldova (excluding Transnistria), Russia (including Asian part), Ukraine.

fact have a long-term relationship with the father of the child(ren). The information included in the FFS about the status of couples at the time of the birth of children is very useful in distinguishing between unmarried parental couples and lone mothers. In Northern Europe and most countries of Western Europe, a majority of extramarital births are planned, intended by both parents, and usually take place within the context of stable cohabiting unions. In Sweden, where the proportion of extramarital births has been the second highest in Europe for many decades (after Iceland), only around one-tenth of births are to single mothers, and many couples marry after having their first or second child (Sweden chapter). In France, where parents who recognise their non-marital child have rights and duties identical to those of parents of children born within marriage, around 94 percent of children are recognised by their fathers (France chapter; see also Munoz-Pérez and Prioux 2000). At the same time, in some countries of Western Europe, a relatively high proportion of first births take place before a woman enters her first union (Table 5). In Central and Eastern Europe, single mothers account for a large portion of all extramarital births (Heuveline, Timberlake and Furstenberg 2003). In some of these countries, non-marital births may still largely be unplanned (Romania chapter), and may meet with disapproval among the majority population (Poland chapter, see also Overview Chapter 6). Coleman (2006) posits that births among single mothers are partly fuelled by specific welfare policies providing support to single mothers (see also Gonzáles 2005 and Salles 2006). The Austria chapter offers the same explanation for the unusually high proportion of children born to lone mothers, who represent one-fifth of all first children (see Table 5). Arguably, some single mothers may intentionally live separately from their partners in order to qualify for the higher parental leave payments granted exclusively to mothers who live alone.

Overall, the proportion of births outside marriage is closely linked to the proportion of women living in unmarried cohabitation. Most non-marital births take place within unmarried unions, and the key explanations of rising non-marital fertility relate to cohabitation; namely, to a combination of the rising number of people entering cohabiting unions, the longer duration of these unions, and the declining propensity of unmarried couples to get married during the pregnancy (Raley 2001, Kiernan 2004, Philipov 2006, Steele et al. 2006). The Netherlands chapter notes a shift that has occurred since the 1960s, when most extramarital children were born to young single women, usually with low levels of education, who had not planned to become pregnant. In contrast, most births to unmarried mothers today take place "within a relationship, usually to a couple in their late 20s or early 30s who have made a conscious decision to have a child and obviously do not (yet) see the necessity to marry" (Fokkema et al. 2008:756). Data for France and England and Wales further illustrate this shift: as the proportion of non-marital births rises, ever higher percentages of these children are recognised by their fathers; these two trends practically mirror and compensate for each other (Munoz-Pérez and Prioux 2000). In England and Wales as well as in France the proportion of children not recognized by their fathers increased slightly during the 1980s, but it has been stable since 1990, while the proportion of extramarital births has continued to increase (Figure 9). In England and Wales, seven percent of children were not recognized by their fathers in 2006, while extramarital births exceeded 40 percent. In France, half of all children were born to unmarried parents, but only seven percent were not recognized at birth and only four percent of children remained unrecognized within a year of birth (Figure 9). A clear sign of a 'normalisation' of non-marital childbearing (but not of 'single motherhood') is given by its spread to different ages and social groups (Russian Federation chapter). This trend is mostly attributable to the diffusion of unmarried cohabitation as a way to live as a couple, and not to the increase in the proportion of women having a child 'with no father.' In many countries, however, the differences between social groups in the frequency of non-marital childbearing remain pronounced (Overview Chapter 6).

Table 5: **Partnership context at first birth, percentage distribution of women with first births at age 20-45 (Northern, Western, and Southern Europe)**

	Before any union	In first cohabiting union	In first marriage	After first union
Northern Europe				
Norway	12	18	65	5
Sweden	7	51	29	13
Western Europe				
Austria	20	22	53	5
France	6	14	74	6
West Germany	10	13	70	7
Switzerland	5	7	77	11
United Kingdom	9	9	75	8
Southern Europe				
Italy	5	3	90	1
Spain	5	3	90	1

Source: Data computed by Kiernan (1999) on the basis of the FFS surveys.

Figure 9: **Proportion of non-marital births in England and Wales and in France, and proportion of children not recognised by their father at birth (or during the year of birth in France), 1965-2006 (percent)**

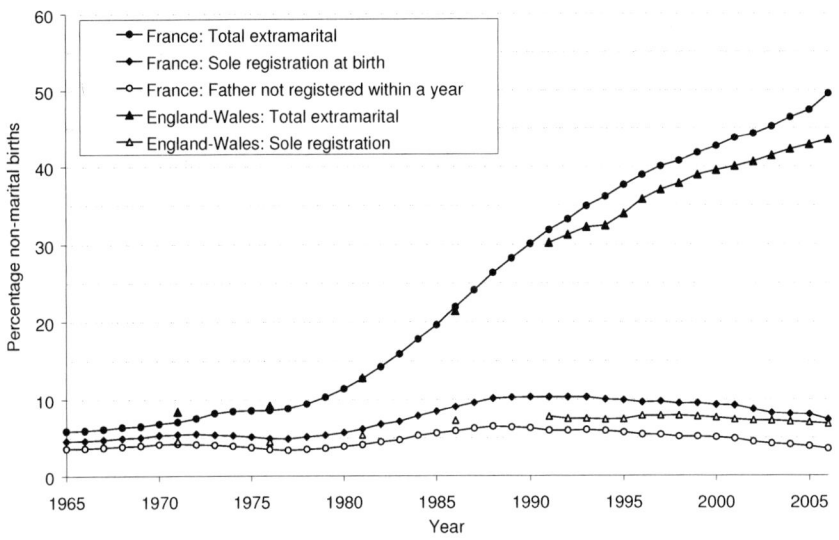

Source: Own computations based on ONS 2007 and Population Trends 2006 for England and Wales; Beaumel et al. 2007 for France.

7.3 Most mothers who remain unmarried do not live with a partner

As a result of rising marriage instability and an increasing prevalence of less-stable living arrangements (cohabitation and LAT partnerships), combined in many countries with a high frequency of single motherhood, there has been an increase in the proportion of one-parent families across Europe. More children live in single families or in stepfamilies, formed when their parents enter a new union (Andersson 2002, Heuveline, Timberlake, and Furstenberg 2003). While unmarried cohabitation has rapidly gained on importance for childbearing, it remains in most countries considerably less frequent than single motherhood when the distribution of living arrangements of younger parents (aged 20-44) is analysed.

According to the census data from 2000-2001, in each of the 21 countries analysed in Table 6, with the exception of France, there were more 'lone mothers' living without a partner than cohabiting mothers at that age. Only in three Nordic countries (Denmark,

Finland, and Norway), did the share of cohabiting mothers (15-17 percent) come close to the share of single mothers (17-19 percent). Assuming that these results reflect reality, they are also surprising given the overall high proportion of mothers living without a partner; more than one-fifth in the Czech Republic, United Kingdom, and Estonia (29 percent). The relatively low importance of cohabitation as a living arrangement among younger parents can be explained by a combination of three factors. First, these data partly mirror past childbearing history; some of these parents had a child in the 1980s, when cohabitation was much less common than at present, and more children were born within marriage. Second, as cohabiting unions remain more fragile than marriages, many cohabiting unions with children dissolve relatively soon after the birth of the child (e.g., Osborne, Manning, and Smock 2007 for the U.S.) Third, many couples who have a child in an unmarried union subsequently marry within several years after childbirth, thereby contributing to the pool of married parents with children.

The data on living arrangements of younger fathers reflect new differences in the family histories of men and women: second unions may be equally frequent for men and women, as in France (Toulemon and Lapierre-Adamcyk 2000); or less frequent for women. In most cases, however, children live with their mothers after a union disruption. Thus, solo parents are almost always single mothers, and stepfamilies are most often made up of a (biological) mother and a stepfather (Prskawetz et al. 2003). Overall, considerably fewer men live with their children or their partner's children at age 20-44, in part also because men become fathers at a later age. While in all the countries studied, except for Ireland and Spain, a majority of women aged 20-44 were living with children, only a minority of men were living with children, with the lowest proportion, just above one-third, registered in Ireland, Greece, Italy, and Spain. Among those living with children, men more often cohabit than women do, and relatively few live as 'single fathers.' This proportion is not entirely negligible, however, and reaches close to four percent in the Czech Republic, Estonia, Norway, and Spain.

Table 6: **Living arrangements of women and men living with children at age 20-44; census data for 2000-2001**

	WOMEN				MEN			
	Percent living with children	Of which:			Percent living with children	Of which:		
		Married	Cohabiting	Single parents		Married	Cohabiting	Single parents
Northern Europe								
Denmark	55.8	67.5	15.4	17.1	39.2	77.8	19.4	2.8
Finland	53.4	67.6	14.5	17.9	37.7	78.5	18.8	2.7
Norway	57.9	64.0	17.0	19.0	39.0	75.6	20.8	3.7
Western Europe								
France	57.5	68.3	17.6	14.1	43.3	76.2	21.7	2.2
Ireland	47.2	76.3	6.8	16.9	34.9	89.2	8.9	1.8
The Netherlands	53.7	78.9	9.3	11.8	40.1	85.9	12.8	1.3
United Kingdom	55.7	64.7	10.8	24.5	39.1	80.9	16.0	3.1
German-speaking countries								
Austria	57.9	73.4	8.4	18.2	40.4	86.2	11.2	2.6
Germany	57.3	79.0	6.9	14.2	41.7	88.3	9.4	2.3
Switzerland	50.6	83.6	5.2	11.2	38.0	90.7	7.7	1.6
Southern Europe								
Greece	53.1	90.1	1.3	8.6	35.1	96.1	1.9	2.0
Italy	50.6	87.6	2.6	9.8	36.1	95.0	3.3	1.7
Portugal	58.9	84.7	5.2	10.1	46.5	93.0	5.6	1.4
Spain	46.1	83.4	3.9	12.6	34.1	91.3	5.0	3.8
Central and Eastern Europe								
Czech Republic	65.1	75.3	2.8	21.8	43.0	92.9	3.6	3.5
Estonia	65.8	56.6	14.6	28.9	45.3	76.4	20.1	3.5
Hungary	61.9	75.5	7.4	17.0	43.6	88.4	9.5	2.1
Poland	63.6	81.1	1.3	17.6	44.9	96.8	1.5	1.7
Romania	65.8	82.7	5.8	11.5	49.1	91.0	6.9	2.1
Slovak Republic	64.4	82.4	1.6	16.0	46.7	96.0	1.9	2.2
Slovenia	60.9	75.1	7.6	17.4	39.2	88.5	8.8	2.7

Source: Own computations based on the 2000-2001 Census data provided by Eurostat (2008) and Insee 2002 for France (1999 census).

Heuveline, Timberlake, and Furstenberg (2003) found that a substantial percentage of children are exposed to living with a single parent before reaching the age of 15. The total exposure ranged from 11-18 percent in Southern Europe (Italy and Spain), Belgium, Poland, and Slovenia; to 39-41 percent in Austria, Germany, and Latvia; and, outside of Europe, to a very high level of 52 percent in the United States (these figures are period life table estimates based on the FFS data). In agreement with the evidence provided by the census data in Table 6 above, the authors argue that, while the pace of family change has varied across countries, the shift of childrearing from married parents to single mothers is universal in Western societies, and has been proceeding faster than the shift to cohabiting parents and stepfamilies.

8. Concluding discussion: marriage, living arrangements, and fertility

Family and marriage behaviours have changed considerably in all the countries of Europe, perhaps with the notable exception of Albania. Different societies are following a similar trajectory of change; namely, towards delayed union formation and further postponement of marriage, a sharp decline in marriage rates, a rise in unmarried cohabitation and in non-co-residential partnerships, and an increase in union instability. Monogamous life-long marriage, which was the 'normative' experience for most Europeans born before 1960, has been progressively eroded by delayed entry into union and increased cohabitation on the one hand, and rising levels of divorce and separation on the other. Marriage has thus lost its two main roles as an institution: first, as a ritual linking the formation of a new couple with their social environment and the society (Heuveline and Timberlake 2004); and, second, as a way to sanction the link between parents and their children. In many European countries, entering a union is now perceived as a private matter, and children born to unmarried parents have the same legal status as children born to married couples. Furthermore, unmarried cohabitation is often becoming a long-term substitute for marriage.

Although some signs of cross-country convergence may be noted—e.g., in the shift to low levels of period first marriage rates, or in a gradual disappearance of marriage from the lives of young adults—most patterns of family behaviour remain widely differentiated across Europe. Such persistent contrasts are manifested in the timing of home leaving, in the importance of cohabitation for union formation and childbearing, in the timing of first unions and first births, and also in the rates of divorce and the frequency of non-marital childbearing. Some of these cleavages follow long-established regional differences (e.g., the North-South contrasts in home-leaving patterns), whereas some other contrasts reflect the persistence of more traditional cultural or religious influences in some societies (e.g., frequency of cohabitation, divorce, and non-marital childbearing). Yet other contrasts have been evolving over time, and do not appear to be closely linked to the established regional and cultural divisions (e.g., the frequency of single motherhood).

In some countries, this shift in family behaviour is associated with low fertility. Presumably, the higher prevalence of more fragile non-marital unions should lead to lower fertility (Sweden chapter). However, such a relationship cannot be identified when all countries are compared. The aggregate-level association seems to shift in the opposite direction: countries where the prevalence of divorce is high had higher total fertility rates in both 2004 and 1990. In a context of very low fertility, conjugal instability may be seen as a potential fuel to fertility, at least when the partners want to have at least one child in their new union, irrespective of their previous fertility

(Prskawetz et al. 2007). Curiously, if more and more couples limit their childbearing aspirations to one child only—as is the case in Southern and Eastern Europe—rising union instability may be seen as a way to raise fertility. As Billari (2005: 80) points out in a slightly provocative way, "If the rule is 'one child per couple', the only way to reach replacement is to have individuals experience two couple relationships!"

Changes in family behaviour and living arrangements are related to many other social and economic changes. The concept of the second demographic transition offers a general interpretation of these changes (see Overview Chapter 6). The relationship between the progression of this transition and the level of fertility is not straightforward. Looking at inter-country correlations may be misleading, as the strength of the relationship may vary between countries (Kögel 2004; Engelhardt and Prskawetz 2004; Billari 2004). Such patterns at the macro level do not necessarily reflect causality in terms of individual behaviour (see e.g., Courgeau 2002). Nevertheless, it is remarkable that the association between the proportion of births outside marriage and the total fertility rate has reversed since 1990, and is now positive; while it was negative, despite many outliers and a strong heterogeneity, during the 1970s and 1980s (Figures 10 and 11). This is also true of the mean age at first marriage and the total divorce rate, while the positive correlation between total first marriage rates and fertility has almost vanished (Figure 11). These changing relationships, however, may not be explained by a change in the causal relationship between fertility and family behaviours at the individual level: such an erroneous inference is known as the "individualistic" or "atomic" fallacy.

Figure 10: **Correlation between the period TFR and the proportion of non-marital births in 1970 and 2004**

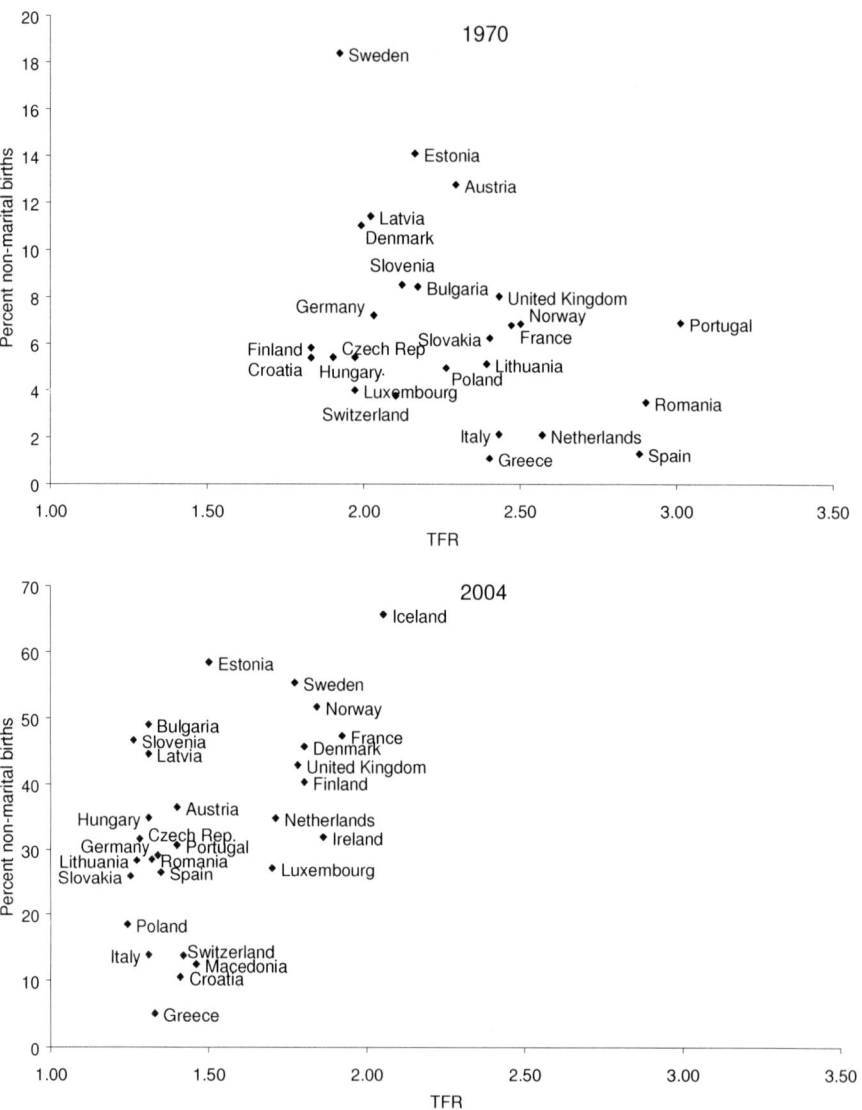

Source: Own computations based on Council of Europe data (2006)

Figure 11:   Correlation between the period total fertility rate and four indicators of family-related behaviours, 1960-2005

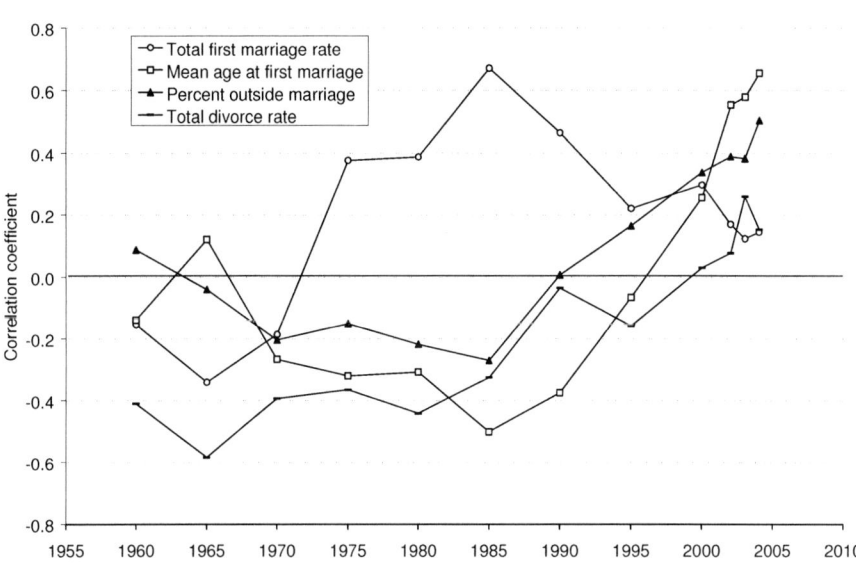

Source: Council of Europe, 2006. Update of computations by Billari (2005).
Note: Unweighted correlations, data include all countries of the Council of Europe.

At the individual level, remaining unmarried or marrying late is undoubtedly and strongly linked with having fewer children: under fixed constraints, the relationship is well established, but it may not be generalised at the macro level. When looking at the time trend within each country, or when comparing several countries at the same period in time, we compare situations with different constraints, family and social policies, and values and norms. Thus the relationship which holds at the micro level may not be linked with the relationships between the changes in these constraints at the macro level. Clearly, complex causal mechanisms not discussed here may be at stake in the country-level relationships between fertility and family and partnership behaviour. However, our key point is that the strong positive relationship which is still present at the individual level between being married and having children is not present at the country level. On the contrary, countries where extramarital births are more common in the early 2000s are the ones where the total fertility rate is at the highest level.

A similar result has been shown for the correlation between mean age at first birth and overall fertility. The negative relationship at the micro level is strong and robust to standardisation by cohort or level of education: late mothers end up having fewer children than young mothers (Billari et al. 2000). Nevertheless, the macro-level trends do not show the same relationship in all countries. For instance, French women born in 1960 have as many children as women born in 1950, despite a later age at first birth, and their parity progression ratios remain stable (France chapter). Furthermore, when we compare cohort fertility from one country to the next we find that the higher the increase in the mean age at first birth, the less pronounced is the decline in fertility (Toulemon 2006).

The positive relationship between period marriage and fertility indices is no longer visible: low marriage rates do not imply low fertility (Figure 11). Among the 1965 cohort, the correlation between marriage and fertility behaviour also appears very weak at the inter-country level (Figure 12). The European countries where the 1965 cohort TFR is the highest include some countries where marriage is still common for these women (Poland, Hungary, Slovak Republic, Czech Republic), as well as countries where many women are unmarried (France, Norway, Sweden).

In most countries, marriage rates declined in parallel with fertility, and it could be assumed that these two trends are part of a consistent change in demographic behaviour. But the evidence leads us to a different conclusion: among European countries, fertility is highest in those countries where marriage is most intensively delayed, where births outside of marriage and unmarried cohabitation are frequent, and divorce rates are high. In most countries, the decline in marriage rates is not related to an increase in the proportion of women and men who chose to remain childless and unmarried, but more to an increase in the number of men and women who decide to enter a union without marriage, and a parallel increase in the number of couples who decide to have children without getting married.

Marriage and partnership behaviour is changing throughout Europe, and countries where fertility is lowest are the ones where the change in partnership behaviour is limited, while fertility is higher and more stable in countries where partnership behaviour has already changed dramatically. In countries where marriage and fertility are no longer linked, fertility is still high; while in countries where the 'traditional family' is still 'strong' as an institution, marriage rates are low (as is the case everywhere), and fertility is also low (see, e.g., chapters on Sweden and Italy). This macro-level relationship will be discussed further in Overview Chapter 6. In our view, the 'big change' in family life and living arrangements discussed in this chapter should not be seen as a reason for the current low level of fertility in Europe.

Figure 12:   Correlation between the proportion never-married at age 50 (horizontal axis) and cohort TFR (vertical axis), among women born in 1965

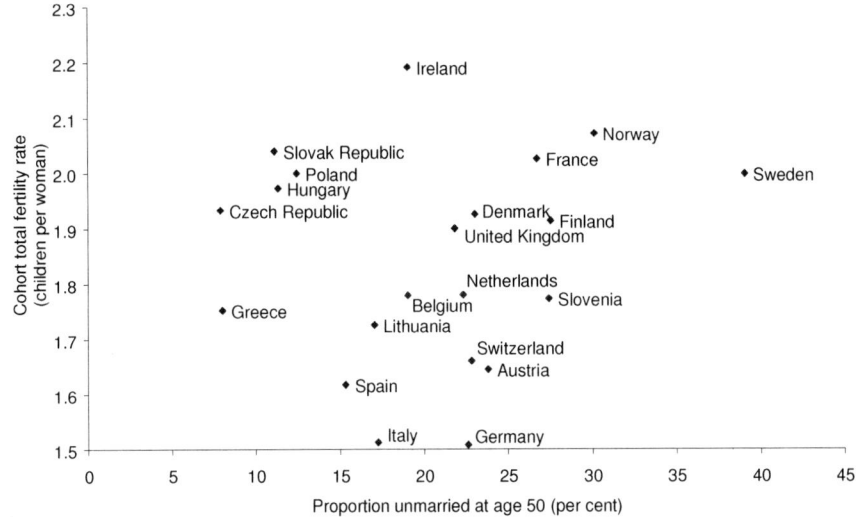

Source: Own calculations from Prioux 2006, Council of Europe 2006.
Note: The proportion of ever married has been partly estimated for the cohorts born in the mid-1950s and later.

References

Aassve, A., F. C. Billari, S. Mazzuco, and F. Ongaro. 2002. Leaving home: a comparative analysis of ECHP data, *Journal of European Social Policy* 12(4): 259–276.

Ahlburg, D. A., and C. J. De Vita. 1992. New realities of the American family, *Population Bulletin* 47(2):1–43.

Andersson, G. 1998. Trends in marriage formation in Sweden, *European Journal of Population* 14(2): 157–178.

Andersson, G. 2002. Children's experience of family disruption and family formation: evidence from 16 FFS countries, *Demographic Research* 7(7): 341–363. http://www.demographic-research.org/volumes/vol7/7/.

Andersson, G. 2003. *Dissolution of unions in Europe: a comparative overview.* MPIDR Working Paper WP2003-004. Rostock: Max Planck Institute for Demographic Research. http://www.demogr.mpg.de/papers/working/wp-2003-004.pdf.

Andersson, G., and D. Philipov. 2002. Life-table representations of family dynamics in Sweden, Hungary, and 14 other FFS countries: a project of descriptions of demographic behaviour, *Demographic Research* 7(4): 67–144.

Bachrach, C. 1987. Cohabitation and reproductive behavior in the U.S., *Demography* 24(4): 623–637.

Barlow, A. 2004. Regulation of cohabitation, changing family policies and social attitudes: a discussion of Britain within Europe, *Law & Policy* 26(1): 57–86.

Beaumel, C., F. Daguet, L. Richet-Mastain, and M. Vatan. 2007. La situation démographique en 2005 - Mouvement de la population, *Insee Resultats* 66. http://www.insee.fr

Blossfeld, H.-P. (Ed). 1995. *The New Role of Women. Family Formation in Modern Societies.* Boulder, Colorado: Westview Press.

Billari, F. 2004. Becoming an adult in Europe: a macro(/micro)-demographic perspective, *Demographic Research* S3(2): 15–44, http://www.demographic-research.org/special/3/2/.

Billari, F. 2005. Partnership, childbearing and parenting: trends of the 1990s, in UNECE/UNFPA (Eds.), *The New Demographic Regime. Population Challenges and Policy Responses.* Geneva: United Nations, pp: 63–94.

Billari F., P. Manfredi, and A. Valentini. 2000. Macro-demographic effects of the transition to adulthood: multistate stable population theory and an application to Italy, *Mathematical Population Studies* 9(1): 33–63.

Billari, F., D. Philipov, and P. Baizán. 2001. Leaving home in Europe: the experience of cohorts born around 1960, *International Journal of Population Geography* 7: 339–356.

Blom, S. 1994. Marriage and cohabitation in a changing society. Experiences of Norwegian men and women born in 1945 and 1960, *European Journal of Population* 10: 143–173.

Bozon, M. 2003. At what age do women and men have their first sexual intercourse? *Population and Societies* 391: 1–4.

Brückner, H., and K. U. Mayer. 2005. De-standardization of the life course. What it might mean? And if it means anything, whether it actually took place?, in R. Macmillan (Ed.), *Structure of the Life Course. Standardized? Individualized? Differentiated?* Series *Advances in Life Course Research* Vol. 9, Amsterdam: Elsevier, pp: 27–53.

Bumpass L., and J. Sweet. 1989. National estimates of cohabitation, *Demography* 26(4): 615–625.

Bumpass L., and H. Lu. 2000. Trends in cohabitation and implications for children's family contexts in the U.S., *Population Studies* 54(1): 29–41.

Castiglioni, M., and G. Dalla Zuanna. 1994. Innovation and tradition: reproductive and marital behaviour in Italy in the 1970s and 1980s, *European Journal of Population* 10(2): 107–142.

Chambaz, C. 2000. Les familles monoparentales en Europe : des réalités multiples, *Etudes et résultats* 66.

Council of Europe. 2006. *Recent Demographic Developments in Europe 2005.* Strasbourg: Council of Europe Publishing.

Corijn, M., and E. Klijzing (Eds). 2001. *Transitions to Adulthood in Europe.* Dordrecht: Kluwer Academic Publishers.

Courgeau, D. 2002. New approaches and methodological innovations in the study of partnership and fertility behaviour, in M. Macura and G. Beets (Eds.), *Dynamics of Fertility and Partnership in Europe. Insights and Lessons from Comparative Research.* Geneva: United Nations, pp: 99–114.

Dalla Zuanna, G. 2001. The banquet of Aeolus: a familistic interpretation of Italy's lowest low fertility, *Demographic Research* 4(5): 133–162. http://www.demographic-research.org/Volumes/Vol4/5/

Delgado, M., Meil, G., and Zamora López, F. 2008. Spain: Short on children and short on family policies, *Demographic Research* 19(27). http://www.demographic-research.org/Volumes/Vol19/27/

Elzinga, C. H., and A. C. Liefbroer. 2007. Destandardization of family life trajectories of young adults: a cross-national comparison using sequence analysis, *European Journal of Population* 23(3): 225–250.

Engelhardt, H., and A. Prskawetz. 2004. On the changing correlation between fertility and female employment over space and time, *European Journal of Population* 20(1): 35–62.

Eurostat. 2006a. *Population Statistics. 2006 Edition.* Luxembourg: Office for official Publications of the European Communities.

Eurostat. 2006b. Population in Europe 2005. First results. Statistics in Focus, Population and Social Conditions, 16/2006. Luxembourg: European Communities.

Eurostat. 2007, 2008. *Population and Social Conditions.* Online database http://epp.eurostat.ec.europa.eu.

Festy, P. 1980. On the new context of marriage in Western Europe, *Population and Development Review* 6(2): 311–315.

Festy, P. 2006. Legal recognition of same-sex couples in Europe, *Population - E* 61(4): 417–453.

Fokkema, T., de Valk, H., de Beer, J., van Duin, C. 2008. The Netherlands: Childbearing within the context of a "Poldermodel" society, *Demographic Research* 19(21). http://www.demographic-research.org/Volumes/Vol19/21/

Giddens, A. 1992. *The Transformation of Intimacy: Sexuality, Love and Eroticism in Modern Societies.* Cambridge: Polity Press.

Gjonca, A., Aassve, A., and Mencarini, L. 2008. Albania: Trends and patterns, proximate determinants and policies of fertility change, *Demographic Research* 19(11). http://www.demographic-research.org/Volumes/Vol19/11/

Gonzáles, L. 2005. *The determinants of the prevalence of single mothers: A cross-country analysis.* IZA Discussion Paper No. 1677, Bonn: Institute for the Study of Labour. http://www.iza.org.

Grünheid, E. 2006. Die demographische Lage in Deutschland 2005 [2005 report on the demographic situation in Germany], *Zeitschrift für Bevölkerungswissenschaft* 31(1): 3–104.

Hajnal, J. 1965. European marriage patterns in perspective, in D. Glass and D. Eversley (Eds.), *Population in History.* Chicago: Aldine Publishing Company, pp: 101-143.

Haskey, J. 1999. Cohabitational and marital histories of adults in Great Britain, *Population Trends* 96: 13–24.

Haskey, J. 2005. First estimates of the number of people 'Living Apart Together' in Britain, *Population Trends* 122: 35–46.

Heinz, W. R., and H. Krüger. 2001. Life course: innovations and challenges for social research, *Current Sociology* 49(2): 29–53.

Heuveline, P., and J. M. Timberlake. 2004. The role of cohabitation in family formation: the United States in comparative perspective, *Journal of Marriage and Family* 66(6): 1214–1230.

Heuveline, P., J. M. Timberlake, and F. F. Furstenberg, Jr. 2003. Shifting childrearing to single mothers. Results from 17 Western countries, *Population and Development Review* 29(1): 47–71.

Hobcraft, J. 1996. Fertility in England and Wales: a fifty-year perspective, *Population Studies* 50(3): 485–524.

Hoem, J. 1986. The impact of education on modern family-union initiation, *European Journal of Population* 2(2): 113–133.

Hoem, J. and B. Rennermalm. 1985. Modern family initiation in Sweden: experience of women born between 1936 and 1960, *European Journal of Population* 1(1): 81–112.

Holdsworth, C. 2000. Leaving home in Britain and Spain, *European Sociological Review* 16(2): 201–222.

Insee. 2002. Recensement de la population de mars 1999. Tableaux thématiques. Exploitation complémentaire: ménages, familles, population totale. France métropolitaine. Paris: Insee.

Kalmijn, M. 2007. Explaining cross-national differences in marriage, cohabitation, and divorce in Europe, *Population Studies* 61(3): 243–263.

Kasearu, K. 2007. *The case of unmarried cohabitation in Western and Eastern Europe.* Draft presented at the conference of European Network on Divorce Comparative and Gendered Perspectives on Family Structure. 17-18 September 2007, London, England: London School of Economics, http://www.eui.eu/Personal/Dronkers/Divorce/Divorceconference2007/Kasearu.pdf.

Kiernan, K. 1999. Cohabitation in Western Europe, *Population Trends* 96: 25–32.

Kiernan, K., 2004. Unmarried cohabitation and parenthood in Britain and Europe, *Law and Policy* 26(1): 33–55.

Kohler, H.-P., F. C. Billari, and J. O. Ortega. 2002. The emergence of lowest-low fertility in Europe during the 1990s, *Population and Development Review* 28(4): 641–680.

Kontula, O. 2003. Trends in teenage sexual behaviour, pregnancies, sexually transmitted infections and HIV infections in Europe, in N. Bajos, A. Guillaume and O. Kontula

(Eds.), *Reproductive Health Behaviour of Young Europeans.* Volume 1. Strasbourg: Council of Europe Population Studies 42, pp: 77–137.

Kuijsten, A. 1996. Changing family patterns in Europe, a case of divergence?, *European Journal of Population* 12(2): 115–143.

Kögel, T. 2004. Did the association between fertility and female employment within OECD countries really change its sign?, *Journal of Population Economics* 17(1): 45–65.

Konietzka, D., and M. Kreyenfeld. 2002. Women's employment and non-marital childbearing: a comparison between East and West Germany in the 1990s, *Population-E* 57(2): 331–357.

Kravdal, Ø. 1999. Does marriage require a stronger economic underpinning than informal cohabitation? *Population Studies* 53: 63–80.

Leridon, H., and C. Villeneuve-Gokalp. 1989. The new couples: number, characteristics and attitudes, *Population-English Selection* 1: 203–230.

Lesthaeghe, R., and G. Moors. 2002. Life course transitions and value orientations: selection and adaptation, in R. Lesthaeghe (Ed.), *Meaning and Choice: Value Orientation and Life Course Decisions.* The Hague, Brussels: NIDI/CBGS Publication, pp: 1–44.

Liefbroer, A. 1991. Choosing between a married and an unmarried first union among young adults: a competing risks analysis, *European Journal of Population* 7: 273–298.

Liefbroer, A., and E. Dourleijn. 2006. Unmarried cohabitation and union stability: testing the role of diffusion using data from 16 European countries, *Demography* 43(2): 203–221.

Macura, M., and G. Beets (Eds.) 2002. Dynamics of Fertility and Partnership in Europe. Insights and Lessons from Comparative Research. Vol. 1. Geneva: United Nations.

Manacorda, M., and E. Moretti. 2006. Why do most Italian youths live with their parents? Intergenerational transfers and household structure, *Journal of the European Economic Association* 4(4): 800–829.

Manting, D. 1994. *Dynamics in Marriage and Cohabitation. An Inter-Temporal, Life Course Analysis of First Union Formation and Dissolution.* Amsterdam: Thesis Publishers.

Mills, M. 2000. *The Transformation of Partnerships. Canada, the Netherlands and the Russian Federation in the Age of Modernity.* Amsterdam: Thela Thesis, Population Studies Series.

Mulder, C., W. Clark, and M. Wagner. 2002. A comparative analysis of leaving home in the United States, the Netherlands and West Germany, *Demographic Research* 7(17): 65–592. http://www.demographic-research.org/Volumes/Vol7/17/.

Munoz-Pérez, F. 1991. Les naissances hors mariage et les conceptions prénuptiales en Espagne depuis 1975. I. Une période de profonds changements, *Population* 46(4): 881–912

Munoz-Pérez, F., and F. Prioux. 2000. Children born outside marriage in France and their parents: recognitions and legitimations since 1965, *Population: An English selection* 12: 139–195.

Munoz-Pérez, F., and F. Prioux. 2005. Filiation des enfants nés hors mariage en France depuis 1950, in C. Bergouignan *et al.* (Eds.), *La population de la France : évolutions démographiques depuis 1946. Vol. 1.* Pessac : CUDEP, pp: 333–354.

Murphy, M. 2000. The evolution of cohabitation in Britain, 1960–95, *Population Studies* 54: 43–56.

Nazio, T., and H.-P. Blossfeld. 2003. The diffusion of cohabitation among young women in West Germany, East Germany and Italy, *European Journal of Population* 19: 47–82.

Ongaro, F. 2001. Transition to adulthood in Italy, in M. Corijn and E. Klijzing (Eds.), *Transitions to Adulthood in Europe.* Dordrecht: Kluwer Academic Publishers.

ONS. 2007. *Birth statistics. Review of the Registrar General on births and patterns of family building England and Wales, 2006.* Series FM1, No. 35, London: Office of National Statistics. http://www.statistics.gov.uk/downloads/theme_population/FM1_35/FM1_No35.PDF.

Oppenheimer, V. 2003. Cohabiting and marriage during young men's career-development process, *Demography* 40: 127–149.

Osborne, C., W. D. Manning, and P. J. Smock. 2007. Married and cohabiting parents' relationship stability: a focus on race and ethnicity, *Journal of Marriage and Family* 69(5): 1345–1366.

Perelli-Harris, B. 2008. Ukraine: On the border between old and new in uncertain times, *Demographic Research* 19(29). http://www.demographic-research.org/Volumes/Vol19/29/

Population Trends. 2006. Vital Statistics Summary, Table 3.2., *Population Trends* 128 (Summer 2007): 57.

Philipov, D. 2006. Portrait of the family in Europe, in L. Hantrais, D. Philipov and F. C. Billari (Eds.), *Policy Implications of Changing Family Formation.* Strasbourg: Council of Europe, Population Studies Series 49: 19–62.

Pinnelli, A. 2001. Determinants of fertility in Europe: new family forms, context and individual characteristics, in A. Pinnelli, H.-J. Hoffmann-Nowotny and B. Fux (Eds.), *Fertility and New Types of Households and Family Formation in Europe.* Strasbourg. Council of Europe, Population Studies Series 35: 47–181.

Prinz, C. 1995. *Cohabiting, Married, or Single.* Avebury: Aldershot, Brookfield, Vermont.

Prioux, F. 1993. The ups and downs of marriage in Austria, *Population: An English Selection* 5: 153–182.

Prioux, F. 2003. Age at first union in France: a two-stage process of change, *Population - E* 58(4-5): 559–578.

Prioux, F., 2006. Cohabitation, marriage and separation: contrasts in Europe, *Population & Societies* 422: 1–4.

Probert, R. 2004. Cohabitation in Twentieth-Century England and Wales: law and policy, *Law and Policy* 26(1): 13–32.

Prskawetz A., A. Vikat, D. Philipov, and H. Engelhardt. 2003. Pathways to stepfamily formation in Europe. Results from the FFS, *Demographic Research* 8(5): 106–149. http://www.demographic-research.org/volumes/vol8/5/.

Prskawetz, A., E. Thomson, M. Spielauer, and M. Winkler-Dworak. 2007. *Union instability as an engine of fertility? A micro-simulation model for France.* Paper presented at the PAA 2007 Annual meeting, New-York, 29-31 March. http://paa2007.princeton.edu/abstractViewer.aspx?submissionId=71738.

Raley, K. 2001. Increasing fertility in cohabiting unions: evidence for the Second Demographic Transition in the United States?, *Demography* 38(1): 59–66.

Reher, D. 1998. Family ties in western Europe: persistent contrasts, *Population and Development Review* 24(2): 203–234.

Rindfuss, R. 1991. The young adult years: diversity, structural change, and fertility, *Demography* 28(4): 493–512.

Rindfuss, R., and A. VandenHeuvel. 1990. Cohabitation: precursor to marriage or an alternative to being single, *Population and Development Review* 16(4): 703–726.

Rosina A., and R. Fraboni. 2004. Is marriage loosing its centrality in Italy?, *Demographic Research* 11(6): 149–172. www.demographic-research.org.

Salles, A. 2006. The effects of family policy in the former GDR on nuptiality and births outside marriage, *Population-E* 61(1-2): 141–152.

Sardon, J.-P. 1991. Mariage et divorce en Europe de l'Est, *Population* 46(3): 547–598.

Sardon, J.-P. 1993. Women's first marriage rates in Europe. Elements for a typology, *Population: An English Selection* 5: 119–152.

Schulze, H.-J., and H. Tyrell. 2002. What happened to the European family in the 1980s? The polarization between the family and other forms of private life, in F.-X. Kaufmann, A. Kuijsten, H.-J. Schulze and K. P. Strohmeier (Eds.), *Family Life and Family Policies in Europe. Vol. 2: Problems and Issues in Comparative Perspective.* Oxford: Oxford University Press, pp: 69–119.

Smallwood, S. 2002. New estimates of trends in births by birth order in England and Wales, *Population Trends* 108: 32–48.

Smock, P. 2000. Cohabitation in the United States: an appraisal of research themes, findings and implications, *Annual Review of Sociology* 26: 1–20.

Sobotka, T., and M. R. Testa. 2008. Attitudes and intentions towards childlessness in Europe, in C. Höhn, D. Avramov and I. Kotowska (Eds.), *People, Population Change and Policies: Lessons from the Population Policy Acceptance Study*, Vol. 1. European Studies of Population, Berlin: Springer Verlag, pp: 177–212.

Steele, F., H. Joshi, C. Kallis, and H. Goldstein. 2006. Changing compatibility of cohabitation and childbearing between young British women born in 1958 and 1970, *Population Studies* 60(2): 137–152.

Stevenson, B., and J. Wolfers. 2007. Marriage and divorce: changes and their driving forces, *Journal of Economic Perspectives* 21(2): 27–52.

Stropnik, N., and Šircelj, M. 2008. Slovenia: Generous family policy without evidence of any fertility impact, *Demographic Research* 19(26). http://www.demographic-research.org/Volumes/Vol19/26/

Thornton A., W. Axinn, and Y. Xie. 2007. *Marriage and Cohabitation.* Chicago: University of Chicago Press, Population and Development Series.

Thomson, E. 2005. Partnership and parenthood: connections between cohabitation, marriage and childbearing, in A. Booth and N. Crouter (Eds.), *The New Population Problem: Why Families in Developed Countries are Shrinking and What It Means.* Mahwah, NJ: Lawrence Erlbaum Associates, pp 129-149.

Toulemon, L. 1995. The place of children in the history of couples, *Population: An English Selection* 7: 163–186.

Toulemon, L. 1997. Cohabitation is here to stay, *Population. An English Selection* 9: 11–46.

Toulemon, L. 2006. La fécondité est-elle encore naturelle? Application au retard des naissances et à son influence sur la descendance finale, in *Entre nature et culture: quelle(s) démographie(s)?* Louvain-la-Neuve: Academia-Bruylant, pp: 15–42.

Toulemon, L., and É. Lapierre-Adamcyk. 2000. Demographic patterns of motherhood and fatherhood in France, in C. Bledsoe, S. Lerner and J. Guyer (Eds.), *Fertility and the Male Life-Cycle in the Era of Fertility Decline.* New York: Oxford University Press, pp: 293–330.

Toulemon, L., and M. Mazuy. 2001. Les naissances sont retardées mais la fécondité est stable, *Population* 56(4): 611–644.

Toulemon, L., Pailhé, A., Rossier, C. 2008. France: High and stable fertility, *Demographic Research* 19(16). http://www.demographic-research.org/Volumes/Vol19/16/

Trost, J. 1979. *Unmarried Cohabitation.* Vasteras: International Library.

Trost, J. 1981. Cohabitation in the Nordic countries, *Alternative Lifestyles* 4: 401–427.

Van de Kaa, D. 1994. The second demographic transition revisited: theories and expectations, in G. Beets *et al.* (Eds.), *Population and Family in the Low Countries 1993.* NIDI/CBGS Publication, No. 30, Lisse: Zwets and Zeitlinger, pp: 91–126.

Villeneuve-Gokalp, C. 1991. From marriage to informal union: recent changes in the behaviour of French couples, *Population: An English Selection* 3: 81–111.

Villeneuve-Gokalp, C. 1997. Vivre en couple chacun chez soi, *Population* 52(5): 1059–1081.

Vikat, A., Z. Spéder, G. Beets, F. C. Billari, C. Bühler, A. Désesquelles, T. Fokkema, J. M. Hoem, A. MacDonald, G. Neyer, A. Pailhé, A. Pinnelli, and A. Solaz. 2007. Generations and Gender Survey (GGS): towards a better understanding of relationships and processes in the life course, *Demographic Research* 17(4): 389–440.

Waaldijk, K. (Ed.) 2005. More or less together: levels of legal consequences of marriage, cohabitation and registered partnership for different-sex and same-sex partners. Documents de travail de l'Ined, 125. http://www.ined.fr/fichier/t_publication/ 1034/publi_pdf1_document_de_travail_125.pdf.

Winkler-Dworak M., and H. Engelhardt. 2004. On the tempo and quantum of first marriages in Austria, Germany, and Switzerland. Changes in mean age and variance, *Demographic Research* 10(9): 231–263. http://www.demographic-research.org/volumes/vol10/9/.

Zeman, K. 2003. *Divorce and Marital Dissolution in the Czech Republic and Austria. The role of Premarital Cohabitation.* Doctoral thesis, Prague: Charles University.

APPENDIX: Methodological note

Imperfect indices are sufficient to show the dramatic trends in marital behaviours since the 1960s in Europe

None of the period measures used in this chapter is a very accurate index. Total first marriage rate (TFMR) is computed from incidence rates by age, and does not take into account the fact that only single women are 'at risk' of a first marriage. In addition, this indicator is based on information on marriages within the country, and does not take account that some inhabitants, especially those of foreign origin, may marry abroad. Finally, it is very sensitive to changes in marriage timing (see, e.g., Winkler-Dworak and Engelhardt 2004): when the age when women marry increases, the number of marriages declines in that period and the period TFMR falls even if the number of marriages that women have over their life course does not change. This distortion is frequently referred to as 'tempo effect'.

In the same way as the total first marriage rate is sensitive to 'tempo effect,' the period mean age at first marriage is also very sensitive to changes in the total first marriage rate: when the latter is declining, the decline is often the strongest for incidence rates at young ages, leading to a strong increase in the mean age.

Total divorce rates (TDRs) are computed from incidence rates of divorce by duration of marriage, and do not take into account the fact that only the existing ('surviving') marriages are 'at risk' of divorce. Thus, the TDRs are subject to 'tempo distortions,' like the total first marriage rate.

The proportion of extramarital births is a simpler index, and it does not take into account the age structure of the population or of the births. The main shortcoming of this index is, however, that it only indicates the legal status of parents at birth, and not their *de facto* living arrangement. It also does not reflect the intensity of childbearing among unmarried women: it can either increase as a consequence of an increase in the number of unmarried women, or as a consequence of an increase in fertility rates among them (or a combination of both factors).

APPENDIX Table A1

Table A1: **Percentage of time spent in different family types at ages 15-39 years (period life table estimates)**

	Period	In parental home (no family) F	M	Single, before union, no child F	M	In consensual union F	M	In marriage F	M	Other (no more in union) F	M
Northern Europe											
Finland	1983–92	22	33	11	13	13	14	47	37	7	3
Norway	1974–89	21	28	9	12	10	10	53	46	7	4
Sweden	1978–93	17	23	13	15	27	25	34	29	9	8
Western Europe											
Austria	1990–96	23	32	7	11	13	14	48	37	9	6
Belgium											
(Flanders)	1985–92	31	40	5	5	5	6	55	47	4	2
France	1988–94	26	34	7	9	15	14	43	37	9	6
West Germany	1986–92	27	34	13	19	9	9	40	30	11	8
Southern Europe											
Italy	1990–95	44	52	4	8	2	1	49	37	1	2
Spain	1989–95	38	48	3	4	3	4	53	42	3	2
Central and Eastern Europe											
Czech	1992–97	25	na	1	na	7	na	60	na	7	na
Hungary	1988–93	26	41	2	2	5	3	63	49	4	5
Latvia	1989–95	25	32	3	4	7	5	53	53	12	6
Lithuania	1989–95	26	30	6	8	2	3	58	56	8	3
Poland	1986–91	30	na	3	na	1	na	59	na	7	na
Slovenia	1989–95	27	30	3	10	9	10	57	47	4	3

Source: Data estimated by Andersson and Philipov (2002: Table 29) on the basis of the FFS surveys.

Demographic Research: Volume 19, Article 7
research article

Overview Chapter 5:
Determinants of family formation and childbearing during the societal transition in Central and Eastern Europe

Tomas Frejka[1]

Abstract

Societal conditions for early and high rates of childbearing were replaced by conditions generating late and low levels of fertility common in Western countries. Central among factors shaping the latter behaviour (job insecurity, unstable partnership relationships, expensive housing, and profound changes in norms, values and attitudes) were the following: increasing proportions of young people were acquiring advanced education, a majority of women were gainfully employed, yet women were performing most household maintenance and childrearing duties. Two theories prevailed to explain what caused changes in family formation and fertility trends. One argues that the economic and social crises were the principal causes. The other considered the diffusion of western norms, values and attitudes as the prime factors of change. Neither reveals the root cause: the replacement of state socialist regimes with economic and political institutions of contemporary capitalism. The extraordinarily low period TFRs around 2000 were the result of low fertility of older women born around 1960 overlapping with low fertility of young women born during the 1970s.

[1] E-mail: Tfrejka@aol.com

1. Introduction

The abrupt termination of the autocratic and centrally planned systems in Central and Eastern Europe, and the ensuing political, social and economic transition, were historically unprecedented. The fast changing societal environment generated rapid changes in family formation, partnership relationships and childbearing. New, different sets of constraints and incentives for childbearing behaviour emerged in the 1990s. How unique and extraordinary these new conditions were can be better understood by exploring and outlining the broad historical context and developments of the past two centuries.

Once European populations had passed through the industrial and technological revolutions and the demographic transition of the 19th and early 20th centuries, the two halves of Europe divided by the Iron Curtain took very different paths. During the latter decades of the 20th century, the consequences of social and economic developments in the West[2] led to an increase in the importance of factors conducive to low fertility rates in many Western European countries. In contrast, during the same period societal conditions in the state socialist authoritarian and centrally planned regimes had developed an environment that was comparatively favourable for early and relatively high rates of childbearing. When the state socialist regimes collapsed in Central and Eastern Europe, the entire societal and institutional system was transformed. Incentives and constraints related to childbearing ended equally abruptly, and were replaced within a period of a few years by a new social, economic and welfare system that is based on the same principles as institutional systems in Western societies. During the 1990s and the early 21st century, young people of prime childbearing age adjusted to these new conditions, which were mirrored by changes in family formation, partnership relationships and patterns of childbearing.

The principal focus of this chapter is to gain a better understanding of the family formation and childbearing determinants during the transition from socialism to capitalism[3]. Section 2 contains a concise sketch of the secular historical context of

---

[2] In this chapter the dichotomy of Western Europe (the West) and Central and Eastern Europe (CEE) is employed. The latter includes all formerly state socialist countries, whereas the former includes the remainder of Europe, namely all countries of Northern, Western and Southern Europe where market economies operated throughout the 20th century.

[3] Intentionally the actual trends and patterns of family formation and childbearing are not described and analyzed in this chapter. A detailed exposition of this topic can be found in the country chapters and an overview was presented, for instance, in chapters 7 and 8 in Sobotka (2004). It would be redundant to essentially repeat such an analysis in this chapter.

European fertility trends up to the second half of the 20th century. Section 3 explores the basic circumstances of the Western European fertility decline from the 1960s through the 1990s. This analysis of Western European developments is justified and relevant because analogous conditions emerged in Central and Eastern Europe after the collapse of state socialism. In section 4, the basic demographic mechanism of fertility trends during the state socialist era is analysed so that these trends can be compared to those of Western countries, as well as to those of Central and Eastern Europe of the 1990s and 2000s. Section 5 characterises the contemporary historical context in Central and Eastern Europe. Section 6 analyses the demographic structural background of the extraordinarily low period fertility rates of the mid- to late 1990s. In section 7, the main reasons for the fertility trends in the contemporary transitional period are discussed. Section 8 deals with the various specific factors modifying childbearing during the transition from socialism to capitalism that were identified in the country chapters. In the final section, the main conclusions are summarized.

2. The secular historical context

By the middle of the 20th century, European societies had experienced major economic and social transformations. General modernization, industrialization and urbanization, which generated the growth of various social strata, especially of the working and the middle classes, were spreading throughout Europe. The timing of these processes was very different from one country to another. There were still a number of populations living in rather underdeveloped economic and social conditions in countries such as Portugal, Macedonia, Bosnia and Herzegovina and, most notably, Albania; as well as in regions of deficient development within these and other countries, such as Poland, Slovakia and Romania.

Almost all European populations had passed through the demographic transition by mid-20th century. Individuals and families had adjusted to the historical, structural, economic and social changes. Childrearing had become costly, children were no longer contributing to the family economy, and children's contribution to old age security was small and decreasing. Economic and psychological costs by far outweighed benefits. According to Caldwell (1976), the net flow of wealth transfer from children to parents in "primitive and traditional societies" had been converted to flows of wealth from parents to children. Ariès (1980) concluded that the family "had turned inward upon itself and organized itself in terms of children and their future. The parents' chief psychological and material investment consisted of children to get ahead. … The fewer the children, the more time and care could be devoted to each and the better the results."

In the wake of the Second World War, "from Stettin in the Baltic to Trieste in the Adriatic an *iron curtain* has descended across the Continent" (Churchill 1946). Countries of Central and Eastern Europe became part of the "Soviet sphere" under the control of Moscow. From thereon for more than 40 years, authoritarian, centrally planned regimes of the type that had been installed in the Soviet Union by the Bolshevik revolution of 1917 were in power in these countries. For these 40-odd years, political, economic and social developments in the countries of Central and Eastern Europe differed in fundamental ways from those of Western countries. Fertility levels and trends were also distinctly different between the two parts of Europe, shaped by varying sets of constraints and childbearing incentives, and by the accompanying changes in values, norms and attitudes.

3. Western Europe

It is crucial to understand the principal determinants of the fertility trends in the West of the second half of the 20th century because analogous conditions were created in the Central and Eastern European countries after the collapse of the state socialist regimes around 1990.

The realization of previously postponed births and marriages were the initial impetus for the post-war rise in fertility in Western Europe. The modern welfare state was established at that time, and became an important factor in sustaining the baby boom through the 1950s and into the early 1960s. Many of the costs of education, health and welfare of children were covered by the state, thus lowering costs of childbearing. This was also a period of extraordinary economic growth. Real wages and salaries were increasing, employment was virtually guaranteed, unemployment was low, and housing destroyed by the war was being reconstructed and expanded. These conditions led people to view parenthood as attractive and affordable (Hobcraft & Kiernan 1995, Hobcraft 1996).

Precipitous declines in period fertility of the 1960s and 1970s, and the persisting sub-replacement fertility of the 1980s and 1990s, were brought about by a number of interacting factors. The underlying demographic mechanism consisted of a gradually declining fertility quantum combined with a postponement of marriages and of childbearing. Among the basic circumstances driving this demographic mechanism were the following:

A. An unprecedented, increasing need for large proportions of the population to acquire more than a basic education,

B. High and increasing labour force participation rates of women, and

C. Increasing roles and responsibilities of women.

There were a host of other circumstances which contributed to the fertility decline and the postponement of parenthood. Generally, it became more difficult for young people to establish a household in the latter decades of the 20th century. It was not easy to find employment or to establish oneself in a career during this period, and housing costs were rising (Hobcraft 1996; Kohler et al. 2002; Billari et al 2002).

The advent of reliable, modern means of contraception; access to safe and legal induced abortion; changing patterns of partnership relations; substantial changes in values, norms and attitudes concerning family formation and childbearing; as well as relatively weak family policies in Western countries were significant in generating the fertility levels and trends of the late 20th century. These latter factors are discussed in overview chapters 3, 4, 6 and 8, respectively, and in the country chapters.

A. The increasing need for a better educated population

The technological advancements of the second part of the 20th century and the restructuring of economies, dominated by the vast expansion of the information and service sectors, required that significant and gradually increasing proportions of the population be well educated. This demand was satisfied by a considerable expansion of educational systems, which absorbed large proportions of young people. The societal demand for a skilled and educated work force was matched by the desire and need of the young to acquire an advanced education, which became a prerequisite for obtaining desirable, well paying positions of gainful employment.

In Europe in 1970, the gross enrolment ratio[4] (GER) was 68 percent at the secondary level and 14 percent at the tertiary level (Table 1). At each level, male GERs were higher than female GERs. At the tertiary level, the GER for males was over 60 percent higher than the female ratio. By 1990, the GERs for men and women combined had increased to 92 and 36 percent, respectively. At both the secondary and the tertiary

---

[4] Regrettably the data are for the whole of Europe, not separately for the West. It does not matter that much for our purpose. Especially the trends between 1970 and 1990 were mostly driven by developments in Western Europe.

levels, female GERs increased faster than male GERs. Thus by 1990, the enrolment ratios for women were higher than those for males. These trends persisted during the 1990s. By 1997, virtually all people of secondary school age were enrolled, but the GERs for women were somewhat higher than those for men. At the tertiary level, the more rapid increase in the enrolment ratio for women was maintained. Consequently, 46 percent of 20-24-year-old women were enrolled, compared to 40 percent of men in this age group.

Table 1:   Gross enrolment ratios[*] at the secondary and tertiary levels of education, Europe 1970–1997

Year	Secondary			Tertiary		
	Total	Male	Female	Total	Male	Female
1970	67.5	69.9	65.1	14.4	17.7	11.0
1990	92.4	91.1	93.7	35.9	35.0	36.9
1997	99.2	97.2	101.3	42.8	39.5	46.3

Source: Unesco Statistical Yearbook 1999, 2005.
*Note: Gross enrolment ratios are crude measures. The denominators are populations of strictly defined age groups whereas the numerators include all individuals enrolled at the respective educational level some of whom can be from outside the age group of the denominator. Thus values higher than 100 can appear and are legitimate

In general, these high levels of enrolment in tertiary education have continued to increase in the early years of the 21st century in most countries of Western Europe (Table 2). These rates have levelled off in some countries, as demonstrated by the trends in Austria. In most countries, enrolments of women have continued to increase faster than those of men, thereby enlarging the gender gap in favour of women in advanced education.

Table 2: **Gross enrolment ratios at the tertiary level of education by sex, selected Western European countries, 1991–2005**

Country	Sex	1991	1999	2002	2005
Austria	M	36	52	44	44
	F	32	55	51	53
France	M	37	47	47	49
	F	43	58	60	63
Italy	M	33	41	47	56
	F	31	53	63	75
Netherlands	M	43	49	54	57
	F	36	50	58	61
Spain	M	36	52	57	60
	F	39	62	68	73
Sweden	M	29	53	60	64
	F	35	75	92	100
United Kingdom	M	30	55	56	50
	F	29	64	70	69

Source: UNESCO 2007.

B. The increase in female labour force participation rates

During the second half of the 20th century, increasing proportions of women in Europe joined the labour force. In the years immediately following the Second World War, the majority of the gainfully employed were men. During the years of the post-war economic expansion, there was a shortage of labour, and women were increasingly drawn into the labour force at all levels and in many professions (ILO 1990). The demand for female labour continued to grow in Western countries throughout the second half of the 20th century, and was still going strong early in the 21st (Table 3). The employment rate of women in the 15 Western countries of the European Union increased by 16 percent between 1995 and 2005, while the employment rate of men grew by only 3 percent.

Table 3:   Employment rates in states of the European Union, 1995–2005

EU-15	EU employment rate		
	1995	**2000**	**2005**
Total	60.1	63.4	65.3
Male	70.5	72.8	72.9
Female	49.7	54.1	57.7

Source: Eurostat Yearbook, 2006-2007.

Women joined the labour force willingly, and for good reasons. For those who were married, an important motive was a second income, making it possible to achieve a higher standard of living for their families. For single women, employment secured the freedom to choose their own course in life. For all women, the psychological benefits of self-realization also played an important role. Thus the demand for additional labour was matched by large proportions of women desiring employment.

C. Increasing roles and responsibilities of women

The male breadwinner family model was gradually replaced by the dual-earner model. Even though women studied longer, became gainfully employed and contributed significantly to family income, the division of labour within the family did not keep pace with these changes. The responsibilities of childrearing and maintaining households continued to be disproportionately carried by women (Table 4).

According to time use surveys conducted by national statistical offices (Aliaga 2006) throughout Europe, employed women spend more time on domestic work than men, from about 50 percent more in Nordic countries, to three times more in Southern Europe. The amount of time employed women spend on domestic work does not differ much between countries. It is the contribution made by men to childrearing and household maintenance that is important. On average, men in Sweden and Norway devote about twice as much time to these activities as men in Italy and Spain (Table 4).

Table 4: **Time use structure of employed women and men (in hours and minutes per day), selected European countries, 1998–2004**

	Spain	France	Italy	Sweden	United Kingdom	Norway
WOMEN						
Gainful work, study	4:57	4:32	4:39	4:05	4:06	3:46
Domestic work	3:29	3:40	3:51	3:32	3:28	3:26
Travel	1:22	1:05	1:28	1:28	1:33	1:17
Sleep	8:11	8:38	8:00	8:05	8:25	8:07
Meals, personal care	2:28	2:57	2:44	2:23	2:07	2:02
Free time, incl. unspecified	3:33	3:08	3:18	4:27	4:21	5:22
Total	24	24	24	24	24	24
MEN						
Gainful work, study	6:11	5:44	6:13	5:17	5:42	4:56
Domestic work	1:20	1:53	1:10	2:23	1:54	2:12
Travel	1:23	1:10	1:40	1:32	1:36	1:23
Sleep	8:15	8:24	7:58	7:52	8:11	7:53
Meals, personal care	2:31	2:58	2:52	2:05	1:55	1:58
Free time, incl. unspecified	4:20	3:51	4:07	4:51	4:42	5:38
Total	24	24	24	24	24	24

Source: Aliaga 2006.

Note: The average time is calculated for the group of all employed persons, and for the whole year including working days and weekends, as well as holiday periods. This explains why time spent on gainful work is significantly less than a normal working day.

These data suggest a correlation between the status of women and men in society and in the family, on the one hand, and fertility, on the other, around the turn of the century in Western Europe. In the Scandinavian countries, where women are involved in many spheres of public life and many of them are gainfully employed, and where men share quite a considerable amount of household responsibilities, fertility is relatively high, close to replacement levels (Oláh and Bernhardt 2008). In contrast, in the Mediterranean countries where women's involvement in public life is rising but still rare, where lesser proportions of women are gainfully employed, and where patriarchal relationships are still quite prevalent in the family, fertility is very low, considerably below replacement rates (De Rose et al. 2008, Delgado et al. 2008).

Summing up this section on Western Europe, we can observe that, towards the end of the 20th century, there were many circumstances making it relatively difficult for young people to establish families and to have children. The situation was very heterogeneous, with national period fertility rates in 1990 ranging from 1.3 in Italy and 1.4 in Spain, to 2.1 in Sweden, Denmark and Ireland. This reflects the numerous differences in the micro and macro conditions that were instrumental in shaping people's childbearing behaviour.

Compared to generations of young people in the 1960s and 1970s, young people in the West in the 1990s spent several more years on average acquiring education. Once they finished school, it was more difficult for them to find employment, and the employment they found was, moreover, less secure than it used to be. It was also more expensive to secure a place to live independently. Much higher proportions of women were studying at the secondary and especially at the tertiary levels, and larger shares of women were gainfully employed. At the same time, however, women retained prime responsibilities for maintaining households and bringing up children. The duration of partnership arrangements --marriages and consensual unions-- became less predictable and increasingly uncertain. Also, modern contraceptive means and liberal abortion legislation made it easier to prevent unwanted and unplanned births (Hobcraft and Kiernan 1995; Lesthaeghe and Moors. 2000).

4. Central and Eastern Europe

In the immediate post-war period, there was a tendency for fertility to increase in the majority of the Central and Eastern European countries. Within a few years, by the late 1940s and early 1950s, fertility started to decline, and this descent was sustained into the 1960s. While fertility was increasing and the baby boom was taking place in Western Europe, fertility in Central and Eastern European countries was on the decline, reaching below replacement levels in a number of countries in the 1960s. Arguably the development strategies adopted by the state socialist governments were the main cause. The central emphasis was on major investments in heavy industries, while consumer industries, housing and services were neglected. Rapid growth of industrial capacity was achieved without sufficient advances in technologies, and with relatively low productivity, creating an environment of high demand for labour. Male labour force participation rates were already high, and so the gap was filled by unprecedented increases in female employment. Moreover, women's employment was promoted on ideological grounds as a basis for gender equality. As a result, in Czechoslovakia, for example, the proportion of women in their prime childbearing years (ages 20-30) in the labour force increased from 30 percent in 1950 to 60 percent by 1961 (Frejka 1980).

The implementation of liberal induced abortion legislation in the mid-1950s in almost all Central and Eastern European countries contributed to the ongoing fertility decline (Frejka 1983). It was frequently modified and often moderately restricted, but, with the notable exception of Romania, access to induced abortion remained in place throughout the state socialist period.

Fertility rates increased in several countries in the late 1960s and early 1970s, and stabilized at close to the replacement level in almost all the Central and Eastern European countries during the 1970s and 1980s. The basic demographic mechanism underlying this fertility level and its stability was universal and early marriage, a low age of childbearing with low rates of childlessness, and high rates of first and second births. Societal circumstances underpinning this demographic regime were generated and sustained by the following factors (Frejka 1980; Sobotka 2004, chapter 8):

A. Predominantly pro-natalist social and population policies,
B. The centrally planned economic system and the socialist welfare state, and
C. A tight authoritarian political system

A. Predominantly pro-natalist social and population policies

Governments throughout Central and Eastern Europe became gravely concerned about the declining and low fertility rates of the 1960s (Macura 1981). This was unexpected and contrary to theoretical and ideological expectations (Besemeres 1980). Under socialism, population was supposed to grow as an expression of the system's strength and superiority relative to capitalism. Yet population growth was faster and fertility levels were higher in the Western capitalist countries. Another reason for concern was the prospect that future generations of young women and men would be too small in numbers to replenish the armed forces and the labour force. Throughout Central and Eastern Europe, social and population policies of a predominantly pro-natalist nature were devised and implemented during the late 1960s and early 1970s (Stefanov and Naoumov 1974, Ziolkowksi 1974, Frejka 1980, Macura 1981, Büttner and Lutz 1990, Kamaras 1996). By and large, these policies generated some of the desired results, and thus brought about moderate fertility increases. These policies were continuously updated and modified during the 1970s and 1980s, and played a role in sustaining fertility at around replacement levels.

The pro-natalist policy measures varied widely, and differed from one country to another. They ranged from various types of financial aid to individuals and families, to the establishment of a network of institutions serving families, to preferential access to housing for young families with children.

The financial aid to families consisted of grants provided at the birth of a child, child allowances up to a certain age, payments during relatively extended maternity leaves, income tax credits, and loans to young couples with favourable terms, such as a provision that a specified amount would be written off upon the birth of a child. The principal component of the institutional networks aiding families were crèches, nurseries and kindergartens. In addition, older children could stay in school after regular classes, and school meals and children's clothing were subsidized. These outlays amounted to a significant redistribution of income, i.e., they resulted in a considerable lowering of the costs of childbearing and child raising[5] (David and McIntyre 1981, Frejka 1980).

The administration of housing policies was a crucial element of social and population policies. Much of the housing stock was state owned and in short supply. To a large extent, access to housing was not governed by the market but by administrative decisions of the government bureaucracy. Young people advanced on waiting lists for housing if they got married and had a child or two. The prospect of gaining access to housing was among the incentives to marry and have a child while young. Starting a family was also a feasible route for young people to leave the parental home and become independent (Frejka 1980, Sobotka 2004).

Sex education was introduced in the 1960s and 1970s, mostly in support of the pro-natalist policies in the form of education for marriage and parenthood. Biological aspects of sex were included in natural science lessons on human anatomy, physiology and hygiene for 8- to 15-year-olds. The classes were usually taught by school physicians, which meant that the health aspects were emphasized, while contraceptive education and many of the broader aspects of partner relationships were neglected (Stloukal 1999).

Extensive reliance on induced abortion, widespread use of inefficient traditional means of contraception, and a lack of modern contraceptive methods were the basic characteristics of practices directly affecting birth regulating behaviour (see also Overview Chapter 3). The state socialist policies in this area originated in the substantial liberalization of abortion legislation in the Soviet Union in 1955. Presumably, the rationale was derived as much from concerns about public health as from ideological considerations (Frejka 1983). Some scholars interpreted this decision

---

[5] In Czechoslovakia in the early 1970s these disbursements amounted to about ten percent of total government expenditures (Frejka 1980).

as an expression of sensitivity to current social problems in the initial years of the post-Stalinist era (Besemeres 1980). The reliance on induced abortion, combined mainly with *coitus interruptus,* developed as the fertility regulation norm in CEE countries during the late 1950s and early 1960s. This was before the introduction of hormonal contraception and before the widespread use of IUDs and sterilization during the 1960s and subsequent years in the West (Westoff and Ryder 1977).

As a rule, governments in Central and Eastern Europe opposed the diffusion of hormonal contraception for a number of reasons, some of them publicly enunciated and purposefully promulgated, especially among physicians, but also among the general public. It was claimed that the risks to women's health associated with oral hormonal contraceptives and IUDs by far outweighed the benefits. Thus, doctors did not promote modern contraception, and the public was suspicious of these methods and did not seek them out. Also, because governments imposed restrictions on their importation and domestic production, modern contraceptives were practically unobtainable and in short supply. In some countries, access to contraceptives was deliberately circumscribed based on pro-natalist intentions of raising fertility (Stloukal 1995). The fact that modern contraceptives were developed and widely used in the capitalist West made them, by definition, unsuitable for use in socialist countries. Nonetheless, the situation was very different from one country to another. For example, authorities in Hungary, the German Democratic Republic and Yugoslavia made the contraceptive pill generally available and encouraged the use of modern contraceptives (see also contributions in David 1999). In 1977, the pill was used by 55 percent of all users in Hungary, compared to 10 percent and 3 percent in Poland and Bulgaria, respectively (Frejka 1983).

B. The centrally planned economic system and the socialist welfare state

The socialist welfare state and the lack of market forces operating in the economy provided further favourable circumstances for childbearing, but also contained several elements that tended to discourage people from having children.

Young people lived in a relatively risk-free environment, created by virtually free education, free health care and guaranteed employment. Full employment and the obligation of all working age population to study or be employed were considered incontrovertible. The inefficient functioning of state-owned enterprises created a large demand for labour, which made full employment possible. Moreover, workers often lacked motivation to work to their full potential, thus reinforcing the inefficiency of the economy (Table 5). Consequently, job security, which was a related, proclaimed goal of the socialist system, was guaranteed.

Table 5: Population, gross domestic product, and GDP per head in Europe and the former Soviet Union 1950 and 2001

Region	Population (millions)			GDP (billion dollars)			GDP per head (dollars)		
	1950	2001	2001/ 1950	1950	2001	2001/ 1950	1950	2001	2001/ 1950
Western Europe	304.9	392.1	1.3	1,396	7,550	5.4	4,579	19,256	4.2
Central & Eastern Europe	87.6	120.9	1.4	185	729	3.9	2,111	6,027	2.9
Former Soviet Union	179.6	120.9	1.6	510	1,343	2.6	2,841	4,626	1.6

Source: Demeny and McNicoll 2006.

A crude measure of the inefficiency of centrally planned economies in contrast to Western economies is expressed by the comparative growth of the respective gross domestic products and GDP/capita during the second half of the 20th century.[6] GDP in Central and Eastern European (CEE) countries increased by a factor of 3.9 times between 1950 and 2001, compared to an increase by a factor of 5.4 times in Western Europe (WE). In addition, per capita income grew at a slower rate in the CEE countries compared to WE, so that the gap between them increased. In 1950, per capita income in the West was more than twice that of the CEE countries; in 2001, the difference was more than threefold. The respective differences between the former Soviet Union and WE were even greater. Moreover, the desire for consumer goods was growing in Central and Eastern Europe, but remained far from satisfied. The inefficient, technologically lagging economies did not produce sufficient quantities of consumer goods, and, in addition, many people operated with a limited purchasing capacity (Table 5). There were long waiting lists for household appliances and furniture, and

---

[6] The period 1950-2001 includes the transition years of the 1990s. A comparison of these indicators for the years 1950-1990 would be slightly more favourable for the former state-socialist countries, due to the economic crisis experienced during that period in most of these countries, but the basic conclusion would be similar.

people often had to wait for years to purchase motor vehicles of inferior quality (Kotowska et al. 2008).

The high demand for labour continued to require that ever growing proportions of women join the labour force. The desire to secure an acceptable standard of living by earning a second income motivated women to seek gainful employment. Practically all women of working age were employed. Their labour force participation rates reached levels almost as high as those of men, particularly if women on maternity leave are taken into account.

Officially, the high female employment rates were heralded as proof of women having achieved equal rights with men. In reality, women became overburdened. The traditional division of responsibilities in the household remained almost unchanged. Women had to maintain households and raise children under rather unfavourable conditions, which frequently included shortages of consumer goods, inadequate services, a lack of labour-saving household appliances, difficulties with child-care facilities and, in some cases, inferior housing. Several surveys of the 1960s documented that women's household duties took up almost as much time as their jobs, leaving only seven or eight hours a day for other activities, including eating and sleeping (Frejka 1980).

A lack of competition and the inefficient economy did not require a highly technically qualified work force, and egalitarian principles were overriding market forces in the demand for labour, and in determining wage levels. Occupations that required advanced education were often rewarded equally, or even less than, manual labour. Physicians earned as much or less than bus drivers and miners. Altogether, there was not much motivation to acquire an advanced education. Compared to the West, smaller proportions of young people were enrolled in institutions of higher learning, and both the quality and the relative size of these institutions lagged behind the West. On average, the part of the life cycle spent in school was shorter in CEE countries than in WE countries.

C. A tight authoritarian political system

Many aspects of citizen's private life were closely watched by the authorities. It was unacceptable to deviate from the official political ideology and positions. A strong security apparatus was maintained to keep people in line. Outside of the family and a circle of close friends, people did not know who could be trusted. The family environment became a safe haven.

There was a major effort to keep the citizenry in isolation from the outside world in order to prevent the infiltration of ideas from abroad. Travel to the West was severely restricted. Authorities were also reluctant to let people travel to some of the other Central and Eastern European countries for fear that liberal ideas or movements could spread. In some countries, people did not have the right to own passports, and for each trip, especially to the West, an exit visa was required. In any case, most people could not afford to travel abroad given their relatively low incomes (cf. Table 5). Moreover, currencies of the state socialist countries were not officially convertible to Western currencies. For the most part, it was very expensive for normal citizens to acquire Western currency, and currency exchanges were mainly done illegally on the black market.

Isolation was severely enforced in limiting contacts of scientists with their counterparts in the West. Many scientific advances developed in Western countries were deemed suspicious and labelled as bourgeois. This was also the fate of progress achieved in human reproductive physiology and the development of modern contraceptives.

The degree to which cultural life and leisure activities were constrained by the authorities also differed very much between countries. In some countries, and during some periods, a certain amount of freedom and creativity were tolerated. But, in general, attractive opportunities to spend meaningful time outside the household were relatively few, the burdens of domestic chores in addition to work were substantial, and, given the relatively low incomes, only limited financial resources were available for these activities in any case.

In sum, the various countervailing forces in the state socialist countries of Central and Eastern Europe during the 1970s and 1980s created a relatively favourable childbearing environment that resulted in a widespread prevalence of the two-child family (cf. overview chapter 2). There was remarkably little variation between CEE countries in terms of period total fertility rates, and there was a conspicuous absence in these countries of fertility postponement that was taking place in other parts of Europe. In the majority of CEE countries, the TFR in 1989 was between 1.9 and 2.1. In a few of these countries, the TFR was at 1.8 or less (Hungary [1.8], Croatia [1.7] and Slovenia [1.5]), while at the other "extreme" it was 2.2 or more (Estonia [2.2], Moldova [2.5] and Romania [2.2]) (Council of Europe 2006).

On balance, the socialist welfare state provided reasonably predictable and reliable risk-free conditions for family life and childbearing based on guaranteed employment, job security, free education and free health care. Couples received direct financial aid (birth grants, child allowances, paid maternity leave, etc.) and benefited indirectly by sending their children to a crèche or kindergarten, receiving free school meals and after-school child care, and by buying subsidized clothing and school equipment. The usual route for young people to acquire a home was to get married and have a child. It could take a long time to gain access to housing, but the cost of maintaining a home was low because rents were state-subsidized. Various other circumstances indirectly contributed to early childbearing, such as limited career options, restricted choice of leisure activities, lack of travel opportunities, and a deficient supply of large-item consumer goods, especially cars. The fact that most women were gainfully employed, yet still burdened by difficult household maintenance and childrearing duties, acted as deterrents to having a larger number of children.

5. The contemporary historical context

By the end of the 1980s, the shortcomings of the state socialist systems in Europe became so acute that the regimes imploded. For a few years under the reform-minded leadership of Mikhail Gorbachev, there was an attempt to cure the existing system from within through economic reforms ("perestroika") and some liberalization of the political structures and conditions ("glasnost"). The general malfunctioning of the system had become so untenable and the discontent of the populations of the CEE countries had become so severe that the authoritarian governments collapsed despite the reform efforts, and new governments sprang up. The primary policies of these governments were to restructure economies and reform state institutions based on the principles inherent in the Western countries. In other words, following the collapse of the state socialist regimes, a full-fledged transition to capitalist political and economic conditions ensued. The process was modified by the specific conditions of each country and thus varied considerably, but, essentially, the social, economic and political conditions of the Western countries were being adopted in CEE countries, and people adjusted to these new conditions. This was true as much for family formation and childbearing as for any other aspect of life.

The transition, i.e., the implementation of the Western societal conditions, turned out to be complex, and was more or less painful in various countries and for various strata of the populations of these countries (cf. all CEE country chapters). The conditions in the labour market changed rapidly as enterprises became concerned with productivity and profitability. Employment was no longer guaranteed and job security ceased. Employment conditions became particularly difficult for women. Demand for highly qualified positions increased, which required a well educated work force.

Institutions of higher learning expanded rapidly, as did tertiary and secondary school enrolment rates. Professional and leisure time opportunities became numerous, and young people started to take advantage of them. Many of the entitlements of the previous socialist welfare state were curtailed or disappeared altogether. Modern contraceptives became readily available, and, for the most part, access to induced abortion was retained (see overview chapter 3).

Family formation and childbearing patterns adjusted to the rapidly changing societal environment. Exit from the parental home, union formation and childbearing were being postponed, various forms of partnership arrangements became acceptable, and cohabitation became more popular (see overview chapter 4). The transformation of family formation and reproductive behaviour in the CEE countries can best be observed by looking at the changing fertility age patterns of successive cohorts.

6. Effects of changing cohort fertility age patterns

At the time of the collapse of the state socialist system, the changes in fertility behaviour affected by the political changes of distinct generations depended largely upon their respective ages (Figure 1).

Those born in or prior to the early 1960s were affected only marginally by the system transition because they had already completed a major part of their family formation and childbearing prior to the central turning point around 1990. They had their children early, and, by their late 20s, they had almost completed their childbearing.

Those born in the late 1960s were in the midst of their childbearing at the time when the state socialist system collapsed, and some of them adopted strategies that differed from those of previous generations. Nonetheless, these cohorts had started their childbearing under the socialist conditions. By their early 20s, they had already borne a considerable share of the total number of children they were likely to have. The effect of the transition was still not very large.

Those born in the early 1970s were starting out in their childbearing careers when communism fell apart, and their family formation and childbearing patterns differed significantly from those of previous cohorts (See the 1975 cohorts in Figure 1). They had fewer births when in their teens and early twenties, and they were starting to delay childbearing.

Finally, those born in the late 1970s and early 1980s entered adulthood in the rapidly changing societal environment. To date, their childbearing behaviour has been very different from that of previous cohorts, with sharply lower fertility while young and with a strong propensity to postpone fertility.

The varying childbearing behaviour of the respective cohorts is a crucial circumstance contributing to the very low fertility rates of the mid- to late 1990s and early 2000s. The birth cohorts of the 1950s and early 1960s had essentially completed their childbearing by that time. Almost all of their children had been born by the early 1990s. On the other hand, many potential parents of the cohorts born during the 1970s and early 1980s were delaying childbearing until their late twenties or early thirties, and thus were not bearing many children during the mid- to late 1990s. Because the former cohorts were no longer having children in the mid- to late 1990s, and the latter cohorts were just gradually starting their childbearing, period fertility was at its lowest.

Let us take one specific example using first births only. The childbearing trajectory of the 1975 birth cohort in Hungary was much lower than that of the 1970 cohort (Figure 1, Panel B). At age 20, the ASFR in the 1975 cohort was almost the same as the ASFR at age 25 in the 1970 cohort. The respective cross-section sums of the cohort age-specific fertility rates of first births for calendar years illustrate the considerable changes that were taking place. The first birth period total fertility rate (PTFR) for the year 2002 was about 0.58, compared to 0.64 for the year 1995, and close to 0.82 in 1990. Starting in the mid- to late 2000s, the PTFRs are likely to increase as age patterns of childbearing in a growing number of birth cohorts start to resemble each other. The confluence of low fertility at different ages in the reproductive cycle will fade away.

During the political and economic transition, childbearing strategies were changing rapidly from one generation to the next. The general patterns of change were common to all the CEE countries. The direction of change is clear, but it is too early to know what the future general age pattern will be, or whether there will be major inter-country differences. One thing is, however, certain: early childbearing, which peaked around age 20 with most children born while women were in their twenties, is a matter of the past.

Figure 1: **First birth cohort age-specific fertility rates[a], birth cohorts 1960, 1965, 1970, 1975 and 1980, Bulgaria, Hungary, Poland and Slovenia, 1975-2003**

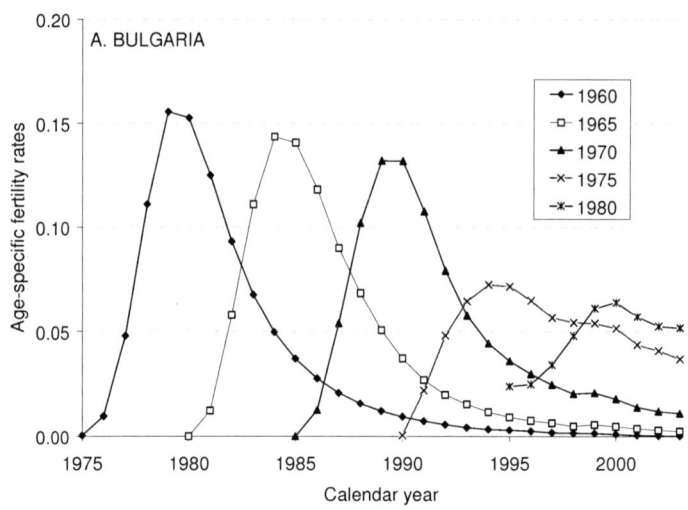

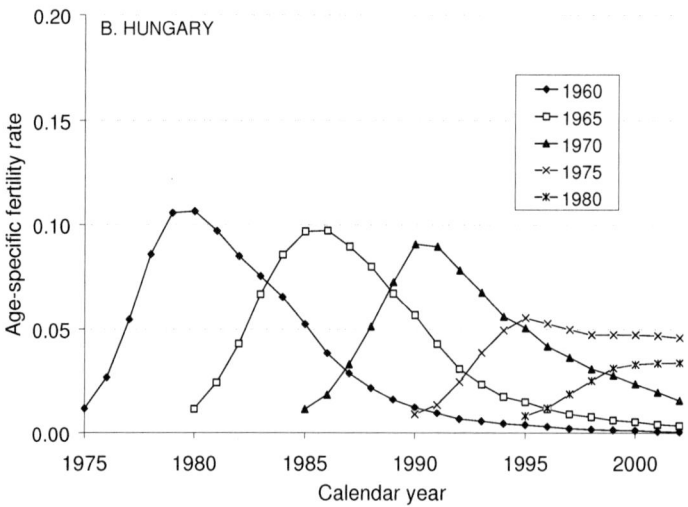

Figure 1: (continued)

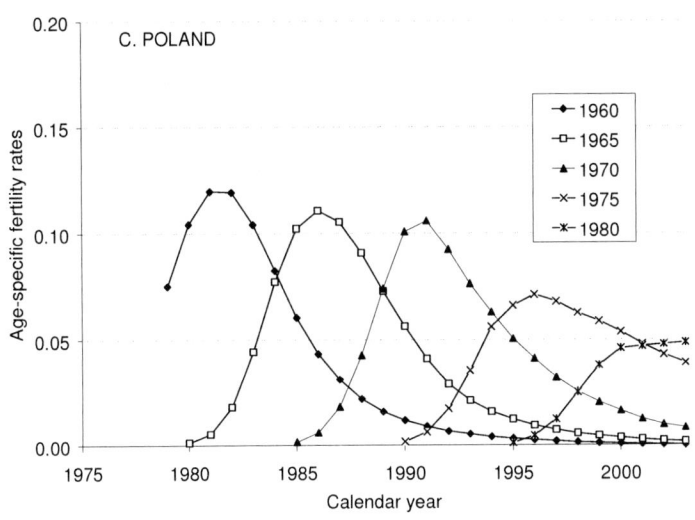

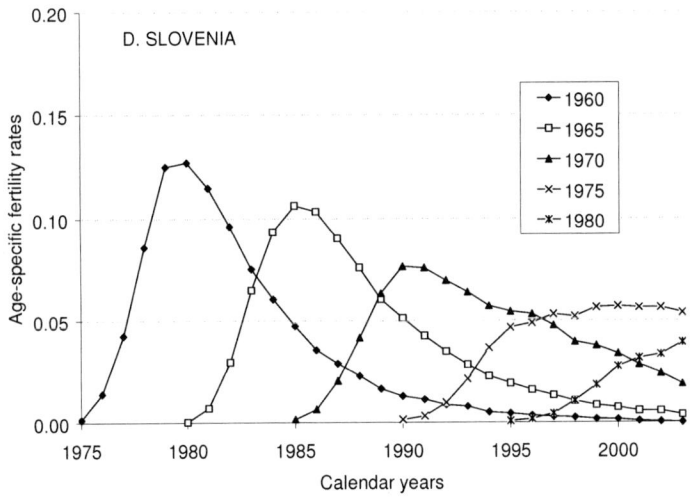

Source: Observatoire Démographique Européen, 2006.
Note: a – Incidence rates, i.e., rates of the second kind.

7. Understanding the causes of the fertility and family formation changes during the 1990s and beyond

Given the magnitude and the velocity of the changes in fertility and family formation, a number of scholars have grappled with the challenge of understanding and describing the mechanisms and causes of these processes (cf., for example, Rychtaříková 1996 and 1999, Rabušic 2001, Kotowska & Jóźwiak, eds. 2003). As Sobotka (2004) and others (e.g., Philipov 2003, Philipov and Dorbritz 2003) have pointed out, attempts to decipher the main determinants of the fertility declines of the 1990s were centred on two theories. The first saw the economic and social crisis of the early 1990s as the principal cause of the respective fertility and family formation trends. The other regarded the diffusion of cultural and ideational developments--namely, the adoption of new, Western norms, values and attitudes--as the main stimulants for the demographic changes. Many authors also recognized that both sets of determinants played crucial roles, with the former being more important early in the transformation process (Lesthaeghe and Surkyn 2002).

Analyses in the country chapters of this project have shown that such a dichotomization between the 'crisis' and the 'cultural and ideational diffusion' theories is a simplification and can lead to confusion, even if both were considered to have operated simultaneously. In addition to the economic crisis factors that impinged on childbearing decisions, a new set of economic factors previously unknown in the state socialist economies emerged, namely, the type that evolve naturally as part of the shift towards a market economy, such as competition in the labour market, job insecurity and rising costs of children. The nature of these factors is primarily economic, yet they do not fit into the category of either 'crisis' or 'cultural and ideational' factors. This suggests that neither of these theories defines the root cause of the demographic changes taking place in the CEE countries during the 1990s and the early 21st century. However obvious and simplistic it may appear, the replacement of the state socialist regimes by market economies and by fledgling democratic institutions of governance is the root cause of the demographic changes and trends during the transition period and beyond.

The crux of the matter is that the economic and political infrastructure of contemporary capitalism is being adopted. The family formation and childbearing environment is undergoing radical change as previous conditions are replaced by the respective conditions prevalent in the West. In individual countries, specific institutional conditions and the character of family policies and welfare support may differ as much as they currently differ in other regions of Europe. It is still unclear whether these conditions and policies will come to resemble the Scandinavian, French, British, Dutch, Central European Germanic or Mediterranean types.

The conditions which were generally conducive for childbearing, such as job security, low-cost housing, free education, free health care, various entitlements associated with child birth and childrearing, as well as a lack of career opportunities and leisure activities; were replaced by the considerably more restraining conditions for childbearing of job insecurity, an increasing pressure to acquire more education, expensive housing, lesser and declining birth and childrearing entitlements, as well as the availability of a variety of career opportunities, consumption attractions and leisure activities. The citizenry of the state socialist countries had grown accustomed to a relatively care-free existence, although the standard living conditions were worse than in the Western countries, and there were numerous unpleasant concomitants to this life-style. All of a sudden, people were submerged into societal conditions which made it more difficult to earn a living, and under which various costs previously borne by the paternalistic state became the responsibility of individuals and families.

This broader explanation does not deny the validity of the 'crisis' or the 'cultural and ideational' theories. Both are inherent in the 'root cause' explanation. The change of the economic systems in the early 1990s generated severe economic crises often accompanied by hyper-inflation and high unemployment rates. These, in turn, led to a diminution of incentives and growth of constraints on childbearing. The radical overhaul of the economic, political and social infrastructure was the basis for emerging changes in the value systems, norms and attitudes regarding family formation and childbearing. The diffusion of western norms, values and attitudes proceeded because a corresponding economic, political and social infrastructure was emerging.

A number of the analyses in the CEE chapters in this book conclude that predominantly economic determinants, rather than ideational ones, were the overriding factors contributing to the fertility decline (e.g., Poland and Lithuania). At the same time, however, to date there has been the general perception that the only two explanatory frameworks for the fertility trends were the 'crisis' and the 'cultural and ideational' theories. Thus, by default, economic determinants were understood to fall into the 'crisis' category. By identifying the replacement of the socialist economic and political system with the capitalist system as the principal explanation – indeed, the root cause – of the contemporary demographic trends, it becomes clear that the observed economic determinants could be signs of emerging market economy conditions which are no longer associated with the initial crisis conditions.

In the Poland chapter it is argued "that for demographic behaviours observed in the 1990s the structural component played a much more important role both in terms of economic restrictions and incentives than it did in [Western] developed countries. ... [I]deational change has not advanced until recently [in Poland] compared with its progress in other European countries" (Kotowska et al. 2008:845). In the Slovenia chapter (Stropnik and Šircelj 2008:1038) it is stated that "the surveys and public discussions in Slovenia repeatedly prove that young people would have children earlier if the two basic preconditions, i.e., a stable job and appropriate housing, were fulfilled". Similarly, in the case of Bulgaria, "Koytcheva (2006) finds that during the 1990s the changes in fertility in Bulgaria were influenced to a higher degree by economic factors than by changes in values and ideas" (Koytcheva and Philipov 2008:392).

Other authors have *de facto* acknowledged the root cause explanation. For instance, Lesthaeghe and Surkyn (2002) summarizing their findings on new patterns of household formation in CEE countries stated *inter alia*:

"In short, a capitalist restructuring leads to greater individual autonomy in the ideational sphere, and this in turn means more convergence of family formation patterns to western types. Rather than the economic crisis per se, it is the entire restructuring of society that is the accelerator of the ideational and demographic changes."

Nevertheless, while acknowledging that "there is nothing mutually exclusive about the operation of both economic and cultural factors" and that "they may be interwoven and mutually reinforcing," Lesthaeghe and Surkyn believe that, in the long run, the cultural factors will become dominant and will eventually "take over."

8. The array of specific factors as identified in country analyses

In the country analyses, numerous specific factors causing and modifying demographic behaviour in the transition countries have been identified and discussed. These are listed because they demonstrate the wide variety of circumstances that played a role. The interplay of these factors was somewhat different from one country to another, and, therefore, some are discussed in almost all CEE country chapters, while others are mentioned only in a few. While some of these factors were predominantly of an economic nature, others were mainly social, cultural, psychological, or political. Due to the instantaneous and rapid change from the state socialist to the capitalist system, particular conditions had an immediate forceful impact, while other factors are of a long-lasting nature. Thus, the economic factors are listed in two general categories: those operating mainly during the initial crisis years, and the long-term factors associated with the development of market economies.

8.1 Economic factors operating mainly during the initial years of the transition

- Massive inflation;
- Considerable unemployment, in particular among women;
- The loss of previously guaranteed rights and entitlements, particularly guaranteed employment and income, as well as the loss of free education and free health care in some countries;
- A decline in social functions and services provided by companies – e.g., health clinics, cafeteria and child day care facilities;
- A decline in real income of individuals and households; a delay in payment or non-payment of earned wages and salaries in a number of countries; the requirement that some employees take unpaid leave, often of long duration;
- Increasing levels of discrimination against women in the economy, in particular in the job market;
- Declining capacity/supply of public child care facilities, especially for children 0-2 years old;
- A lack of housing coupled with increasing costs of housing; lack of credit opportunities, particularly for young people;
- Increasing disparities in the income distribution, with some segments of the population becoming impoverished while others became more affluent and acquired wealth;
- A state of deprivation and anomie in some segments of the population.

8.2 Economic factors associated with the development of market economies

- A restructuring of the market with an increasing availability of consumer goods and services;
- A tightening job market and growing degree of labour market competition that resulted in an increase in required qualifications, and which, in turn, necessitated the acquisition of appropriate skills;
- Rising job insecurity;
- New career opportunities, especially for individuals with higher education;
- Rising direct costs for child care, education and health, an increasing proportion of which had to be borne by users;
- Rising indirect costs of children.

8.3 Social, cultural and psychological factors

- Changing norms, values and attitudes regarding marriage, cohabitation, separation, divorce, extra-marital childbearing, modern contraception (see overview chapter 6);
- A largely continuing traditional perception of gender roles in the family, although a more egalitarian modern perception is also starting to spread;
- Continued unequal division of responsibilities and work within households between genders (shopping, maintenance, child care, laundry, cooking, etc.);
- Continuing or further deepening marriage and union instability;
- Significantly enhanced access to, and increasing utilization of, modern contraception;
- Temporary and permanent emigration for work- and study- generated income/remittances, but with an accompanying destabilization of family relations;
- Amplified social stratification with more pronounced differences between the lower, middle and upper strata;
- A massive expansion of education, especially at the tertiary level;
- An expansion of consumerist behaviour;
- Increased opportunities in education, leisure activities and international travel.

8.4 Political factors

- A disarray in family policies; no clear family policy goals and strategies; curtailed family policy benefits;
- Legalization of induced abortion in Albania and Romania;
- Severe restriction of abortion legislation in Poland, and the possibility of some restrictions in other countries.

There are no definite dividing lines between the two types of economic factors. For example, the fact that various types of educational, health and child care costs borne by the state under the socialist regimes became the responsibility of the family might have initially been perceived as part and parcel of the crisis determinants. In a market economy, however, it is natural that some of these costs are mainly the responsibility of households, although specific policy measures can mitigate their burden.

In some of the country chapters, the discrimination against women and the continued unequal division of responsibilities and work within households between genders are considered important circumstances curtailing childbearing. "Female emancipation during the years of transformation progressed in a highly controversial way in Lithuania. It was, and still is, developing, along with the preservation of the traditional/patriarchal attitudes towards gender roles .... Society's delay in adapting to the new female roles forces women to work out certain new strategies, which they use to the best of their needs and abilities, to solve the problem of reconciling the varied challenges of daily life. They postpone childbearing for a later period, have fewer children, or refuse to have children altogether" (Stankuniene and Jasilioniene 2008:731). "In Slovenia, the traditional gender division of roles in the family persists, leading to a double burden for employed women. Having less children may thus constitute a coping strategy for young women" (Stropnik and Šircelj 2008:1039). A peculiar perception on gender roles exists in the Czech Republic. "The continuing inequality in the gender division of housework has been documented in a number of research studies. ... Czech women contribute two thirds of the total time necessary for doing the housework ... Interestingly, even women who work full-time, as do their partners, opine that it is fair to work more in the home than their partners" (Sobotka et al. 2008:438).

Ukraine and the Czech Republic are vivid examples of how different the transition experience was in individual countries. According to the Ukraine chapter, "[a]fter the dissolution of the Soviet Union, Ukraine experienced a grave economic crisis, leading to individual level economic uncertainty" (Perelli-Harris 2008:1162). ... "This instability has led to social anomie, or a breakdown in social norms ... The negative change has caused individuals to feel they have lost control over their lives, resulting in high levels of stress and anxiety" ... "Social anomie, as opposed to simple economic uncertainty, may be one of the main reasons for the rapid decline in fertility in Ukraine" (Perelli-Harris. 2008:1163). The country chapters on Russia (Zakharov 2008), Romania (Muresan et al. 2008) and Bulgaria (Koytcheva and Philipov 2008) provide evidence of similar developments in those countries.

In contrast, in the Czech Republic "extreme shocks or turbulence as experienced in many other post-communist societies" were avoided. "Thanks to the existence of an extensive social security net, combined with a rapid expansion of small enterprises, the economic transformation did not entail severe consequences for the majority of the population" (Sobotka et al. 2008:404). However, the Czech Republic also experienced a considerable fertility decline during the 1990s. "The rapidity of observed changes can be explained as the outcome of a simultaneous occurrence of several factors, especially the expansion of higher education, the emergence of new opportunities competing with family life, increasing job competition, rising economic uncertainty in young adulthood, and changing partnership behaviour" (Sobotka et al. 2008:403). Apparently Slovenia and, to a large extent, also Hungary and other countries of Central Europe had similar experiences.

9. Conclusions

By historical standards, the rapid changes in family formation and childbearing levels in the CEE countries during the 1990s were unprecedented. To date, two theories have been elaborated to provide an understanding of the determinants that brought about these trends. The first theory argues that the economic and social crises which occurred in the wake of the transition from the state socialist centrally managed economies to capitalist market economies in the early 1990s were the principal causes of the rapid demographic changes. The other theory claims that it was the diffusion of western norms, values and attitudes regarding family formation and childbearing that were instrumental in causing the observed demographic trends. The two theories were not considered mutually exclusive, and it was accepted that the economic crisis and the diffusion factors could be operating simultaneously.

Both theories make valid observations, but they do not reveal the principal underlying or root cause of the respective demographic trends, namely, the replacement of the state socialist regimes by market economies and by fledgling democratic institutions of governance. The former created the relatively favourable conditions for childbearing of job security, low-cost housing, free education, free health care, and a variety of entitlements associated with child birth and childrearing, as well as shortages of career opportunities, leisure activities, and consumer goods. These were replaced by the more restraining conditions for childbearing of job insecurity, an increasing pressure to acquire more education, expensive housing, lesser and declining birth and childrearing entitlements, as well as the availability of a variety of career opportunities, leisure activities and consumer goods. The populace of the CEE countries had grown accustomed to the socialist paternalistic welfare state circumstances over several decades, and, all of a sudden, young people were confronted with the need to deal with a whole new Western type of family formation and childbearing environment. Market economy principles and Western democratic institutions provided the framework for family formation and childbearing, and they also provided the basis for the adoption and diffusion of western type norms, values and attitudes regarding demographic behaviour.

Individual generations were affected by the changing incentives and constraints on childbearing in very different ways. This turned out to reinforce the declines and extraordinarily low levels of the period total fertility rates during the 1990s. The birth cohorts of the 1960s had borne almost all their children when in their twenties, and, consequently, had very low fertility rates when in their thirties, i.e. during the 1990s. In contrast, the birth cohorts of the mid- to late 1970s were delaying many births into their late twenties and thirties, and thus had low fertility when starting out on their childbearing careers during the 1990s. Thus the low fertility rates of the former when ending their childbearing overlapped with the relatively low fertility rates of the latter when they were in the initial years of childbearing, resulting in the total period fertility rates of around 1.1 to 1.3 births per woman observed around the year 2000 in most countries of Central and Eastern Europe. In the foreseeable future, cohorts with similar age patterns of childbearing will, in all likelihood, overlap. This fact alone is likely to cause an increase in total period fertility rates. Any increase in period fertility will also depend upon the extent of recuperation of delayed births, which is likely to vary from one country to another.

References

Aliaga, C. 2006. How is the time of women and men distributed in Europe?, *Statistics in Focus* 4, Eurostat.

Ariès, P. 1980. Two successive motivations for the declining birth rate in the West, *Population and Development Review* 6(4): 645–650.

Besemeres, J. F. 1980. Socialist Population Politics: The Political Implications of Demographic Trends in the USSR and Eastern Europe. Armonk. NY: Sharpe.

Billari, F.C., M. Castiglioni, T. Castro Martín, F. Michielin and F. Ongaro. 2002. Household and union formation in a Mediterranean fashion: Italy and Spain, in E. Klijzing and M. Corijn, (Eds.), Dynamics of Fertility and Partnership in Europe: Insights and Lessons from Comparative Research, vol. II. Geneva/New York: United Nations, pp. 17-41.

Büttner, T., and W. Lutz. 1990. Estimating fertility responses to policy measures in the German Democratic Republic, Population and Development Review 16(3): 539–555.

Caldwell, J. C. 1976. Toward a restatement of demographic transition theory, *Population and Development Review* 2(3–4): 321–366.

Churchill, W. 1946. Sinews of Peace (the Iron Curtain speech), reprinted in Kishlansky, M. A. ed. 1955. *Sources of World History.* New York: Harper Collins, pp. 298–302.

Council of Europe. 2006. *Recent demographic developments in Europe 2005.* Strasbourg: Council of Europe Publishing.

David, H. P., and R. J. McIntyre. (Eds.) 1981. *Reproductive Behavior: Central and Eastern European Experience.* New York: Springer.

David, H. P. (Ed.) 1999. *From Abortion to Contraception: A Resource to Public Policies and Reproductive Behavior in Central and Eastern Europe from 1917 to the Present,* Westport, Connecticut: Greenwood Press.

Delgado, M., Meil, G., and Zamora López, F. 2008. Spain: Short on children and short on family policies, *Demographic Research* 19(27). http://www.demographic-research.org/ Volumes/Vol19/27/

Demeny, P., and G. McNicoll. 2006. World population 1950–2000: perception and response, in P. Demeny and G. McNicoll (Eds.), *Population and Development Review, a supplement to* vol. 32*:* 1–51.

De Rose, A., Racioppi, F., and Zanatta, A-L. 2008. Italy: Delayed adaptation of social institutions to changes in family behaviour, *Demographic Research* 19(19). http://www. demographic-research.org/Volumes/Vol19/19/

Eurostat. 2007. *Eurostat Yearbook 2006–2007.* http://epp.eurostat.ec.europa.eu/cache/ ITY_OFFPUB/KS-CD-06-001-05/EN/KS-CD-06-001-05-EN.PDF.

Frejka, T. 1980. Fertility Trends and Policies: Czechoslovakia in the 1970s, *Population and Development Review* 6(1): 65–93.

Frejka, T. 1983. Induced abortion and fertility: a quarter century of experience in Eastern Europe, *Population and Development Review* 9(3): 494–520.

Hobcraft, J., and K. Kiernan. 1995. *Becoming a Parent in Europe, Evolution or Revolution in European Population.* Proceedings of the European Population Conference. Milano, pp: 27–65.

Hobcraft, J. 1996 Fertility in England and Wales: a fifty-year perspective, *Population Studies* 50(3): 485–524.

ILO. 1990. *Yearbook of Labour Statistics: Retrospective edition on population censuses, 1945-89.* Geneva: ILO.

Kamarás, F. 1996. Birth rates and fertility in Hungary, in P. P. Tóth and E. Valkovics (Eds.), *Demography of Contemporary Hungarian Society.* Boulder, Colorado: Social Science Monographs, pp: 55–88.

Kohler, H.-P., F. C. Billari, and J. A. Ortega. 2002. The emergence of lowest-low fertility in Europe during the 1990s, *Population and Development Review* 28 (4): 641–680.

Kotowska, I. E., and J. Jóźwiak. (Eds.) 2003. *Population of Central and Eastern Europe. Challenges and Opportunities.* Warsaw: Statistical Publishing Establishment.

Kotowska, I., Jóźwiak, J., Matysiak, A., and Baranowska, A. 2008. Poland: Fertility decline as a response to profound societal and labour market changes?, *Demographic Research* 19(22). http://www.demographic-research.org/Volumes/Vol19/22/

Koytcheva, E. 2006. *Social-Demographic Differences in Fertility and Family Formation in Bugaria Before and After the Start of the Societal Transition.* Working Paper. Rostock: Max Planck Institute for Demographic Research.

Koytcheva, E., and Philipov, D. 2008. Bulgaria: Ethnic differentials in rapidly declining fertility, *Demographic Research* 19(13). http://www.demographic-research.org/Volumes/Vol19/13/

Lesthaeghe, R., and G. Moors. 2000. Recent trends in fertility and household formation in the industrialized world, *Review of Population and Social Policy* 9: 121–170.

Lesthaeghe R., and J. Surkyn. 2002. New forms of household formation in Central and Eastern Europe: are they related to newly emerging value orientations, in *Economic Survey of Europe 2002/1.* New York and Geneva: United Nations, Economic Commission for Europe, pp: 197–216.

Macura, M. 1981. Evolving population policies, in H. P. David and R. J. McIntyre (Eds.), *Reproductive Behavior: Central and Eastern European Experience.* New York: Springer, pp: 30–52.

Muresan, C., Hărăgus, P.T., Hărăgus, M., and Schröder, C. 2008. Romania: Childbearing metamorphosis within a changing context, *Demographic Research* 19(23). http://www.demographic-research.org/Volumes/Vol19/23/

Observatoire Démographique Européen. 2006. *Personal Communication.*

Oláh, L., and Bernhardt, E. 2008. Sweden: Combining childbearing and gender equality. *Demographic Research* 19(28). http://www.demographic-research.org/Volumes/Vol19/28/

Philipov, D. 2003. Fertility in times of discontinuous societal change, in I. E. Kotowska and J. Jóźwiak (Eds.), *Population of Central and Eastern Europe. Challenges and Opportunities.* Warsaw: Statistical Publishing Establishment, pp: 665–689.

Perelli-Harris, B. 2008. Ukraine: On the border between old and new in uncertain times, *Demographic Research* 19(29). http://www.demographic-research.org/Volumes/Vol19/29/

Philipov, D., and J. Dorbritz. 2003. Demographic consequences of economic transition in Countries of Central and Eastern Europe, *Population Studies* 39. Strasbourg: Council of Europe Publishing.

Rabušic, L. 2001. *Kde ty všechny deti jsou?* (Where have all the children gone?) Praha: SLON.

Rychtaříková, J. 1996. Current changes of the reproduction character in the Czech Republic and the international situation, *Demografie* (Czech) 38(2): 72–89.

Rychtaříková, J. 1999. Is Eastern Europe experiencing a second demographic transition?, *Acta Unuversitatis Carolinae, Geographica* 1:19–44.

Sobotka, T. 2004. *Postponement of childbearing and low fertility in Europe.* Doctoral thesis, University of Groningen. Amsterdam: Dutch University Press.

Sobotka, T., Šťastná, A., Zeman, K., Hamplová, D., and Kantorová, V. 2008. Czech Republic: A rapid transformation of fertility and family behaviour after the collapse of state socialism, *Demographic Research* 19(14). http://www.demographic-research.org/Volumes/Vol19/14/

Stankuniene, V., and Jasilioniene, A. 2008. Lithuania: Fertility decline and its determinants, *Demographic Research* 19(20). http://www.demographic-research.org/Volumes/Vol19/20/

Stefanov, I., and N. Naoumov. 1974. Bulgaria, in B. Berelson (Ed.), *Population Policy in Developed Countries.* New York: McGraw-Hill, pp. 149–170.

Stloukal, L. 1995. *Demographic Aspects of Abortion in Eastern Europe: A Study with Special Reference to the Czech Republic and Slovakia.* Ph.D. thesis. Australian Canberra: National University.

Stloukal, L. 1999. Understanding the 'abortion culture' in Central and Eastern Europe, in H. P. David (Ed.), *From Abortion to Contraception: A Resource to Public Policies and Reproductive Behavior in Central and Eastern Europe from 1917 to the Present.* Westport, Connecticut: Greenwood Press, pp. 23-47.

Stropnik, N., and Šircelj, M. 2008. Slovenia: Generous family policy without evidence of any fertility impact, *Demographic Research* 19(26). http://www.demographic-research.org/Volumes/Vol19/26/

UNESCO. 2005. *Unesco Statistical Yearbook 1999.* http://www.uis.unesco.org/en/stats/statistics/yearbook/tables/Table_II_S_5_Region(GER).html.

UNESCO. 2007. Unesco Institute of Statistics, Data Centre. http://stats.uis.unesco.org/unesco/TableViewer/document.aspx?ReportId=143&IF_Language=en

Westoff, C. F., and N. B. Ryder. 1977. *The Contraceptive Revolution.* Princeton: Princeton University Press.

Zakharov, S. 2008. Russian Federation: From the first to second demographic transition, *Demographic Research* 19(24). http://www.demographic-research.org/Volumes/Vol19/24/

Ziolkowski, J. A. 1974. Poland, in B. Berelson (Ed.), *Population Policy in Developed Countries.* New York: McGraw-Hill, pp. 445–488.

Demographic Research: Volume 19, Article 8
research article

Overview Chapter 6:
The diverse faces of the
Second Demographic Transition in Europe

Tomáš Sobotka[1]

Abstract

This chapter discusses the concept of the second demographic transition (SDT) and its relevance for explaining the ongoing changes in family and fertility patterns across Europe. It takes a closer look at the shifts in values and attitudes related to family, reproduction, and children, and their representation in different chapters in this collection. It re-examines the link between the second demographic transition and fertility, highlights its strong positive association with fertility at later childbearing ages, and suggests that the transition does not necessarily lead to sub-replacement fertility levels. Subsequently, it provides an extensive discussion on the progression of the SDT behind the former 'Iron Curtain.' To explain some apparent contradictions in this process, it employs a conceptual model of 'readiness, willingness, and ability' (RWA) advocated by Lesthaeghe and Vanderhoeft (2001). It also explores the multifaceted nature of the second demographic transition between different social groups, and points out an apparent paradox: whereas lower-educated individuals often embrace values that can be characterised as rather traditional, they also frequently manifest family behaviour associated with the transition, such as non-marital childbearing, high partnership instability, and high prevalence of long-term cohabitation. This suggests that there may be two different pathways of the progression of the second demographic transition. The concluding section points out the role of structural constraints for the diffusion of the transition among disadvantaged social strata, highlights the importance of the 'gender revolution' for the SDT trends, and discusses the usefulness of the SDT framework.

---

[1] Vienna Institute of Demography. E-mail: tomas.sobotka@oeaw.ac.at

1. Introduction: the fluidity of the 'second demographic transition'

The idea of the *second demographic transition* was first suggested by Ron Lesthaeghe and Dirk van de Kaa in 1986, when it referred to interrelated changes in fertility, family formation, and partnership behaviour, which started in the late 1960s in many countries of Western and Northern Europe. The term *transition—* initially used with a question mark reflecting uncertainty about it (van de Kaa 2002: 9)—shows that its proponents became convinced that a long-lasting change in demographic regime was under way. This change was closely related to substantial shifts in values related to family life and children, and was marked by the weakening of the 'traditional' family as an institution. Decline in fertility rates well below the replacement level, facilitated by the spread of modern contraception, was perceived as the main feature of the transition (van de Kaa 1987: 4). The concept of the second demographic transition (SDT) has been subsequently elaborated upon in numerous publications (e.g., Lesthaeghe 1995; van de Kaa 1994, 2001 and 2002; Lesthaeghe and Surkyn 2002 and 2004). It has tentatively incorporated mortality and migration, and has been broadly linked to numerous structural changes (modernization, the growth of the service economy and the welfare state, the expansion of higher education), cultural changes (secularization, the rise of individualistic values, the importance of self-expression and self-fulfilment) and technological changes (the adoption of modern contraception, the advances in assisted reproduction, the explosion of new information technologies) (see van de Kaa 1994). According to van de Kaa (1996: 425), the second demographic transition has become a "quintessential narrative of ideational and cultural change," whose main distinction from the first demographic transition is the "overwhelming preoccupation with self-fulfilment, personal freedom of choice, personal development and lifestyle, and emancipation, as reflected in family formation, attitudes towards fertility regulation and the motivation for parenthood." A stylised discussion of the development over time of the second demographic transition concept, and of associated ideas, is provided by van de Kaa (2002) in a paper entitled "The idea of a Second Demographic Transition in industrialized countries."

The widening scope of the second demographic transition concept and its evolution over time imply that it has become broadly used as a label, description, and even explanation for a plethora of diverse changes in fertility and family-related behaviours and attitudes, to the point where its usage "has escaped the control of its initial proponents" (Billari and Wilson 2001: 3). Considerable ambiguity prevails among demographers about the concept, its main facets and its main underlying mechanisms: to many observers, it remains unclear what the transition really is and how to define it. Adding to this definition problem, the crucial elements of the transition may change over time: for instance, van de Kaa (2002: 29) suggests that "while below replacement fertility currently is a crucial element of the Second Transition, this need not be a permanent state." Different facets of the SDT idea have attracted considerable amount of criticism. Cliquet argued that there is no apparent discontinuity between the first and the second demographic transition; he views demographic changes of the last decades as "a new acceleration in relational and reproductive patterns, associated to modernization" (Cliquet 1991: 28, see also counter-arguments by Lesthaeghe and Neels 2002 and Lesthaeghe and Surkyn 2004). The timing of the onset of the SDT can be disputed as well. For instance, van Bavel (2007) has shown using an example of low fertility between the First and Second World Wars that contemporary interpretations of below-replacement fertility centred on the factors frequently associated with the second demographic transition, such as secularisation, changes in the character of marriage, consumerism, increased economic aspirations, and the conflict between employment and motherhood. The idea of a 'transition' seemingly suggests that there is a 'final state,' a new demographic regime on which different societies eventually converge. However, Lesthaeghe and van de Kaa neither formally define a starting point, nor envision any quantifiable endpoint of the transition.[2] What matters in their arguments is not an envisioned 'end-of-transition' equilibrium, but rather a direction of changes and trajectories, which are generally shared across countries.

But even the idea of such widely shared behavioural and value changes raises a question about the eventual convergence among countries and diverse social groups in their family patterns and demographic characteristics. While on an individual level the transition may be expected to lead to an increased variability in fertility and family behaviours, and result in a 'pluralisation of family forms,' the notion of common cross-country trends suggests that the differences between countries are likely to diminish. However, many researchers emphasise the persistent diversity in family patterns and living arrangements across Europe (e.g., Kuijsten 1996), which has historical roots (e.g., Reher 1998). Consequently, some scholars argue that different types of changes in family and fertility "cannot simply be interpreted in one model of the second demographic transition" (de Beer, Corijn and Deven 2000: 124, see also Micheli 2004: 80). Micheli (2004) proposes that family patterns in Europe remain strongly regionally embedded, and that, in contrast to Northern Europe, modernisation has led to a revitalisation of the 'kinship-alliance family

---

[2] Noting that the outcome of the second demographic transition cannot be predicted with any certainty, and that it is unlikely to lead to any sort of equilibrium, van de Kaa (2004b: xiii) suggested that the term 'revolution'—which does not imply a shift from one steady state to another—would probably have been a better label for the ongoing "change in demographic regime."

patterns' in the South.[3] Also, the hypothesised synchronicity between the behavioural and value changes occasionally attracts criticism. Rotariu (2006: 19), for instance, suggests that in Romania the behavioural change manifested by falling fertility rates, fertility postponement, and rising proportion of non-marital births "appears to precede the shift in the system of values and attitudes toward family and children." Another common criticism of the SDT concept is its anchoring in European, or, when viewed from an even narrower perspective, Northwestern European patterns of demographic changes, which make it far from certain that it will spread to other parts of the world (Coleman 2004). Some contributions indicate that the SDT, or at least many of its features, is well underway in non-European advanced societies (see Lesthaeghe and Neidert 2006 for the U.S. and Matsuo 2001 and Rindfuss et al. 2004 for Japan), but the differences in family-related behaviours and attitudes between North-western Europe and most advanced Asian countries, like Japan or Korea, remain enormous. Finally, there may be a problem with the term itself: Coleman (2004) claims that the second demographic transition concerns mostly changes in living arrangements, and can therefore hardly be labelled 'demographic.'

The broadness and the fluidity of the transition narrative have, to some extent, hindered empirical studies examining its validity and the spread of the transition in different societies and regions. With a rising acceptance of the concept, the number of articles investigating the SDT in different countries has increased (e.g., de Beer, Corijn and Deven 2000; Sobotka, Zeman, and Kantorová 2003, Lesthaeghe and Neidert 2006, Kertzer et al. 2006, Rotariu 2006, Gerber and Berman 2006, and Gerber and Cottrell 2006). Despite valid criticisms of the 'transition' framework, it is worthwhile to discuss the spread of the second demographic transition in Europe, and outline how it is reflected in the country-specific chapters in this collection. The various reasons for focusing on the second demographic transition can be summarised as follows. First, the fact that the SDT has become a rather established concept, which is often used to understand changes in demographic behaviour (Liefbroer and Fokkema 2008) and which is also discussed in many country chapters, warrants specific attention. Second, the significance of a substantial shift in family-related behaviour and attitudes in advanced societies in the last four decades has been recognised not only by numerous demographers, but also by

---

[3] Lesthaeghe and van de Kaa acknowledge huge cross-country heterogeneity in the SDT progression. Van de Kaa (2002: 31) concludes, nevertheless, that the persistent differences "are variations on the common themes: major changes in fertility, a redefinition of the model of the family, improvements in mortality, and becoming countries of immigration." He then concludes that "[i]t is our inability to explain these changes as a purely temporary disturbance, which convinces me that describing them as a 'Second Demographic Transition' is warranted."

researchers from other disciplines. Some of the well-known sociological books, including Inglehart's (1990) *Culture shift in advanced industrial society,* Gidden's (1992) *The transformation of intimacy,* or Bauman's (2000) *Liquid modernity* provide convincing arguments about the intensity of changes in the character of partnerships, family, and childbearing, and the values attached to them. Many family economists have also recognised that the 'Western' family has entered a period of rapid change (Lundberg and Pollak 2007); Goldin (2006) speaks about the 'quiet revolution' in women's lives, and emphasises the link between the spread of the contraceptive pill, extended education, postponement of marriage, and the change in women's identity and career orientation. Third, an examination of the second demographic transition sheds light on different factors affecting the shifts in demographic behaviour, and on the relation between changing values and attitudes, and changing family-related behaviours. Fourth, the discussion about the second demographic transition is particularly illuminative in the case of the post-communist societies of Central, Eastern, and South-eastern Europe, all of which have experienced numerous 'symptoms' of the SDT behaviour. Scholars disagree, however, on the extent and significance of the diffusion of individualistic value orientation in this region. This debate, which has been often simplistically reduced to 'cultural change' vs. 'economic crisis' arguments (see Overview Chapter 5[*]), may also contribute to our ability to foresee future family changes in the former state-socialist societies. It is not by coincidence that most chapters on Central and Eastern Europe explicitly discuss the relevance of the second demographic transition model for explaining recent changes in family behaviour.

This chapter is closely related to Overview Chapter 4, which outlines changes in family life and living arrangements in Europe since the 1960s, illustrating many trends that constitute the backbone of the second demographic transition. Taking profound family transformation as a starting point, this chapter looks at the relevance of the SDT concept for explaining the ongoing changes in fertility patterns and takes a closer look at the shifts in values and attitudes related to family, reproduction, and children. It re-examines the link between the second demographic transition and sub-replacement fertility, and pays special attention to the 'progression' of the second demographic transition behind the former 'Iron Curtain.' To explain some apparent contradictions in this process, it employs a conceptual model of 'readiness, willingness, and ability' (RWA) advocated by Lesthaeghe and Vanderhoeft (2001). It also discusses the multifaceted nature of the

---

[*] All overview and country chapters referred to herein are part of Special Collection 7: *Childbearing Trends and Policies in Europe*, and can be found online at: http://www.demographic-research.org/special/7/.

second demographic transition between different social groups, and points out an apparent paradox: whereas lower-educated individuals often embrace values that can be characterised as rather traditional, they also frequently manifest most pronounced features of family behaviour associated with the transition, such as non-marital childbearing, high partnership instability, and high prevalence of long-term cohabitation. The concluding section summarises the main findings, speculates on two possible pathways of the progression of the second demographic transition, and provides notes on selected factors fuelling this transition. Finally, a brief reflection on the usefulness and validity of the SDT concept is provided. Throughout this chapter, I use interchangeably the terms 'transition,' 'second transition,' 'second demographic transition,' as well as an acronym, 'SDT.' I use these terms in a rather broad sense, trying to avoid their narrow deterministic interpretation.

2. Changes in values and attitudes related to family life, childbearing, and sexuality

Diverse contributions provide strong support for the notion of a profound change in attitudes and values related to childbearing, family life, living arrangements, and sexuality; as well as a relative decline of the importance of family in the hierarchy of values everywhere in Europe. Albania, a country which had been almost isolated from the rest of Europe until 1990, constitutes a notable exception: early marriage and childbearing remain universal, cohabitation is rare, and traditional contraception, especially withdrawal, still constitutes the dominant mode of birth control (Albania chapter).[4] Although the profound change in family-related values appears to be universal, the diversity between countries is enormous, shaped by their culture, history, family policies, and different pace of secularisation. One important aspect of family attitudes provides continuity with the era preceding the SDT: whereas the acceptance of voluntary childlessness and non-family living arrangements has risen rapidly, and marriage and family life have increasingly become 'optional,' attitudes towards parenthood remain overwhelmingly positive in practically all the analysed societies. This is in parallel with similar findings in the United States, where not only parenthood, but also marriage remain valued, desired, and centrally significant to the vast majority of Americans (Thornton and Young-DeMarco 2001).

---

[4] As Albania is a notable outlier in many of the trends discussed throughout this chapter, most of the conclusions and generalisations in this chapter do not apply to this country.

The value attached to children and parenthood

Remarkably, children and parenthood continue to be almost universally valued even in societies that have progressed furthest in the second demographic transition (e.g., France chapter; see also Fokkema and Esveldt 2008). A number of chapters in this collection indicate that voluntary childlessness remains rather marginal[5], and parenthood is still at the top of people's life priorities (Liefbroer and Fokkema 2008). Despite rising instability of partnerships, family life often continues to be strongly valued and idealised (the Czech Republic chapter). But behind this general picture, a number of subtle shifts can be recognised. Parenthood gradually ceases to be the main goal in the lives of men and women (e.g., Austria chapter). Concomitant to that, the importance of leisure and friends increases, and the acceptance of voluntary childlessness spreads (Sweden chapter) – having children is no longer considered a precondition to achieving happiness and self-fulfilment (van de Kaa 2004a). The unwillingness to give up leisure activities scores prominently among the reasons for not having a(nother) child, especially among childless women (Austria, Lithuania, and Germany chapters). In line with van de Kaa's (1987) and Ariès' (1980) reasoning, the motivation for parenthood changes profoundly: childbearing is less frequently seen as a 'duty towards society,' and instead becomes a result of a carefully planned decision of a couple, who may consider various potential positive and negative effects of parenthood on their relationship, lifestyle, and economic wellbeing (Slovenia and Sweden chapter; see also Liefbroer 2005). Having children ceases to be a normatively-bound decision, and it increasingly serves individual self-fulfilment and private joy (Fokkema and Esveldt 2008). The Netherlands chapter quotes Beets et al. (2001), who emphasise the importance of modern contraception in this process, which led to the change in the perception of 'having children' to the decision of 'taking children' (*kinderen nemen*). Importantly, this shift also implies more demanding prerequisites of parenthood and a greater emphasis on the norm of responsible parenthood (Slovenia and Spain chapters).[6]

---

[5] However, Sobotka and Testa (2008) found a significant level of intended childlessness and relatively high uncertainty about parenthood plans among childless women and men of reproductive age in 13 European countries that participated in the Population Policy Acceptance Survey in 2001-2003. The intention to remain childless was most frequently expressed by West German respondents, suggesting an emergence of a 'culture of childlessness' in this region.

[6] These increasing demands on parent's ability to raise a child seem to run contrary to the notion that the second transition implies a shift from 'altruistic' to 'individualistic' motivations for parenthood, i.e., a shift from child-centred to parent-centred perspective (van de Kaa 1987, Ariès' 1980). Present-day parents need to sacrifice a substantial amount of resources (especially time, but also money) to raise and educate their children in conformity to the norm of responsible parenthood. At the same time, successful

Consequently, the stress and the difficulties connected with the proper upbringing of children may emerge as important reasons for not having an additional child (Spain chapter). Finally, the position of children in the family changes as well, as educational practices are based less on strict discipline, and focus more on "rational reasoning with children," who become equal members of the family (Toulemon et al. 2008:524).

More tolerant attitudes towards non-marital childbearing

Across Europe, childbearing outside marriage has experienced an explosive increase (Overview Chapter 4) and is "becoming socially acceptable at all ages and in all social strata" (Zakharov 2008:934). More positive attitudes towards extramarital childbearing are typical of younger persons and the residents of big cities (Poland chapter). Arguably, the enactment of legislation that provided equal rights to married and unmarried parents might have contributed both to an increase in non-marital childbearing, and to a wider acceptance of this phenomenon (Slovenia and Spain chapters). However, a distinction should be made between the acceptance of childbearing within a stable cohabiting union, which often receives general approval, and childbearing among single mothers, which is frequently seen as undesired behaviour linked to an unstable socio-economic situation.

The rising popularity of cohabitation and non-family living arrangements

Unmarried cohabitation, especially as a pre-marital living arrangement, is perceived positively in most European countries, even when the actual prevalence of cohabitation remains relatively low (Pongrácz and Spéder 2008). Liefbroer and Fokkema (2008) have noted that, as early as 1994, a majority of younger respondents (aged 18-35) in 20 countries participating in the International Social Surveys Program agreed that it is acceptable for a couple to live together without intending to get married. Remarkably, at that time cohabitation was rather rare in some of the countries participating in this survey, particularly in Italy, Poland, and Spain. Furthermore, a majority of respondents in all these countries except Poland also agreed that "it is a good idea to cohabit prior to entering marriage." In most cases, the approval of cohabitation further increased between 1994 and 2002,

---

though demanding childrearing brings satisfaction to parents, and may be seen as a part of an individualistic motivation for 'self-fulfilling' parenthood.

especially in regions where it was relatively low in 1994 (Liefbroer and Fokkema 2008: Table 1).

Despite being granted general approval, cohabitation in many countries is still perceived as a pre-marital stage of a short duration, a sort of 'trial marriage' (chapters on Romania, Russia, Slovakia, and Spain). Some contributions show that, over time, pre-marital cohabitation becomes established as a new norm (the Czech Republic, the Netherlands and Sweden chapters), whereas 'direct marriage' becomes a minority option typical of specific religious and ethnic communities.

Even in countries where unmarried cohabitation has become recognized as equal to marriage, a large majority of people do not see marriage as an outdated institution, and most unmarried couples eventually plan to get married. Whereas the superiority of marriage is commonly rejected, marriage remains a desirable and generally preferred living arrangement (Pongrácz and Spéder 2008). Family life continues to be highly and almost universally valued. This pattern is most clearly outlined in the Sweden chapter: although Sweden is frequently categorised as a country with a 'weak family system,' where individualism and residential autonomy play a very important role, Swedes "are somewhat more likely than the 'average European' to say that the family is very important in their life" (Oláh and Bernhardt 2008:1120). Lifelong cohabitation or a 'living apart together' (LAT) relationship is preferred by a relatively small minority of younger respondents (Sobotka and Testa 2008), but there is also evidence of a rising popularity of these living arrangements over time (the Netherlands chapter). In particular, leaving the parental home to live independently without a partner has become increasingly common among young adults (the Netherlands chapter).

Attitudes towards sex and contraception

As Overview Chapter 3 shows, the use of modern contraception has reached relatively high levels in most regions of Europe, and, recently, it has been spreading rapidly in Central, Eastern and South-eastern Europe. Contraceptive use is broadly accepted by all segments of the population; there is significant opposition to contraception only in some Catholic countries with a large proportion of conservative religious people, such as in Poland and Slovakia. The Poland chapter notes that, for almost one-tenth of respondents, contraceptive use remains unacceptable. Similarly, deeply religious women in Slovakia have negative attitudes towards birth control and premarital sex (Slovakia chapter). In Italy, the strong opposition of the Catholic Church to modern contraception and its continuing influence on many institutions, including the media, may partly explain a slow diffusion of the pill (Dalla Zuanna, De Rose, and Racioppi 2005).

The spread of modern contraception, especially of the pill, has helped to separate sex, procreation, and marriage; and arguably had a direct impact on the norms regarding sexual and reproductive behaviour (van de Kaa 1987 and 1994). In the majority of 'Western' societies, sexual activity among unmarried people of all ages, including young adults, is now considered a normal part of a satisfactory life. For instance, the Sweden chapter notes a "positive attitude towards sexual activity among young people, including those not living in co-residential partnerships" (see also Bracher and Santow 1998). This seems to be in contrast to the United States, where many people embrace restrictive attitudes towards premarital sex, and towards sex among teenagers in particular (Thornton and Young-DeMarco 2001). However, most people continue to disapprove of extramarital (or extra-partnership) affairs; such sexual contacts have, in fact, become generally less accepted over time (see Kraaykamp 2002 for the Netherlands and Thornton and Young-DeMarco 2001 for the U.S.).[7] This trend seemingly goes against the current of rising sexual permissiveness, but it is concomitant with the idealisation of marriage and the shift in the character of intimate partnerships, which have become increasingly based on trust and mutual affection, and on the notion of 'exclusivity' of sexual relationships (Giddens 1992).

3. Is sub-replacement fertility a necessary feature of the second demographic transition?

The concept of the second demographic transition, as formulated by its proponents, is related to fertility levels and trends in three distinct respects. First, the SDT brings a massive postponement of parenthood, which is facilitated by the widespread use of modern contraception, and which enables couples to concentrate on pursuing other goals earlier in life. Second, as a result of spreading cohabitation and rising union instability, the SDT leads to a marked rise in the proportion of non-marital births. Third, the transition leads to "structural long-term subreplacement fertility" (Lesthaeghe and Neidert 2006: 669). The fall in period fertility rates is first fuelled by a reduction in higher-order fertility, and later by the postponement of

---

[7] Kraaykamp (2002: Table 1) documents a brief and strong upward shift between 1965 and 1970, and a subsequent gradual decline in the percentage of Dutch respondents agreeing with the statement, "A single affair can do no harm to a good marriage," from a high value of 45% in 1970 to 19% in 1995.

parenthood.[8] Although some fertility recuperation usually occurs once women who had postponed births have children later in life, most often this recovery is not sufficient to bring fertility back to the replacement level and, as a result, the "cohort fertility of currently reproducing women is expected to reach a maximum value well below replacement" (van de Kaa 2002: 10). While the SDT constitutes a complex narrative of demographic change, low fertility is often – and rather simplistically – perceived as a main symptom of this transition. Since this collection primarily focuses on fertility changes and their determinants, I discuss the SDT-fertility link in greater detail.

The relationship between delayed childbearing and the second demographic transition has been relatively firmly established; the onset of the recent long-standing fertility postponement also constitutes a suitable indicator of the onset of the SDT (Sobotka 2004: 58). A number of indicators capturing different aspects of the shift towards late timing of childbearing are closely correlated with the second demographic transition. This can be illustrated with the use of an SDT index constructed on the basis of characteristic changes in values and attitudes, as captured in the 1999 round of the European Values Surveys (data reported in Halman 2001). This index, termed SDT2, ranges from 0 to 10 (10 represents the highest possible score on 'SDT-related' values and attitudes). It is introduced in more detail in Sobotka (2008), and its components are listed in the Appendix. The SDT2 index is relatively closely correlated with the timing of the onset of fertility postponement, with the mean age at first birth (in 1999 and in 2006), and negatively correlated with fertility rates below age 25 (see also below). A close correlation ($r = -0.78$) also emerges with the calendar year when the mean age at first birth among women increased by two years since the onset of first birth postponement (Figure 1; the onset of postponement is measured since the year when the period mean age at first birth started a long-term rise; see Sobotka 2004: 57-58). In other words, the timing of the onset of first birth postponement, combined with the initial pace of this postponement, can serve as rather reliable 'predictors' of SDT-related values in 1999: the earlier the first birth postponement started, and the faster it subsequently progressed, the higher the SDT score that was reached in 1999.

Surprisingly, among different demographic manifestations of the SDT, the often emphasised association with (very) low fertility has become most questionable. Whereas the 'model countries' of the spread of the SDT values and behaviour, such as the Netherlands and Sweden, have experienced a prolonged

---

[8] In addition, an increasing importance of immigrants for childbearing discussed in Overview Chapter 7 may be seen as another, not initially envisioned, trait of the second demographic transition.

Figure 1: **Index of the second demographic transition in 1999 (index SDT2)
and the year when the mean age of mothers at first birth increased
by 2 years since the onset of first birth postponement**

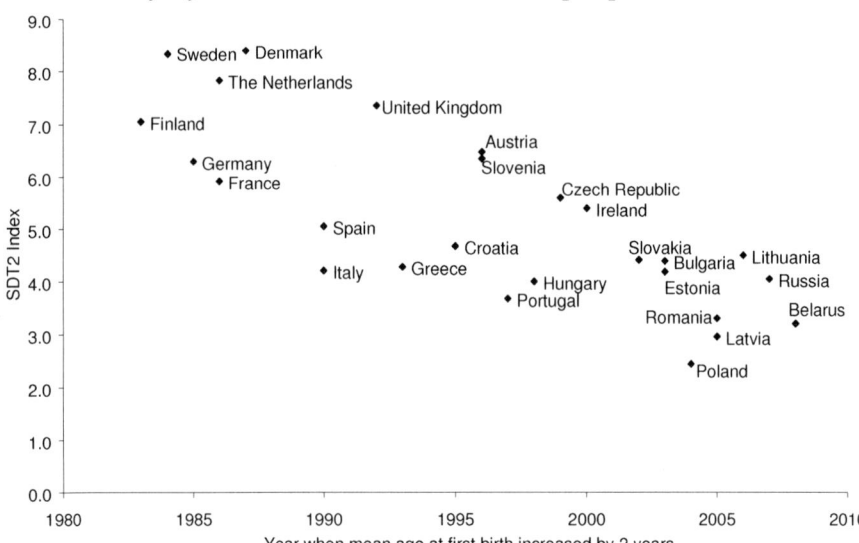

SOURCE: Own computations based on Council of Europe (2006), Eurostat (2008), Sobotka (2004), France and Russia
chapters, and Halman (2001).

period of first birth postponement and an intensive rise in the proportion of children
born outside marriage, their period fertility rates surpass fertility in most other parts
of Europe, and their cohort fertility remains relatively close to the replacement level
threshold (see also Overview Chapters 1 and 4). Several distinct findings and
arguments that cast doubt on the second demographic transition – low fertility
connection may be outlined:

- Some countries retain cohort fertility close to the replacement level. The
  most 'notorious' example is that of the United States, where both period
  and completed cohort fertility remain around this threshold. Lesthaeghe
  and Neidert (2006) attribute this 'American exceptionalism' mainly to the
  'ethnic factor,' namely, high fertility among Hispanic immigrants. Several
  European countries, including Denmark, France, Norway, and Sweden,
  also retain completed fertility close to the replacement level (see also
  Overview Chapter 1). For instance, recent projection of cohort fertility in

France suggests that the cohorts born in the early 1970s will have 2.0 children on average (trend projection in Prioux 2006: 351, T. 5). This finding indicates that the second demographic transition does not necessarily lead to below-replacement cohort fertility levels. This argument, which I further elaborate in another publication (Sobotka 2008), is also reflected in several country chapters. For example, the authors of the chapter on France note that this country has maintained a relatively high level of fertility in spite of experiencing many characteristic social and demographic changes commonly thought as conducive to low fertility, such as delayed entry into parenthood, rising couple instability, increasing number of births outside marriage, or the spread of modern contraception (Overview Chapter 4). Similarly, the Sweden chapter mentions a puzzling contradiction that Sweden, which is often viewed as a forerunner of the second transition, also "exhibits one of the highest fertility levels in Europe, with a completed fertility close to replacement."

- This finding is also linked to another distinct line of reasoning, which emphasises the lack of cross-sectional correlation between the second demographic transition and low fertility in contemporary Europe (Coleman 2004). In fact, my analysis (Sobotka 2008) of cross-country association between selected behavioural and values components of the SDT and fertility indicates that there is a *positive* correlation between the second transition and fertility in contemporary Europe. This positive association emerges most clearly with respect to the period total fertility rate (TFR, Figure 2a), which is a very problematic indicator of the fertility level (Overview Chapter 1, Lutz and Sobotka 2008), but it also holds for the TFR adjusted for changes in the timing of childbearing and, to a smaller extent, for desired family size (Sobotka 2008). In contrast, there was no detectable association between the SDT index based on family-related behaviour (SDT1 index[9]) and the TFR level in 1990 for Europe as a whole (Figure 2b). Only the group of 'Western' countries (i.e., all European countries except the post-communist societies of Central and Eastern Europe) exhibited as early as 1990 a positive association between the

---

[9] The SDT1 index is constructed in analogy to the SDT2 index introduced above. It combines six components of family-related behaviour in 2004: mean age at first birth, mean age at first marriage, teenage fertility rate, proportion of non-marital births, total divorce rate, and total first marriage rate for women (see Appendix). To account partly for the spread of cohabitation, this index was adjusted upward by 0.5 for countries where cohabiting unions account for more than one-tenth of all unions (according to the 2001 census data assembled by Philipov 2006: 31, Table 2 and national data sources).

SDT1 index and fertility, an association which was also found to be strong in 2004. This finding potentially suffers from all the weaknesses linked to such a simple bivariate cross-country analysis conducted at one point of time, such as the danger of ecological fallacy, an ignorance of country-specific trajectories over time, and the lack of adequate controls for important factors affecting this association. Nevertheless, it seems safe to conclude that the recent shift to low and very low fertility in Europe appears to be driven more by the structural factors (family and social policies, economic trends, employment patterns; see also Liefbroer and Fokkema 2008, Sobotka 2008, Adsera 2004), which are only indirectly linked to the second demographic transition.[10]

- The absence of a negative cross-sectional correlation between the second demographic transition and desired family size among younger women (Sobotka 2008) is also significant. Van de Kaa's (2001) analysis showed that, in a number of European countries, young women with a post-materialist value orientation had higher family size ideals than those with 'materialist' values, whereas fertility intentions did not differ between these two groups. Apparently, the spread of the second demographic transition may not lead to the spread of sub-replacement fertility intentions. In most of the countries that made the biggest advances along the SDT trajectory, the fertility desires of younger women remain at or above two, and the two-child family norm continues to enjoy an uncontested popularity. There are countries where fertility intentions declined below the replacement level among the younger cohorts (see, for example, the chapters on the Czech Republic, Poland, and Spain), but it remains unclear to what extent this is a reflection of new values, perceived obstacles to childbearing, or a delay in accommodation to the previous fall in fertility rates.

- Finally, some studies point out that the fall in period fertility rates in numerous countries had preceded changes in the underlying attitudes towards family life and children. This is an especially common assertion in discussions of the former communist countries (see Section 4.2 below).

---

[10] The association between the second demographic transition and fertility would become more convincing if it were manifested also for cohort fertility. However, the fertility level among the cohorts that are currently close to completing their reproductive life, i.e. those born in the late 1960s, relates to the periods when the SDT had not yet fully taken off in Central, Eastern, but also Southern Europe.

Figure 2a: Index of the second demographic transition ('behavioural' index SDT1) and the total fertility rate in Europe in 2004

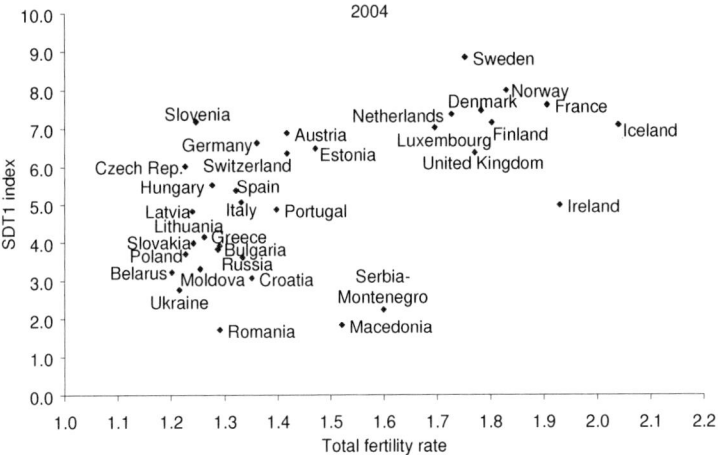

Figure 2b: Index of the second demographic transition ('behavioural' index SDT1) and the total fertility rate in Europe in 1990

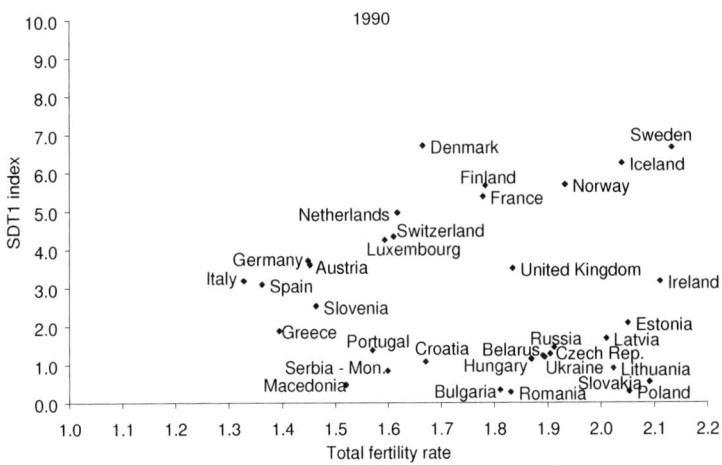

NOTE: See footnote 9 and the text for a definition of the SDT1 index. More details are provided in the Appendix and in Sobotka (2008).

SOURCES: Own computations based on Council of Europe (2006), Eurostat (2008), Philipov 2006, and national statistical offices.

The surprising positive association between the second demographic transition and fertility can be better understood when the transition is related to fertility rates at younger and older childbearing ages. Specifically, the values and attitudes-based index SDT2 is negatively correlated with fertility rates of women below age 25, and positively correlated with fertility rates above age 35. This is illustrated in Figure 3, which looks at this association in 2000 for young-age fertility, and in 2006 for later-age fertility.[11] The figure excludes Southern Europe and Ireland, where this association was particularly weak, probably because factors other than SDT-linked values and attitudes were more relevant for fertility rates at younger and later childbearing ages. This simple analysis of the SDT-fertility link offers the following interpretation: the second demographic transition leads to a marked decline of fertility at younger ages ('postponement' component), but later becomes positively linked to fertility rates at higher childbearing ages ('recuperation' component). This recuperation is strong enough to bring an overall positive association between SDT and fertility, despite some fertility-inhibiting effects of progressively delayed childbearing. This association becomes clearly manifested only if and when fertility in the analysed countries falls to relatively low levels.

In sum, the low and very low fertility rates in contemporary Europe stand on three legs: fertility postponement, which is a long-lasting trend that should eventually come to an end[12], numerous structural and institutional constraints that negatively influence fertility decisions of individuals, and, in some cases, a shift in family-size norms and desires towards sub-replacement fertility (see also Overview Chapter 4). While the first factor ('postponement') has been losing in importance in many of the countries that advanced the most in the SDT progression, and the third factor ('sub-replacement desires') is far from universal, it seems that the impact of the second set of factors (different 'constraints') constitutes the most important explanation for very low fertility. These factors are not central to the changes in the

---

[11] The SDT2 index is used here because its demographic (behavioural) counterpart SDT1 includes period TFR that is linked with the analysed age-specific fertility rates. The selection of a later year, 2006, for a comparison of the SDT2 index and fertility rates at higher ages was motivated by the 'recuperation' argument: If the SDT is linked to fertility recuperation of cohorts that had postponed childbearing at younger ages, this link can be established only with a time lag, i.e., at the time when these cohorts actually reach later childbearing ages. If this argument holds, the positive association between SDT and late fertility may become even more apparent in the future.

[12] Recently an increasing number of countries have recorded a slowing-down or even a stopping in an increase of the mean age at childbearing (see also Overview Chapter 1). The Netherlands was the first European country where fertility postponement has, at least temporarily, come to an end in the late 1990s (Sobotka 2004). Consequently, there was a stabilisation of cohort fertility trajectories among women born in the 1970s (Frejka and Sardon 2006: 357).

Figure 3: **Association between the 'attitudinal' index of the second demographic transition (SDT 2, 1999) and the sum of age-specific fertility rates below age 25 in 2000 and above age 35 in 2006**

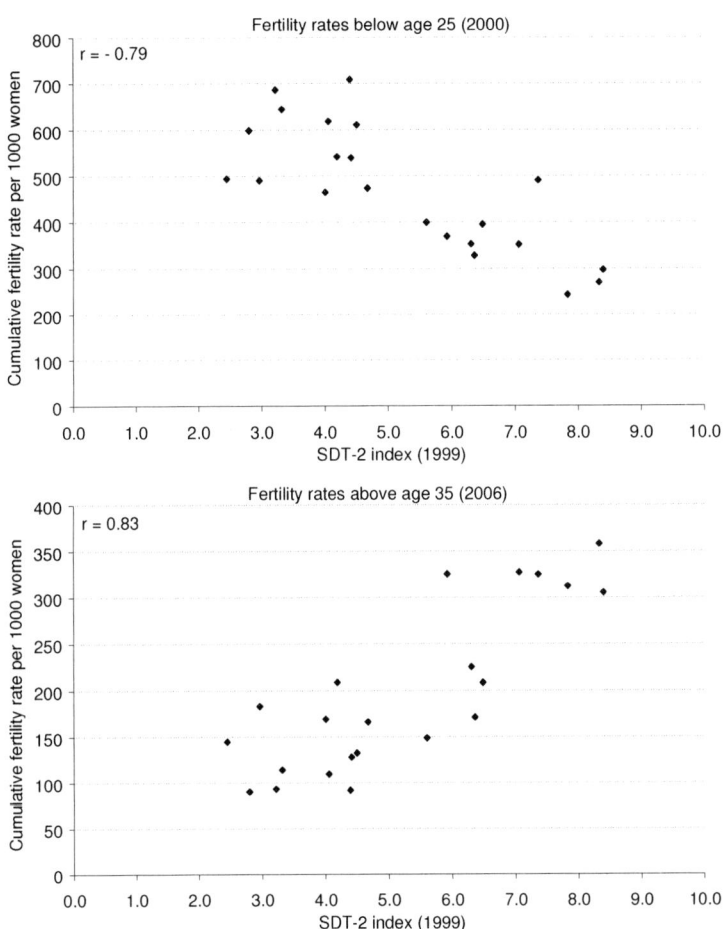

NOTES: See the text and the Appendix for a definition of the SDT2 index (see also Sobotka 2008). The figure includes all European countries that participated in the European Values Study survey of 1999, except Ireland, Southern European countries (Greece, Italy, Portugal, and Spain) and countries with small population size (Luxembourg and Iceland).
SOURCES: Own computations based on Council of Europe (2006), Eurostat (2008), Sobotka (2004), Halman (2001), Russian Federation chapter, and national statistical offices.

values of family and children and, therefore, may not be seen as a part of the SDT 'package'.[13] Their importance may explain an unexpected outcome, namely, the current positive association between the SDT and fertility 'recuperation' at higher childbearing ages, and hence also period fertility rates. This association is consistent with recent research by Myrskylä, Kohler, and Billari (2008), who reported a positive association between 'development' (as measured by the widely used human development index, HDI), and period total fertility for the countries that reached high levels of HDI (above 0.8).

However, at least one aspect of low fertility – the rise in childlessness – is closely linked to the transition. As parenthood ceases to be a 'natural' part of individual biographies and the main goal in a woman's life, voluntary childlessness becomes a broadly accepted option. This has led to a rise in the proportion of people who are undecided about whether they will have children later in life. Sobotka and Testa (2008) show that a substantial proportion of childless men and women in Europe do not intend to have a child, or are uncertain about their parenthood intentions. So far, voluntary childlessness has spread most in western Germany, where it has become a broadly accepted lifestyle, and where childlessness, especially among higher-educated women, has reached the highest level in Europe (Germany chapter; see also Overview Chapter 2 and Sobotka 2005). The Germany chapter points out that there is a small group in the population that "does not regard children as an enrichment to life," and for whom "children do not fit with their own identity" (Dorbritz 2008:590).

4. The second demographic transition in Central and Eastern Europe

4.1 Regional economic and social differentiation and the changes in family-related behaviour after 1989

The discussion on the diffusion of the second demographic transition in the former state-socialist countries of Europe is closely linked to the analysis of the factors responsible for rapid changes in fertility and family patterns observed in this region

---

[13] However, changes in values and attitudes that take place during the second demographic transition may bring to the fore different structural and institutional factors that had not affected fertility decisions substantially in the past, when a strong normative pressure for parenthood and traditional family norms prevailed. Once the timing of childbearing as well as the choice of parenthood as such become more optional parts of individuals' biographies, many factors that had not played an important role in the past emerge as powerful constraints affecting fertility.

since the early 1990s (see Overview Chapter 5). A number of specific questions regarding the occurrence of the SDT in this region arise repeatedly: Are behavioural changes since the early 1990s qualitatively comparable to those that took place earlier in 'Western' societies? If so, are the underlying mechanisms similar as well, or are there constraining factors related to the political and economic changes prominent in Central and Eastern Europe? Do the typical normative and value changes accompany the changes in family and reproductive behaviour in these countries, or do changes in norms and values 'lag' behind behavioural changes? And, finally, how can shifts in values and attitudes that are typical of affluent societies take place in countries that have often been severely affected by economic crisis and political turmoil? Before delving deeper into any of these issues, it is important to stress the enormous cultural and economic diversity of the region, which is often overlooked in broad comparative studies (Sobotka 2003, Manning 2004). The region consists of countries that are very secularised and culturally rather 'liberal' (e.g., the Czech Republic, Estonia, Slovenia, the former GDR or East Germany, and, in many respects, also Hungary) and countries that are more culturally conservative, where people attach higher importance to traditional family values, and where religion often continues to play an important role (e.g., Poland, Romania, or Slovakia). It also consists of societies that are culturally close to Western Europe, and that considered themselves part of the 'Western world' before the Second World War (e.g., the Czech Republic and the Baltic countries); and of countries that had been historically distinct from the 'West', a category that includes most of the predominantly Christian Orthodox and Muslim countries. Finally, the economic restructuring of the 1990s led to widely divergent outcomes and a vast differentiation in the overall economic performance and living standards, despite many comparable pathways and policies, including large-scale economic privatisation, opening of the economy, and market reforms. For instance, the GDP per capita in US Dollars in 2005 (constant 2000 level) varied from 429 in Moldova, to 959 in Ukraine, 2,071 in Bulgaria, and up to 6,515 in the Czech Republic and 11,382 in Slovenia. (World Bank 2007).[14] Keeping this diversity in mind, I review the evidence of the typical changes in fertility, family, and living arrangements, as well as in values and attitudes to children, sexuality, and family life, and subsequently suggest an interpretation of the ongoing second demographic transition in Central and Eastern Europe.

---

[14] This enormous difference becomes smaller when the GDP level is adjusted for purchasing power parity. Then, the difference between the poorest country, Moldova, and the most affluent country, Slovenia, reduces to 1,908 and 22,292 US Dollars, respectively.

A number of country chapters provide strong evidence of massive behavioural changes typically associated with the second transition. Although some of these changes started well before 1990 (Hungary chapter, Stankuniene and Maslauskaite 2008, Hoem et al. 2007, Katus et al. 2007, Gerber and Berman 2006)[15], the period after 1990 has seen a rapid acceleration of all the characteristic trends: first births and first marriages have been postponed (less intensively in Eastern and South-eastern Europe, more vigorously in Central Europe and the Baltic countries), fertility levels have fallen, the percentage of non-marital births has surged, marriage rates have plummeted, and divorce rates have remained high, or have further increased. Cohabitation has been spreading as well, although its significance differs widely across countries.[16] Whereas in many countries, cohabitation mostly retains the character of a 'trial marriage,' it has been rising fast in Bulgaria, the Czech Republic, Estonia, Hungary, Latvia, Russia, and Slovenia; often becoming a standard part in a partnership 'career' among younger cohorts (see the respective country chapters, Gerber and Berman 2006, Hoem et al. 2007, Katus et al. 2007, Spéder 2005, Philipov and Jasilioniene 2007). In other countries, such as Lithuania, Poland, Romania, and Ukraine, the diffusion of cohabitation has been rather slow, and is often typical of people in disadvantaged economic positions (Poland and Romania chapters, Muresan 2007). In almost all countries, however, cohabitation has been spreading most rapidly among younger people below age 30, and it has increasingly replaced marriage as a dominant form of the first union (Czech Republic and Hungary chapters, Spéder 2005, Katus et al. 2007, Hoem et al. 2007). In addition, the duration of cohabitation has risen over time, suggesting that it is gradually becoming a lasting alternative to marriage (Hungary chapter, Spéder 2005, Philipov and Jasilioniene 2007; see also Overview Chapter 4).

Following the collapse of the restrictive state-socialist regime in 1989, the countries of Central and Eastern Europe have experienced a full-blown sexual and contraceptive revolution, bringing a boom of information and messages on contraception, sex, and pornography (the Czech Republic chapter). This trend has also affected more traditional and more religious societies. For instance, in 1997,

---

[15] Some behavioural features typical of the SDT have spread widely in Central and Eastern Europe between the 1960s and the 1980s: premarital sex, marriage instability, and, in some countries, cohabitation (especially among divorced and separated people), and also a one-child family model (especially in urban areas of Russia; see Avdeev and Monnier 1995).

[16] In several countries, including Estonia, Latvia, Hungary, Slovenia, and the former GDR, cohabitation had already become more common during the state-socialist period. In other countries, such as Bulgaria, it was rather common as a very short period of living together before marriage (e.g., Philipov and Jasilioniene 2007), often only once the marriage has been agreed upon. Among the Roma ethnic group, cohabitation (or rather a marriage not officially registered with the authorities) was common prior to 1990 for the reasons entirely unrelated to the second demographic transition (see also Bulgaria chapter).

three-quarters of Slovak women of reproductive age were found to have a positive attitude towards premarital sex (Potančoková et al. 2008:997). An increasing acceptance of sex outside marriage is also noted in the Poland chapter. In many countries, the actual prevalence of premarital sex had already become almost universal during the post-war decades (the Czech Republic chapter) or increased rapidly after 1990: in Romania, the proportion of sexually experienced young adult women who began their sexual life prior to marriage rose from about one-half in 1993 and 1996, to 77% in 1999, and to around 90% in 2004 (RHS 2005). It is important to emphasise, however, that a 'stealthy' liberalisation of sexual morals and behaviour started in Central and Eastern Europe well before 1990, despite the limited spread of modern contraception there. As the Russia chapter notes, this sexual revolution "proceeded more quietly and less noticeably to the observer, by virtue of the taboo placed on the theme for research," and also due to a general avoidance of this subject by the media (see also Binyon 1983). Sexual debut and regular sexual relations occurred at younger ages, and usually prior to marriage. In the absence of proper knowledge and availability of modern contraception, an early start of sexual life led to the surge in premarital conceptions, which gave rise to shotgun marriages at an early age (chapters on Russia, the Czech Republic, and Slovakia).[17]

4.2 Factors fuelling the changes in family behaviour

Individual chapters take a more nuanced view when discussing the factors responsible for the observed changes in family behaviour. Some of them emphasise the lack of evidence for a marked change in values that would progress in parallel with the changes in family-related behaviour, or that would precede it. The Poland chapter raises the question of whether the transition can explain family-related developments in Poland when "ideational change has not advanced until recently compared with its progress in other European countries" (Kotowska et al. 2008:845). The absence of a link between behavioural and value changes in fertility behaviour has been similarly noted by Rotariu (2006) in the case of Romania, and by Gerber and Cottrell (2006) in the case of Russia. The Romania chapter suggests that both 'post-modern' and conservative values have been advancing there: people

---

[17] It is remarkable that the officially published advice literature on partnerships, sexuality, and family often provided very little practical information on sex and contraception. Potančoková (2007) shows that in Czechoslovakia this literature often portrayed contraception and pre-marital sexual relations as problematic, and even linked contraceptive use with promiscuity.

started to "adopt Western values and to imitate modern and post-modern behaviour," but, at the same time, material insecurity enhanced the importance of traditional values and favoured "conservative behaviour" (Muresan et al. 2008:895). In the absence of strong evidence of ideational changes, several chapters stress the importance of structural factors for initiating the change in family behaviour (e.g., the Bulgaria, Poland, and Ukraine chapters). The Ukraine chapter suggests that "the new trends may be the result of economic or cultural factors that have little to do with a shift towards SDT" (Perelli-Harris 2008:1165). Gerber and Cottrell (2006) posit that, despite the rapid increase in the proportion of non-marital births in Russia, there is a continuing traditionalism towards fertility (but not towards marriage, see Gerber and Berman 2006), and no clear evidence of a greater tolerance of extramarital childbearing. In contrast, the Hungary chapter points out that specific changes in values affecting family life, such as rise in consumer aspirations and social atomisation, had taken place during the period preceding the change of political regime in 1989. The Czech Republic chapter, on the other hand, emphasises the abrupt and multifaceted nature of social change after 1989, which makes it impossible to separate the contribution of different economic, structural, and cultural factors to fertility changes.[18]

Three distinct findings support the idea that long-lasting changes in both family-related values and behaviour are reinforcing each other. First, both country-level evidence, as well as the research on household positions and value orientations in Central and Eastern Europe, show that, as is the case in 'Western' countries, there is a consistent relationship between changes in family behaviour and value orientations. Countries that have made greater progress on the SDT dimension also exhibit most clearly values and attitudes typical of the SDT (see also Section 4.5 and Figure 4 below). The profiles of 'non-traditional' value orientation are closely patterned by the living arrangements in which individuals live, with those who are divorced or who had ever cohabited displaying the most 'non-conformist' values, both in post-communist countries and in other regions of Europe (Lesthaeghe and Surkyn 2002). Second, as the Russian Federation chapter points out, the end of the economic crisis and an improvement in living conditions beginning in 1999 did not bring any signs of return to the previous pattern of family behaviour. Rather, very low fertility levels persisted, and the trend towards delayed family formation, decline in marriage, and the rise in cohabitation continued (see also Gerber and Cottrell 2006). Similar evidence for other countries casts doubt on the validity of the

---

[18] Because of the emphasis on different sets of values and attitudes in various country chapters, and also due to a lack of comparable surveys on family-related values prior to 1990, these evaluations of ideational changes in individual countries are to a large extent subjective.

'economic crisis' explanation of the intensive demographic changes in Central and Eastern Europe after 1989 (see Overview Chapter 5 and Russia chapter). Finally, there are signs of a transformation in values and attitudes towards family and children, and the spread of individualism across the whole region, especially among the younger, better-educated, and urban populations. Lesthaeghe's and Surkyn's (2002: Table 6.7.2) analysis of European Values Study surveys in 1990 and 1999 shows that some of the family-related attitudes in Central and Eastern Europe moved in the expected direction envisioned by the SDT concept (while some other attitudes, especially acceptability of divorce and adultery, remained rather stable). This shift has been particularly notable in the Czech Republic, where the majority of people have become highly tolerant of abortion, premarital sex, divorce, or same-sex partnerships (Sobotka, Zeman, and Kantorová 2003 and the Czech Republic chapter). The Lithuania chapter suggests that Lithuanians have been "absorbing and adopting the life styles, value orientations, and norms of behaviour" typical of Western European societies (Stankuniene and Jasilioniene 2008:706; see also Bulgaria chapter). The Poland chapter has noted that younger generations are "less altruistic, more inclined to strive for self-fulfilment and appreciation outside the family," and they attach less importance to family life and children (Kotowska et al. 2008:837). Several chapters emphasise that the 'value change' explanation best fits the highly educated group of the younger population (Romania and Ukraine chapters; see also below).

How can we reconcile the somewhat conflicting evidence on the progression of the second demographic transition in Central and Eastern Europe? As proposed by de Beer, Corijn, and Deven (2000), there indeed seems to be more than one model of the transition. Moreover, given the complexity and the fluidity of the SDT narrative, the assessment of its progression as reflected in individual country chapters is necessarily rather subjective. The 'Central-Eastern European' model of the transition is as diverse as the post-communist societies and their cultural heritage. Nevertheless, several shared features in their SDT may be outlined:

1) Late occurrence of many of the behavioural and value changes typical of the transition, especially those related to alternative living arrangements;

2) Rapidity with which many features of this transition emerged during the 1990s;

3) The importance of structural and economic factors, especially in the early stage of the transition; and

4) The importance of disadvantaged social groups in the spread of some of the new types of family behaviour, especially non-marital childbearing and, in many cases, unmarried cohabitation.

4.3 Explaining the peculiar progression of the SDT using the *Readiness – Willingness – Ability* framework

To get a better understanding of the peculiar and, at times, puzzling progression of the SDT in Central and Eastern Europe, I adopt a conceptual model proposed by Lesthaeghe and Vanderhoeft (2001), which elaborates on an idea first put forward by Coale (1973).[19] This model, called *RWA* (an acronym for *Ready, Willing,* and *Able*), is built around the idea that widespread behavioural change occurs only if three different preconditions are simultaneously met. 'Readiness' (*R*) reflects the 'cost-benefit calculation,' namely, the economic, social, and psychological advantages of adopting a new behaviour. 'Willingness' (*W*) refers to the cultural and ethical acceptability, and thus also the legitimacy of the new form of behaviour. Finally, the 'ability' (*A*) refers to the technical or legal means that enable individuals to adopt new behaviour. The attractiveness of this model lies in its recognition of the joint importance of economic/structural factors (*R*), norms, values, and attitudes (*W*), as well as technology and legal regulation (*A*). This makes it particularly appropriate for understanding recent shifts in fertility and family behaviour in Central and Eastern Europe.

The RWA scheme makes it possible to outline the factors that had been conducive to the SDT, and that had already spread in the state-socialist countries between the 1950s and the 1980s, as well as the factors that had prevented the onset of a full-blown second demographic transition prior to 1990. With respect to *readiness*, the creation of a relatively broad social security net during the decades following the Second World War had diminished in many countries the economic consequences for women of divorce or single motherhood. Similarly, the shift towards an almost universal employment of women enhanced their economic position, and reduced their dependence on male partners and relatives. On the other hand, the stalled expansion of tertiary education, the lack of alternatives for self-realisation outside the family, as well as the peculiar system of preferential housing distribution to married couples with children, discouraged cohabitation and supported early marriage and childbearing (see also Overview Chapter 4 and Chapter 8 in Sobotka 2004). Women's emancipation had stalled halfway between tradition and modernity. On the one hand, women gained similar levels of education as men, they were entitled—and even pressed[20]— to participate in paid labour, and

---

[19] Most recently, Lesthaeghe, Neidert and Surkyn (2006) have used this model to explain spatial differences in the second demographic transition in the United States.

[20] This pressure for employment was circumstantial, motivated by 'financial necessity,' as one income could not secure a decent standard of living in the families, but also ideologically motivated (the

their economic activity was "ideologically supported by equating emancipation with employment" (Kotowska et al. 2008:825). On the other hand, they were confronted with very traditional norms and expectations about their family and childrearing roles, and they were expected to take care of the household, shopping, cleaning, cooking, and childcare. Despite gaining more economic independence, women frequently worked in low-pay occupations (Bulgaria chapter) and they faced multiple burdens that were a far cry from the ideas of gender equality and 'women's liberation.' Family life became highly idealised. Family relationships enhanced the well-being of individuals, as the mutual help of family members substituted for a deficient service economy (the Czech Republic and Hungary chapters). Moreover, family life provided a "shelter from the politicised public scene" (Potančoková et al. 2008:1001), and from the omnipresent eyes of the state (see also Sobotka 2004).

Concerning *willingness*, the official Communist ideology was strongly anti-religious, and thus helped to erode some of traditional norms related to marriage, family, and sexuality, which had previously been anchored in religious teachings. The destruction of various religious and civic organisations led to an 'atomisation' of the society (Hungary chapter). Despite the shortage of consumer goods, consumerist orientation had spread well before 1990 (Spéder 2005; Sobotka 2004). Moreover, even the media censorship and the limits placed on travel to 'Western' countries were not sufficient obstacles against the spread of new fashions, ideas, and aspirations associated with 'Western' culture, often progressing in a rather bizarre and deformed way.[21] However, the new values were embraced in a selective fashion. Even the relatively 'conservative' official ideology supporting traditional family values could not prevent the stealthy progress of the sexual revolution and the increase in family instability. At the same time, official 'puritanism' related to sexuality, gender roles, and the family probably helped to preserve the overwhelmingly positive image of marriage, childbearing, and family life, as well as widespread negative attitudes to feminism, homosexuality, and extramarital childbearing. This led to the development of a special form of secularised and pragmatic familism: family was of a paramount importance to individuals, but family dissolution through divorce or separation was increasingly accepted.

'emancipation' argument), and economically motivated by the permanent shortage of labour in an ineffectively organised economy (e.g., Poland chapter).

[21] The spread of 'Western' culture can be best illustrated by a widespread adoration of 'Western' pop music and fashion among teenagers and young adults. In Russia, for instance, teenagers were willing to invest enormous amount of money to obtain a pair of jeans that were neither produced in state-socialist countries, nor available in ordinary shops (Binyon 1983). Jeans thus constituted a powerful symbol of 'Western' fashion and affluence, and jeans ownership gave teenagers higher status among their peers.

The picture is similarly mixed with respect to the *ability dimension*. On the one hand, legislative changes enabled some of the family changes typical of the SDT, for example, through relatively good access to divorce, and a wide availability of abortion in most state-socialist countries. At the same time, the widespread reluctance towards the production and distribution of the contraceptive pill, combined with a discouragement of abortion among childless young women (often explained on the grounds of the potential pregnancy complications later in life), and a lack of comprehensive education on sexuality and contraception, helped to sustain a pattern of early pregnancies and shotgun marriages, and of overall higher fertility due to unwanted and mistimed pregnancies.

On balance, the peculiar combination of the *R-W-A* factors during state socialism helps to explain why some types of family-related changes, such as an increase in divorce, had spread rapidly in many countries, while other behaviours typical of the SDT could not spread much because at least one factor of the *R-W-A dimension* acted as a bottleneck, preventing the diffusion of the new behaviour. For example, a combination of preferential housing distribution and special marriage loans (*R dimension*), the strong persistence of norms supporting traditional family (*W dimension*), and the low access to modern contraception, especially the pill (*A dimension*) helped to sustain an early and almost universal pattern of first marriage and first birth, with a pronounced peak among women in their late teens and early twenties.

A specific combination of *R-W-A* factors in Central and Eastern Europe prior to 1990 also affected the changes in family behaviour after the collapse of communism. The early erosion of some traditional norms related to the family helps to explain why the new demographic trends have spread with such intensity after the breakdown of the state-socialist system.[22] In an environment in which traditional norms had diminished, and the more recent communist ideology had been discredited, there was relatively little resistance to forms of behaviour that would have been deemed inappropriate in more traditional settings. Philipov (2003) stresses the importance of discontinuity and the resulting disorientation and anomie (normlessness) after the regime change around 1990. The lack of generally recognised norms of behaviour supported the diffusion of the less stable forms of partnership, and the postponement of union formation and parenthood (see also Bulgaria chapter). These factors explain why the *W dimension* did not constitute a

---

[22] It should be noted, however, that the official Communist ideology gradually espoused a rather conservative model of the family, pursuing the idea of parental 'duty' and the responsibility of women to the society to bear children. Paradoxically, this ideology has in some instances developed into a morality similar to the orthodox teachings of the Catholic Church (Ferge 1997).

strong barrier to the spread of many new forms of behaviour. As was the case in Western and Northern Europe, many 'traditional' family norms had already eroded or had diminished in importance during the decades following the Second World War, or their importance had weakened significantly during the turbulent period of the late 1980s and the early 1990s.[23] In this environment, many people openly embraced values and living standards characteristic of Western European countries (see also below).

4.4 Emerging cultural and family divides in Central and Eastern Europe

A new family divide has (re-)emerged among post-communist countries after 1990, reflecting varying degrees of secularisation, modernisation, and traditionalism (especially in countries with a predominantly Roman Catholic tradition), as well as historical regional divisions (e.g., Fux 2008).[24] These differences appear to have a lasting impact on the progression of the second demographic transition, and, more generally, on demographic patterns there. Selected chapters express a contrasting evaluation of the importance of religion, and the reputation enjoyed by religious authorities in the respective countries. On the one hand, a majority of the population in Romania believes that the (Orthodox) church provides the "right answers to family issues" (Muresan et al. 2008:895), the Catholic Church in Poland continues to enjoy "the highest ranks of social trust" (Kotowska et al. 2008:838), and the Catholic Church in Slovakia "plays an important role in the society and has an influence on reproductive behaviour" (Potančoková et al. 2008:1007). On the other hand, in Slovenia, the "position of the [Catholic] Church and the clergy on the confidence scale is low" (Stropnik and Šircelj 2008:1039) and religious affiliation, church attendance and the support of traditional religion are at very low levels in the Czech Republic (Sobotka et al. 2008:436; see also Stankuniene and Maslauskaite 2008). On an individual level, religiosity still exerts a substantial impact on the attitudes to marriage and childbearing. Less religious people in Europe tend to reject

---

[23] Unfortunately, very little comparable data exist on family-related values and attitudes in Central and Eastern Europe during the state-socialist era. Thus, most of the literature on changes in values and attitudes in this region take the early 1990s as a starting point, often implicitly assuming that the surveys conducted in the early 1990s also provide a portrait of values prevalent before the collapse of state socialism.

[24] Fux (2008) discusses the links between historically dominant religious traditions, developments of welfare state, modernisation, and differentiation in demographic behaviour in Europe. His study is one of the few that address emerging differences in welfare regimes and family patterns in Central and Eastern Europe.

the benefits and exclusivity of marriage as a form of partnership (Pongrácz and Spéder 2008), and consider children less essential to their lives (Fokkema and Esveld 2008).

On a country level, the prevalence of different family trajectories can be interpreted in conjunction with different levels of secularisation. Stankuniene and Maslauskaite (2008), while cautioning against simply equating religiosity with 'conservative' attitudes towards family changes, also attribute the huge differences in the acceptance of the changes in family formation in Central and Eastern Europe to a combination of the early onset of these changes, and different levels of individualisation and secularisation. Among the six societies analysed, respondents were found to evaluate selected family changes most positively in highly individualised, secularised and non-Catholic East Germany, and, to a lesser extent, in the strongly secularised Czech Republic. On the other hand, respondents in religious and conservative Polish society assessed recent changes in family formation most negatively. The correlation between religiosity and family behaviour is often clearly detectable on a regional level. In the Czech Republic, for example, the proportion of people who declare their religious affiliation is negatively linked to the proportion of extramarital births on a district level (Czech Republic chapter). Thus, the new family behaviour spreads most intensively in the most secularised regions, where it meets little resistance. In the more religious regions, church and other moral authorities, as well as a significant portion of the population, oppose the new family behaviour. In these countries, the *W factor* may constitute a bottleneck that slows down the spread of the second demographic transition.[25]

With a general decline in the importance of the *willingness dimension* before 1990, the *readiness factor* increased in prominence. A number of chapters emphasise the role of economic and structural constraints as the main driving forces of the SDT behaviour among post-communist countries during the 1990s (e.g., Bulgaria, Lithuania, Poland, and Ukraine chapters). Although the initial spread of rapid behavioural changes was indeed primarily facilitated by structural and economic factors in many societies, these shifts have in part rested on peculiar 'atomisation' of society progressing before 1990 (Hungary chapter). Emerging

---

[25] Two countries positioned on the western side of the former Soviet Bloc, the Czech Republic and Poland, illustrate this point. In the secularised Czech Republic, cohabitation and non-marital childbearing have spread rapidly after the regime change in 1989, births and marriages have been postponed massively, the divorce rate has further increased, the contraceptive pill soon became the dominant means of birth control, and, since 2006, homosexual couples may register their partnerships (the Czech Republic chapter). In contrast, in Poland, which remains a highly religious society where the Catholic Church retains considerable influence, abortions were severely restricted since 1993, the use of the contraceptive pill has only spread gradually, cohabitation remains relatively marginal, and acceptance of cohabitation is lower than in most other countries (Poland chapter).

changes in family behaviour have in turn greatly contributed to the rising acceptance and popularity of the new partnership and family forms (thus leading to a further decline in the importance of *W dimension*). Consequently, even when many constraints typical of the transition era diminished, the new trends had become firmly established, and were preferred, or were at least accepted, by a majority of young people. As Lesthaeghe and Surkyn (2002: 215) posited, "[R]ather than the economic crisis per se, it is the entire restructuring of society that is the accelerator of the ideational and demographic changes." This argument suggests that the distribution of the *R dimension* has shifted in favour of the new family behaviour, marked by delayed family formation, rising popularity of less stable types of partnerships, rising numbers of childless individuals and one-child families, and the decline in the importance of marriage. The disappearance of specific factors sustaining the early and almost universal pattern of childbearing and marriage (e.g., the system of preferential housing distribution and pronatalist policies), together with the emergence of many new structural factors favouring late family formation and less traditional living arrangements (e.g., an expansion of tertiary education, delayed home leaving, rapid rise of economic uncertainty in early adulthood, and low availability of housing), have shifted the cost-benefit calculation in favour of the less traditional family behaviour typical of the second demographic transition. As Overview Chapter 5 argues, this shift is long-lasting and cannot be explained by a temporary economic crisis in the early 1990s; rather, it is consistent with the whole transition towards a market economy and adoption of democratic institutions. An additional important element further reinforcing the diffusion of the new family patterns was a conscious adoption and imitation of 'Western' lifestyles and social norms, facilitated partly by the belief that such norms are intrinsically linked to modern life and the economic affluence typical of Western and Northern Europe (Thornton and Philipov 2007).[26] An increasingly common experience of working or studying abroad has further supported the diffusion of new values and lifestyles among the younger population.

As for the *ability dimension*, the rapid spread of modern contraception, especially the pill (see Overview Chapter 3 and some country-specific chapters) has further facilitated the delay of family formation and the rise of cohabitation and other non-traditional living arrangements. Teenagers and young adults are also far

---

[26] Using the example of Albania, writer Slavenka Drakulić (1996: 56) notes the crucial role of foreign TV channels, which were frequently received through satellite dishes, in transmitting idealised images of the life in the 'West' to a population that has never travelled outside the country: "This is where the vision of the future life came from, as well as the idea of what revolution is all about: it should bring not only a change in political power, but also better standard of living."

better informed and educated about contraception and sexuality than their older counterparts growing up in the 1970s and 1980s.

4.5 Diversity in the second demographic transition in Central and Eastern Europe

Overall, the huge differences between Central and Eastern European countries in the current spread and acceptance of SDT behaviours, and of 'post-modern' value orientations, can be explained by a combination of many factors, of which the level of secularisation, the actual welfare and family policies, and historical family patterns appear to be most important. Economic prosperity and affluence are also among the obvious candidates for explaining the cross-country differences in the spread of the SDT. Individualistic values of self-expression and self-fulfilment can thrive only in societies where people experience sufficiently high levels of affluence so that they do not need to worry much about the satisfaction of their basic needs. Finally, the importance of history cannot be overstated. In several Central European countries, 'history' may be seen as a factor explaining the 'return' to the late marriage, late childbearing, and higher childlessness pattern, typical in the past of the populations positioned to the west of Hajnal's (1965) line running between Trieste and St. Petersburg. Such a 'return' to the previous ('Western') demographic patterns has been mentioned by Možný and Katrňák (2005) as an important explanation of demographic changes in the Czech Republic. The breakdown of the 'Eastern Bloc' has led to an emergence of new regional demographic divides (Sobotka 2003), some of which may lead to a reappearance of historical cleavages across Europe (e.g., Fux 2008). But 'history' may also refer to the influence of cultural changes and policies during communism. For instance, Salles (2006) has argued that the policies enacted to help lone mothers, but also to promote marriage in East Germany since the 1970s, eventually had a negative effect on marriage in the long run: "East German family policy instrumentalized marriage and stripped it of all the appeal once the associated material advantages were withdrawn. The family policy of the GDR thus played a key part in weakening of the role of marriage in the family and in East German society" (Salles 2006: 149).

Commenting on the pervasive character of changes in Central and Eastern Europe, Lesthaeghe and Surkyn (2004: 10) concluded that the SDT is emerging there "as a feature that is here to stay, just as in the West. Once more it is emerging as a salient characteristic of capitalist economies and of cultures that recognize the primacy of individual autonomy and that develop the higher order needs." While the findings on behavioural trends—and, to some extent, also on value changes—

generally support this view, it is also important to reiterate vast cross-country differences in the progress of the SDT in this region, and the complexity of different structural and cultural factors fuelling changes in family behaviour (see also the concluding section). Figure 4, showing the score of selected behavioural components of the SDT (SDT1 index), as well as the attitudinal and values components of the SDT (SDT2 index) in 29 European countries, show that the differences in the second demographic transition between post-communist countries of Europe have become large enough to blur any clear distinction between the 'East' of Europe and the other European regions (see Appendix and Section 3 for the definition of SDT indexes). Whereas some post-communist societies reach the lowest SDT score with respect to the behavioural component (Romania and Belarus) and the values component (especially Poland and Latvia), three central European societies (Estonia, Hungary, and the Czech Republic) occupy an intermediate position, while Slovenia scores high on both the behavioural and values component of the SDT. In contrast with this diversity, the clustering of the Nordic countries, German-speaking countries (only data for Austria and Germany are available), and Southern and Western European countries is considerably more compact, broadly corresponding to welfare state typology developed by Esping-Andersen (1990; see also Liefbroer and Fokkema 2008). Remarkably, the behavioural and the values factors are strongly correlated, suggesting that, in line with the theoretical arguments, changes in family and reproductive behaviour progress hand in glove with the characteristic changes in values and attitudes in practically all the countries in which the second demographic transition emerges.

5. Social status differences in behavioural and value changes typical of the transition

Lesthaeghe and Surkyn (1998) stress the importance of education for the spread of post-materialist values that form an essential component of the second demographic transition. Education, when perceived as a proxy for cultural endowment, is linked to non-conformism, decline of traditional religious beliefs, higher permissiveness in personal matters (such as homosexuality or abortion), openness about sexuality, and high values placed on personal self-fulfilment from work (Lesthaeghe and Surkyn 1998: 18). Some earlier studies, especially those conducted in the Low Countries, provided strong support for the idea that highly educated individuals have been the forerunners in the values and behaviour associated with the transition. De Feijter (1991) showed that, alongside age and religious affiliation, having a high level of

Figure 4: **Behavioural (SDT1) and values (SDT2) components of the second demographic transition in Europe**

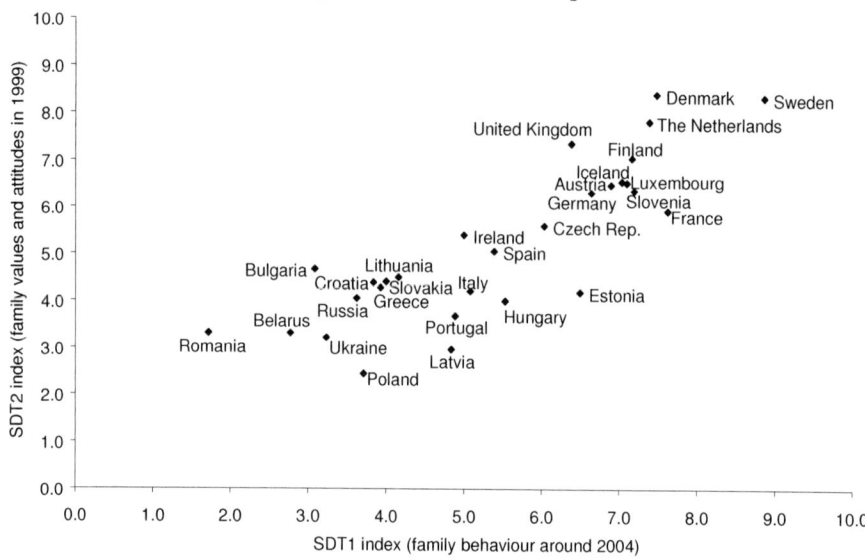

NOTES: A brief description of the SDT indexes is provided in Appendix; see also Section 3 and Sobotka (2008).
SOURCES: Own computations based on vital statistics data in 2004 for the SDT1 index (Council of Europe 2006 and Eurostat 2006) and the data from the European Values Study in 1999-2000 for the SDT2 index (Halman 2001).

education was a powerful determinant of more liberal attitudes towards cohabitation, sexuality, and parenthood in the Netherlands. Cohabitation and voluntary childlessness there were initially most typical of women with higher levels of education. These findings conformed well to the 'classic' theories of cultural innovation, whereby higher-educated and economically advantaged social strata first adopt a new behaviour, which subsequently spreads through 'imitation' to other social groups (e.g., Lesthaeghe and Surkyn 1988). Contemporary research documents wide and often increasing social status heterogeneity in the timing and trajectories of parenthood, union formation and family life (see England and Wales chapter). These trajectories do not, however, always follow a predictable pattern. One paradox, discussed below, appears puzzling: while, as expected, the lower-educated individuals display more 'traditional' or 'conservative' values, they are often the early adopters in the spread of cohabitation, non-marital childbearing, and unstable living arrangements. This is especially true in the case of the post-communist countries of Europe.

If the concept of the second demographic transition is understood as predicting greater diversity in individual behaviour as a result of increased freedom from traditional norms and constraints, then such diversity is closely following educational lines. The connection between different events that typically took place in young adulthood (finishing education, leaving home, entering first job, marrying, and having a first child) has weakened considerably in the Western countries among the post-1950 cohorts. Consequently, a "large majority of individuals do not follow the 'normal' succession of events and ages" (Bourdelais and Gordon 2006: 257). Among younger cohorts higher education implies a progressive delay of most early life transitions, especially of parenthood, while lower-educated women often become parents as teenagers (chapters on the Czech Republic, Slovakia, Spain, and Ukraine; see also McLanahan 2004). In addition, highly educated women still frequently follow the normatively preferred path to childbearing, marked by the succession of school graduation, work, marriage, and first birth. In contrast, women with lower levels of education often "go through shorter routes to motherhood," frequently 'bypassing' regular work and marriage (Ravanera and Rajulton 2004: 11).

In most countries, ultimate family size and childlessness are also clearly differentiated by education, with higher-educated women having the highest levels of childlessness and the lowest levels of fertility.[27] This pattern is most pronounced in countries where career attachment, which is stronger among the higher-educated women, is incompatible with motherhood due to lack of childcare facilities, low level of labour flexibility, low gender equality within the family, or the prevailing normative pressure on mothers to interrupt their work career. The work-childrearing incompatibility, as well as an institutionalised pattern of an extended withdrawal from work among mothers of small children, are frequently cited as the reasons for particularly high childlessness among university-educated women in Austria and Germany (see the respective country chapters). In contrast, in countries where the 'motherhood penalty' is less pronounced, there are smaller or narrowing educational differentials in childlessness and family size (France and Sweden chapter; see also Ekert-Jaffé et al. 2002).[28] In France, childlessness is somewhat higher among the more educated women, but once they become mothers they are more likely to have three children than women of medium educational levels (France chapter). In sum, there seems to be a consistent pattern of fertility differentials by education, which

---

[27] In contrast to women, highly educated men frequently have the lowest level of ultimate childlessness (Sweden chapter).

[28] The Sweden chapter also emphasizes the importance of the field of education, which has a greater impact on fertility than the level of education or the length of education (Hoem, Neyer and Andersson 2006).

are conditional on entering parenthood: the structural and cultural incompatibility of childbearing and pursuing a career usually leads to pronounced education differentials in fertility that are typically attributable to higher childlessness among the more educated women. Once they have their first child, higher-educated women usually display equally high, or even higher, progression rates to second and third births than their less-educated counterparts (e.g., Neels 2006 for Flanders; Rendall and Smallwood 2003 for England and Wales).

Data on fertility intentions suggest that the gap in intended fertility between the higher- and the lower-educated women might become narrower among the 1970s cohorts (see de Graaf and van Duin 2007 for the Netherlands). When controlling for factors like partnership and employment status, and the partner's characteristics, the association of higher levels of education with lower fertility intentions disappears altogether: van Peer and Rabušic (2008) have found that highly educated people in Europe desire a larger family size. Similarly, Sobotka and Testa (2008) show that, net of selected factors[29], an intention to remain childless is expressed most frequently by the lower-educated women.

In line with Lesthaeghe and Surkyn's (1998) argument, individuals with a higher level of education usually display higher acceptance of non-traditional family forms. For instance, Pongrácz and Spéder (2008) show that the attitudes towards unmarried unions are most positive among highly educated men and women, and Fokkema and Esveldt (2008) find that the value attached to children declines with the level of education. For the United States, Pagnini and Rindfuss (1993) found that better-educated women were more tolerant toward non-marital childbearing when responding to three different questions related to it. Several chapters in this collection, especially those on the more 'conservative' societies of Central and Eastern Europe, suggest that young, urban, and better-educated people have developed more positive attitudes towards cohabitation and 'alternative lifestyles' (Poland and Romania chapters), have embraced individualistic values (Lithuania chapter), and spearheaded fertility postponement (Slovakia and Ukraine chapters).

The role of education in the spread of cohabitation differs greatly between countries. Historically, cohabitation in Europe had been practised especially by working-class people and by the poor (Kiernan 2004). More recently, some countries have seen cohabitation spreading as a new lifestyle, especially among the highly educated, and later being adopted by the lower-educated couples.[30] This

---

[29] The model controls for the following factors: Partnership status, employment, religiosity, attitudes towards children, preferred living arrangement, and partner's employment and educational level.
[30] Kalmijn's (2007) cross-country analysis of cohabitation, marriage, and divorce in Europe in the 1990s found a positive effect of tertiary education on cohabitation, but, at the same time, also on marriage rates.

pattern of a modern diffusion of cohabitation, documented for the Netherlands (de Feijter 1991), England and Wales (England and Wales chapter), Italy (Rosina and Fraboni 2004), and Spain (Baizán, Aasve, and Billari 2003), supports the notion of highly educated individuals as open-minded forerunners heralding the changes in family formation.[31] However, in a number of other societies, cohabitation had initially spread among the less-educated and economically disadvantaged people. In Sweden, cohabitation has spread first in the working-class environment, rather than as a 'campus movement' (Hoem 1986). In the United States, cohabitation had been historically most common among the lower-educated (Bumpass and Sweet 1989), and in the 1980s and the 1990s it still remained more prevalent among women who had not completed high school (Bumpass and Lu 2000).[32] Similarly, in a number of Central and Eastern European societies, cohabitation had initially proliferated among the lower-educated, particularly after divorce (see Spéder 2005 for Hungary and Romania chapter). This pattern was also evidenced for Bulgaria, where, according to the Bulgaria chapter, cohabitation had spread in the 1990s as an an arrangement without a long commitment, especially among lower-educated women, who typically have disadvantaged occupational and earning status, and are thus less attractive on the marriage market (Koytcheva and Philipov 2008:377). Such diversity in the spread of cohabitation can be partly explained by the diversity of cohabitation as a living arrangement (see Overview Chapter 4). A cross-country comparison of divorce by Härkönen and Donkers (2006) shows that divorce rates among women are also not systematically patterned by education. Whereas nine out of 17 analysed countries did not have a significant education gradient of divorce, five countries (France, Greece, Italy, Poland, and Spain) had higher divorce rates among higher-educated women, whereas three countries (Austria, Lithuania, and the United States) had higher divorce propensity among lower-educated women. In addition, higher prevalence of divorce and non-traditional family behaviour (cohabitation and extramarital births) was associated with a shift towards a negative educational gradient.

Whereas the role of higher levels of education in the diffusion of cohabitation and prevalence of divorce differs across countries, the evidence on the spread of non-marital childbearing and lone motherhood, in particular, is relatively uniform:

This suggests that educational expansion may be positively linked to the diffusion of cohabitation, but does not necessarily lead to a decline in the popularity of marriage.

[31] Rosina and Fraboni (2004) have also detected a strong significant effect of father's education on a young woman's propensity to enter cohabitation before marriage (model based on data for Northern and Central regions of Italy).

[32] However, in line with the SDT arguments cohabitation in the U.S. is also linked to less traditional value orientation. It is more typical of people who are "slightly more liberal, less religious, and more supportive of egalitarian gender roles and nontraditional family" (Smock 2000: 4).

highly educated women have the highest propensity to marry before childbearing, and therefore have the lowest ratio of extramarital births. Even in a country like Sweden, where cohabitation has become almost indistinguishable from marriage (Heuveline and Timberlake 2004), and where more than half of all births take place outside marriage, women and men with a university degree have the highest rates of marriage (Bracher and Santow 1998). This finding holds irrespective of whether they are cohabiting or not, although the latter case – direct marriage – is rather unusual there (Sweden chapter). The association of low educational levels with a high frequency of extramarital childbearing is illustrated in Table 1 with data from selected countries of Central Europe (Austria, the Czech Republic, Hungary and Poland). Except in Austria, the educational gradient is very steep: for women with the lowest levels of education, non-marital childbearing has become a common experience and the percentage of out-of-wedlock births among this group exceeds by a factor of 5-10 the share among university-educated women. In Austria, where unmarried parenthood has a long tradition in many Alpine regions (Austria chapter), this educational gradient is only moderate, and women who achieved only a primary level of education have a below-average percentage of extramarital births. This finding is attributable to a high proportion of immigrant women with more traditional and religious background among the lowest-educated group, for whom extramarital childbearing is not morally acceptable.

Table 1: **Percentage of extramarital births by the highest educational attainment of mother in selected countries of Central Europe, 1990-2005**

| | Year | Highest educational attainment | | | | | |
		Basic (including incomplete)	Apprentice-ship and basic vocational	Lower secondary	Higher Secondary	Tertiary	Total
Austria	1996	26.9	32.6	25.7	24.7	19.7	28.0
Austria	2005	28.7	43.3	38.6	35.3	30.6	36.5
Czech Republic	1990	26.6	7.7		4.1	3.3	8.6
Czech Republic	1995	44.5	14.4		7.8	5.7	15.6
Czech Republic	2005	67.6	37.2		23.8	13.7	31.7
Poland	2003	39.4	16.9	12.6		6.6	15.8
		Completed years of education					
		0-7	8	9-12	13+		Total
Hungary	1990	49.1	16.2	6.3	4.5		13.1
Hungary	1998	63.5	33.0	16.9	10.4		26.6

SOURCES: Statistics Austria 1997 and 2006, FSO 1991, CZSO 1996 and 2006, GUS 2004 and Pongrácz 2002 (Table 3)

However, in all cases, the trend over time is uniform, towards a higher share of non-marital births among women of all educational levels. Thus, extramarital childbearing (and, frequently, also cohabitation) constitutes a peculiar feature of the second demographic transition, which spreads from the lowest-educated population to the more affluent and higher-educated social groups. It is plausible that, among the higher-educated women, non-marital childbearing usually takes place in the context of stable cohabiting unions, whereas lower-educated women frequently experience lone motherhood or childbearing within unstable partnerships. Kiernan's (1999) analysis of the FFS data indicates that non-graduate women are more likely than graduate women to have a child before experiencing any partnership. Numerous studies conducted in the United States show that non-marital childbearing and unstable unions are concentrated especially among the women at the bottom of the educational and income distribution, and that this group increasingly differs from the higher-income and higher-educated group (Lundberg and Pollak 2007). McLanahan (2004) argues that the rising divergence in partnership, family, and work trajectories of lower-educated and higher-educated women and their partners is linked to an increasingly disadvantaged economic position of the former group. This argument, which is likely to hold for most societies of Europe as well, suggests that some behaviours associated with the STD spread first as a reaction or an accommodation to economic and social disadvantages, rather than as an alternative lifestyle of highly educated individuals.

6. Summary and conclusions

The progression of the characteristic changes in family behaviour

Chapters in this collection demonstrate that wide-sweeping changes in partnership and family behaviour have spread to all parts of Europe. More recently, this trend has been particularly pronounced in Southern Europe and in the post-communist countries of Central and Eastern Europe (see also Lesthaeghe and Surkyn 2004), which had been often perceived as rather 'immune' to the rapid diffusion of the transition. In country after country, births and marriages have been postponed intensively. Cohabitation has become a common choice for a first union, and has increasingly emerged as a substitution for marriage. Meanwhile, marriage rates have plummeted, and the connection between marriage, sexual life, and childbearing has rapidly eroded. The spread of cohabitation and LAT arrangements have been connected with an increase in partnership instability, which is also signalled by persistently high or increasing divorce rates. Some 'traditional' pathways to first partnership and first birth have become unusual in the countries that have progressed furthest in the second demographic transition (see Overview Chapter 4). Sexual initiation takes place well before the formation of a first partnership, not only because of an earlier onset of sexual activity, but also owing to a postponement of partnership formation. 'Direct' marriage not preceded by cohabitation has become in some countries an unusual pathway typical of specific religious and ethnic groups. Furthermore, having a first child within marriage is becoming a 'minority experience' in a rising number of countries. Symptomatic of this change is a marked decline in the normative pressure to marry in the case of out-of-wedlock pregnancies, leading to a gradual disappearance of the once relatively common phenomenon of 'shotgun marriages.' If not permanent, the new family behaviour appears to be a long-standing trait of the European demographic landscape, which is here to stay for many decades.

In the post-communist countries of Europe, where the new behavioural trends are often thought of as arising in response to the economic crisis and 'anomie' of the early 1990s, these changes have been further intensifying during the recent period of higher prosperity and economic recovery. While fertility and marriage postponement, as well as voluntary childlessness, have been heralded by higher-educated women, lower-educated individuals are often at the forefront of the rise of unstable living arrangements and non-marital fertility. Paradoxically, higher-educated people, who have generally more positive attitudes towards the new family forms, resist longest the erosion of the 'bourgeois family,' especially when they decide to have children.

Changes in family-related values and attitudes

Attitudes towards children, family, and sexuality remain widely differentiated across Europe, to an extent which is impossible to portray accurately in this review. However, a common direction of changes can be clearly detected across all countries (perhaps with the exception of Albania), which is generally in agreement with the second demographic transition hypothesis:

- a move towards tolerant and generally positive attitudes regarding intimate relationships among unmarried and un-partnered people, including young adults and teenagers
- a positive regard for cohabitation as a specific premarital stage, and its rising recognition as an alternative to marriage

- a higher tolerance of non-family living arrangements and voluntary childlessness

Marriage and childbearing have increasingly become optional parts of individual biographies, even in countries that have been until recently considered rather 'conservative.' For example, the Spain chapter emphasises the increasing freedom in the design of individual life projects: "inherited models of family organization have ceased to be binding; the form that family life eventually adopts have thus come to depend on the negotiation" (Delgado et al. 2008:1087). These shifts do not imply, however, that family has become an obsolete institution. It has undergone a remarkable transformation: "feelings and love have become the centre of the family, a trend that explains the weakening of the conjugal bond, the loss of popularity of marriage, and the growing complexity of marital trajectories" (Toulemon et al. 2008:524). At the same time, the family appears to have adapted well to the increase in individual autonomy (France chapter). Perhaps the most important indication of the continuing strength of the family is the persistent high value attached to family and children and the overwhelmingly positive attitude towards parenthood. This may partly explain the absence of a negative association between the second demographic transition, and fertility level as well as childbearing intentions in contemporary Europe.

Structural constraints may facilitate some SDT trends among disadvantaged social groups

The experience of the post-communist countries of Central and Eastern Europe highlights the importance of structural factors in facilitating the trends associated with the SDT. The initial contributions (e.g., van de Kaa 1987) tended to emphasise the prominence of normative and value changes for an initiation of the second demographic transition. When economic factors entered the SDT narrative, economic prosperity was perceived as an engine of cultural dynamics: it leads to an increase in individual aspirations and to the accentuation of higher-order needs and individual self-fulfilment (for a more detailed elaboration see Lesthaeghe and Surkyn 1988). This mechanism seems to be instrumental for explaining value changes symptomatic of the SDT. However, some characteristic behavioural changes, such as the rapid rise in cohabitation and non-marital childbearing, can also be driven by the emergence of new structural factors that make such behaviour more attractive for people with a socially disadvantaged background. This was often the case during the transition process in Central and Eastern Europe: the rapid restructuring of society towards a capitalist market economy led to much social and economic turbulence, as well as to increased anomie, which most affected the lowest-educated individuals. As many structural characteristics of capitalist economies, such as huge income disparities, unstable working conditions, and a need for more lifestyle flexibility (see also Mills and Blossfeld 2005) are not compatible with the 'bourgeois ideal' of a stable family consisting of a married couple with (a) child(ren), lower-educated individuals were often at the forefront of a shift towards extramarital childbearing and cohabitation. Perhaps unwillingly, disadvantaged segments of the population may thus become trendsetters of new behaviour, paving the way to a wider legitimisation and acceptance of the new family forms, which are later openly embraced by the rising number of highly educated individuals.

Two pathways of the SDT diffusion

Such a mechanism of change is consistent with the *Ready-Willing-Able (RWA)* model of diffusion of new behaviour, which has been advocated by Lesthaeghe and his colleagues (e.g., Lesthaeghe, Neidert and Surkyn 2006), and which has also been adopted in this chapter for explaining the diffusion of the second demographic transition in the post-communist countries of Europe. If the arguments sketched above are valid, we are left with two pathways of behavioural and value changes in the course of the second demographic transition. The first one, consistent with the 'classical' narrative of the SDT, sees cultural and value changes as factors driven by economic affluence and characterised by secular individualism, and by an orientation towards personal self-fulfilment as a precondition to large-scale changes in family behaviour. In this case, the new behaviour is first heralded by the more educated and economically more privileged social groups, who adopt new preferences with respect to their living arrangements and childbearing and their 'coordination' with other domains of life (education, employment, leisure). The second pathway may first lead to an emergence of new family behaviour, especially among the disadvantaged strata, as a response to changed structural conditions in the society, frequently marked by economic crisis. In this case, the new behaviour is less driven by new choices and personal preferences, and may constitute a reaction to adverse life circumstances. Consequently, as this behaviour spreads, it gradually becomes accepted and adopted by other social groups, which in turn leads to the changes in attitudes towards it and its continuous diffusion. This diffusion becomes self-reinforcing and continues even at the time when the conditions which had facilitated an emergence of the new behaviour decline in importance (Kohler,

Billari, and Ortega 2002). Needless to say, changes in values and behaviour are reinforcing each other (e.g., Rindfuss et al. 2004), and none of these pathways occurs in a 'pure form.' In real life, a mixture of cultural and structural changes may lead to differentiated responses and feedback effects among various social groups, whose values and life histories may also differ markedly.

The importance of the 'gender revolution' for the spread of SDT and for fertility recuperation

The '*gender revolution*' was marked by a huge expansion of higher education among women, their increasingly perfect ability to prevent unwanted pregnancies, women's massive and almost universal participation in the labour market and their resulting economic independence, and also their higher aspirations, in which an employment career constitutes an expected and essential part of their life biographies (Goldin 2006). This 'revolution' ended what Keyfitz (1986) described as a societal 'conspiracy' that maintained the image of women as mothers and wives, enforced a strong socialisation of girls towards these roles and where various elements converged to "maintain women in a position where their time was available for reproduction and for not much else" (Keyfitz 1986: 150). The gender revolution in a broad sense appears to be one of the most important factors driving the trends associated with the second demographic transition. Countries that were first to embrace the principles of gender equality, particularly the Nordic countries, now score highest in the SDT progression (Sweden chapter). Macro-level analysis by Kalmijn (2007) shows that the proportion of women in paid employment is linked to lower marriage rates, higher divorce rates, and higher levels of cohabitation. 'Women's liberation' might possibly also explain the positive association between the second demographic transition and fertility. Countries where many people adhered early to egalitarianism and women's emancipation also enacted at an early stage different policies supporting gender equality, which subsequently reduced the incompatibility of work and childrearing. These policies are conducive for the 'recuperation' of fertility at later childbearing ages, especially among more-educated women, which I found to be strongly associated with the transition. In addition, the ideology of gender equality nurtures more equal division of household and childcare tasks between partners, reducing gender asymmetries within the family that may strongly contribute to low fertility in many parts of Southern, Central, and Eastern Europe (Esping-Andersen 1999, McDonald 2000; see also Lithuania chapter).

As women increasingly outnumber men in tertiary education in most OECD countries (OECD 2005), their economic and employment position is poised to improve further in the future, whereas more men will probably become unemployed, unemployable, and economically disadvantaged. This may bring yet unforeseen consequences for the course of future family and fertility change, some of which may be linked to the rising inability of many women to find a suitable partner matching their level of education and income.

Further progression of the transition and the likely future trends in fertility

The experiences of the Nordic countries, of France, and also of the United States, indicate that the SDT does not inevitably lead to long-term sub-replacement fertility, especially when fertility rates are analysed in a cohort perspective. The future of the fertility – SDT relationship remains open. It is possible that the progression of the SDT in countries with currently very low fertility, such as Italy and Spain, will lead to a wider acceptance and the further spread of very low fertility, and of a one-child family norm even when the structural constraints initially responsible for a pronounced fertility decline eventually diminish. In other words, low fertility rates in the last two decades would engender low family size preferences among younger cohorts that were socialised under the new low-fertility regime, a possibility envisioned by Lutz, Skirbekk, and Testa (2006). But an alternative outcome is possible as well: some structural factors that are arguably affecting fertility behaviour in many countries may be seen as an outcome of a delayed societal adaptation to the progressing second demographic transition. In this view, the persistence of the traditional family norms and expectations, the continuation of family policies tailored to support the 'male breadwinner model,' and the persistence of marked gender inequality within the family in many low-fertility societies may be seen as temporary features of societies that failed to adapt to the changing character of family and partnership behaviours. Then, the very low fertility observed in Southern Europe, Central-Eastern Europe, and the German-speaking countries may be perceived as a temporary outcome of the second demographic transition (see also Sobotka 2008), whose importance may diminish if the society embraces gender equality and adapts to the new patterns of family behaviour. This view is voiced in the chapter on Italy, which suggests that the slow spread of non-marital fertility in Italy is a syndrome of an "uncompleted second demographic transition," (De Rose et al. 2008:678) which is in part responsible for very low fertility in Italy. More generally, the authors view "a lack of modernity" as "a main cause of the current depressed childbearing level" (De Rose et al. 2008:679).

On the usefulness of the second demographic transition concept

In conclusion, the second demographic transition seems to be particularly useful as an umbrella concept that encompasses a broad range of interrelated changes in sexuality, family, and partnership behaviours and attitudes, as well as a massive postponement of parenthood. This chapter has shown that, despite widely different social and economic contexts, the SDT provides a powerful narrative reflecting well the shared trajectories in the evolution of the new model of family and reproduction in Europe during the last four decades. As the relationship of the SDT to fertility levels is shown to diverge from the originally envisioned negative association, the term itself may be seen as problematic—it is too suggestive of an irreversible and predictable shift in reproductive behaviour, similar to the concept of the (first) demographic transition. However, as the term has become firmly established, it would be fruitless to attempt to change it. The SDT is also potentially problematic as a scientific theory. On one hand, it appears to hold quite well on a very general level: if, for instance, the SDT concept were used to foresee the trends in family and fertility behaviours after the establishment of democracy and market capitalism in Central and Eastern Europe after 1989, it would have provided a very sound projection of general change. On the other hand, the SDT is too fuzzy as a theory when scrutinised on a finer level. By definition, historical contingency, context-specific institutions, and multiple interactions between ideational and behavioural changes always make it extremely difficult to construct a theory that can precisely specify conditions under which a certain change in behaviour takes place. But the experience of many countries of Central and Eastern Europe, which can be seen as a giant demographic laboratory, indicates that much more research needs to be done in order to pinpoint the most important structural and cultural factors that stand at the root of the SDT in diverse settings, and to specify how different facets of SDT behaviour are initiated, and later progress across social groups.

7. Acknowledgements

I am thankful to Arland Thornton, Ron Lesthaeghe and three anonymous reviewers for their useful comments and suggestions. An initial version of this chapter was discussed at the workshop on "Family changes in industrialised countries" at Cumberland Lodge in Windsor in May 2008.

References

Adsera, A. 2004. "Changing fertility rates in developed countries. The impact of labour market institutions." *Journal of Population Economics* 17(1): 1-27.

Ariès, P. 1980. "Two successive motivations for the declining birth rate in the West." *Population and Development Review*, 6(4): 645-650.

Avdeev A. and A. Monnier. 1995. "A survey of modern Russian fertility". *Population: An English selection* 7: 1-38.

Baizán, P., A. Aassve, and F. C. Billari. 2003. "Cohabitation, marriage, and first birth: The interrelationship of family formation events in Spain". *European Journal of Population* 19 (2): 147-169.

Bauman, Z. 2000. *Liquid modernity.* Polity Press, Cambridge.

Beets, G., E. Dourleijn, A. Liefbroer, and K. Henkens. 2001. *De timing van het eerste kind in Nederland en Europa.* Raport No. 59, NIDI, Den Haag.

Billari, F. C. and C. Wilson. 2001. "Convergence towards diversity? Cohort dynamics in the transition to adulthood in contemporary Western Europe". *MPIDR Working paper* WP 2001-39, Max Planck Institute for Demographic Research, Rostock. www.demogr.mpg.de/Papers/Working/WP-2001-039.pdf

Binyon, M. 1983. *Life in Russia.* New York: Pantheon Books.

Bourdelais, P. and V. Gourdon. 2006. "Demographic categories revisited. Age categories and the age of the categories." In.: C. Sauvain-Dugerdil, H. Leridon, and N. Mascie-Taylor (eds.) *Human Clock. The Bio-cultural Meanings of Age.* Vol. 5, Population, Family, and Society. Peter Lang, Bern, pp. 245-269.

Bracher, M. and G. Santow. 1998. "Economic independence and union formation in Sweden." *Population Studies* 52: 275-294.

Bumpass, L. and H.-H. Lu. 2000. "Trends in cohabitation and implications for children's family context in the United States." *Population Studies* 54(1): 29-41.

Bumpass, L. L. and J. A. Sweet. 1989. "National estimates of cohabitation." *Demography* 26(4): 615-625.

Cliquet, R. L. 1991. *The second demographic transition: fact or fiction?* Population Studies, Vol. 23. Council of Europe, Strasbourg

Coale, A. J. 1973. "The demographic transition reconsidered." In: IUSSP, Proceedings of the International Population Conference, Liège, Editions Ordina, Vol. 1, pp. 53–72.

Coleman, D. 2004. "Why we don't have to believe without doubting in the "Second demographic transition"—some agnostic comments." *Vienna Yearbook of Population Research* 2004: 11-24.

Council of Europe. 2006. *Recent demographic developments in Europe 2005.* Strasbourg: Council of Europe Publishing.

CZSO. 1996. *Pohyb obyvatelstva v České republice v roce 1995* [Population movement in the Czech Republic in 1995]. Český statistický úřad / Czech Statistical Office, Prague.

CZSO. 2006. *Demografická ročenka České republiky 2005* [Demographic yearbook of the Czech Republic 2005]. Český statistický úřad / Czech Statistical Office, Prague. http://www.czso.cz/csu/2006edicniplan.nsf/p/4019-06

Dalla Zuanna, G., A. De Rose, and F. Racioppi. 2005. "Low fertility and limited diffusion of modern contraception in Italy during the second half of the twentieth Century." *Journal of Population Research* 22(1): 21-48.

de Beer, J., M. Corijn and F. Deven. 2000. "Summary and discussion." In: J. De Beer and F. Deven (eds.) *Diversity in Family Formation. The 2nd Demographic Transition in Belgium and in the Netherlands.* Kluwer Academic Publishers, Dordrecht, 115–130.

De Rose, A., Racioppi, F., and Zanatta, A-L. 2008. Italy: Delayed adaptation of social institutions to changes in family behaviour, *Demographic Research* 19(19). http://www.demographic-research.org/Volumes/Vol19/19/

de Feijter, H. 1991. *Voorlopers bij demografische veranderingen.* NIDI Reports No. 22, NIDI, The Hague.

de Graaf, A. and C. Van Duin. 2007. "Bevolkingsprognose 2006–2050: veronderstellingen over de geboorte." *Bevolkingstrends*, 1e kwartaal 2007: 45-55. www.cbs.nl/nl-NL/menu/themas/bevolking/publicaties/artikelen/archief/2007/2007-k1-b15-p45-art.htm

Delgado, M., Meil, G., and Zamora López, F. 2008. Spain: Short on children and short on family policies, *Demographic Research* 19(27). http://www.demographic-research.org/Volumes/Vol19/27/

Dorbritz, J. 2008. Germany: Family diversity with low actual and desired fertility, *Demographic Research* 19(17). http://www.demographic-research.org/Volumes/Vol19/17/

Drakulić, S. 1996. *Café Europa. Life after Communism.* London: Abacus.

Ekert-Jaffé, O., H. Joshi, K. Lynch, R. Mougin, and M. Rendall. 2002. "Fertility, timing of births and socio-economic status in France and Britain". *Population-E* 57 (3): 475-508.

Esping-Andersen, G. 1999. *Social foundations of postindustrial economies.* Oxford University Press, Oxford.

Esping-Andersen, G. 1990. *The three worlds of welfare capitalism.* Polity Press, Cambridge.

Eurostat. 2006. *Population statistics. 2006 edition.* Luxembourg: Office for official Publications of the European Communities.

Ferge, Z. 1997. "Women and social transformation in Central-Eastern Europe". *Czech Sociological Review* 5 (2): 159-178.

Fokkema, T. and I. Esveldt. 2008. "Motivation to have children in Europe" In: Ch. Höhn, D. Avramov, and I. Kotowska (Eds.) *People, Population Change and Policies: Lessons from the Population Policy Acceptance Study – Volume 1.* Berlin: Springer, pp. 141-155.

Frejka, T. and J.-P. Sardon. 2007. "Cohort birth order, parity progression ratio and parity distribution trends in developed countries." *Demographic Research* 16, Article 11, pp. 315-374. www.demographic-research.org

FSO. 1991. *Pohyb obyvatelstva v České a Slovenské Federativní republice v roce 1990: část 1.* Federální statistický úřad (Federal Statistical Office), Český statistický úřad, Slovenský statistický úřad, Praha.

Fux, B. 2008. "Pathways of welfare and population-related policies. Towards a multidimensional typology of welfare state regimes in Eastern and Western Europe". In: Ch. Höhn, D. Avramov, and I. Kotowska (Eds.) *People, Population Change and*

Policies: Lessons from the Population Policy Acceptance Study – Volume 1. Berlin: Springer, pp. 59-90.

Gerber, T. P. and D. Berman. 2006. "Economic Crisis or Second Demographic Transition? Trends and Correlates of Union Formation in Russia, 1985-2001." Updated version, Paper presented at the Annual Meeting of the Population Association of America 2005, Philadelphia.

Gerber, T. P. and E. B. Cottrell. 2006. "Fertility in Russia, 1985-2001. Insights from individual fertility histories." Paper presented at the Annual Meeting of the Population Association of America, Los Angeles, March 2006.

Giddens, A. 1992. *The transformation of intimacy. Sexuality, love & eroticism in modern societies.* Polity Press, Cambridge.

Goldin, C. 2006. "The quiet revolution that transformed women's employment, education, and family." *American Economic Review* 96(2): 1-21.

GUS. 2004. *Rocznik demograficzny. Demographic Yearbook of Poland 2004.* Główny urząd statystyczny / Central Statistical Office, Warsaw.

Hajnal, J. 1965. "European marriage patterns in perspective". In.: D. V. Glass and D. Eversley (eds.) *Population in history.* London, pp. 101-143.

Halman, L. 2001. *The European Values Study. A third wave.* Source book of the 1999/2000 European Values Study surveys. WORC, Tilburg University.

Härkönen, J. and J. Dronkers. 2006. "Stability and change in the educational gradient of divorce. A comparison of seventeen countries." *European Sociological Review* 22(5): 501-517.

Heuveline, P. and J. M. Timberlake. 2004. "The role of cohabitation in family formation: The United States in comparative perspective." *Journal of Marriage and Family* 66: 1214-1230.

Hoem, J. 1986. "The impact of education on modern family initiation." *European Journal of Population* 2: 113-133.

Hoem, J., A. Jasilioniene, D. Kostova, and C. Muresan. 2007. "The second demographic transition in selected countries in Central and Eastern Europe: Union formation as a demographic manifestation." Research note, Max Planck Institute for Demographic Research, Rostock.

Hoem, J., G. Neyer, and G. Andersson. 2006. "Education and childlessness: the relationship between educational field, educational level, and childlessness among Swedish women born in 1955-59." *Demographic Research* 14, Article 15: 331-380. http://www.demographic-research.org

Inglehart, R. 1990. *Culture shift in advanced industrial society.* Princeton University Press, Princeton, New Jersey.

Kalmijn, M. 2007. "Explaining cross-national differences in marriage, cohabitation, and divorce in Europe." *Population Studies* 61(3): 243-263.

Katus, K., A. Puur, A. Põldma, and L. Sakkeus. 2007. "First union formation in Estonia, Latvia, and Lithuania: Patterns across countries and gender." *Demographic Research* 17, Article 10: 247-300. http://www.demographic-research.org

Kertzer, D. K., M. W. White, L. Bernardi, and G. G. Gabrielli. 2006. "Italy's path to very low fertility. The adequacy of economic and second demographic transition theories." MPIDR Working Paper WP-2006-049, Max Planck Instittue for demographic research, Rostock. http://www.demogr.mpg.de/papers/working/wp-2006-049.pdf.

Keyfitz, N. 1986. "The family that does not reproduce itself." In.: *Below-Replacement Fertility in Industrial Societies: Causes, Consequences, Policies.* Supplement to Vol. 12, *Population and Development Review,* pp. 139-154

Kiernan, K. 2004. "Unmarried cohabitation and parenthood in Britain and Europe". *Law & Policy* 26(1): 33-55.

Kiernan, K. 1999. "Childbearing outside marriage in Western Europe." *Population Trends* 98 (Winter 1999): 11-20.

Kohler, H.-P., F. C. Billari, and J. A. Ortega. 2002. "The emergence of lowest-low fertility in Europe during the 1990s". *Population and Development Review* 28 (4): 641-680.

Kotowska, I., Jóźwiak, J., Matysiak, A., and Baranowska, A. 2008. Poland: Fertility decline as a response to profound societal and labour market changes?, *Demographic Research* 19(22). http://www.demographic-research.org/Volumes/Vol19/22/

Koytcheva, E., and Philipov, D. 2008. Bulgaria: Ethnic differentials in rapidly declining fertility, *Demographic Research* 19(13). http://www.demographic-research.org/Volumes/Vol19/13/

Kraaykamp, G. 2002. "Trends and countertrends in sexual permissiveness: Three decades of attitude change in thye Netherlands." *Journal of Marriage and the Family* 64: 225-239.

Kuijsten, A. C. 1996. "Changing family patterns in Europe: A case of divergence?" *European Journal of Population* 12(2): 115-143.

Lesthaeghe, R. 1995. "The second demographic transition in Western countries: An interpretation". In.: K. O. Mason and A.-M. Jensen (eds.) *Gender and family change in industrialized countries.* Oxford, Clarendon Press, pp. 17-62.

Lesthaeghe, R. and K. Neels. 2002. "From the first to the second demographic transition: An interpretation of the spatial continuity of demographic innovation in France, Belgium and Switzerland". *European Journal of Population* 18(4): 325-360.

Lesthaeghe, R. and L. Neidert. 2006. "The second demographic transition in the United States: Exception or textbook example?" *Population and Development Review* 32(4): 669-698.

Lesthaeghe, R., L. Neidert and J. Surkyn. 2006. "Household formation and the 'Second demographic transition' in Europe and the U.S. Insights from middle range models." http://sdt.psc.isr.umich.edu/pubs/online/rl_romantic_unions_paper.pdf

Lesthaeghe R. and J. Sukyn. 1988. "Cultural dynamics and economic theories of fertility change."*Population and Development Review* 14(1): 1-45.

Lesthaeghe, R. and J. Surkyn. 2002. "New forms of household formation in Central and Eastern Europe: Are they related to newly emerging value orientations?" In.: *Economic Survey of Europe 2002/1.* Economic Commission for Europe, United Nations, New York and Geneva, pp. 197-216.

Lesthaeghe, R. and J. Surkyn. 2004. "When history moves on: The foundations and diffusion of a second demographic transition" Paper presented at the seminar on "Ideational perspectives on international family change", Population Studies Center, Institute for Social Research (ISR), University of Michigan, Ann Arbor. http://sdt.psc.isr.umich.edu/pubs/online/WhenHistoryMovesOn_final.pdf.

Lesthaeghe, R. and D. J. van de Kaa. 1986. "Twee demografische transities?" In.: D. J. van de Kaa and R. Lesthaeghe (eds.) *Bevolking: groei en krimp.* Van Loghum Slaterus, Deventer, pp. 9-24.

Lesthaeghe, R and C Vanderhoeft. 2001. "Ready, willing, and able: a conceptualization of transitions to new behavioral forms." In.: J. B. Casterline (ed.) *Diffusion processes and fertility transition. Selected perspectives,*. Washington, D.C.: National Academy Press, pp. 240-264.

Liefbroer, A. C. 2005. "The impact of perceived costs and rewards of childbearing on entry into parenthood: Evidence from a panel study." *European Journal of Population* 21(4): 367-391.

Liefbroer, A. C. and T. Fokkema. 2008. "Recent developments in demographically relevant attitudes and behaviour: New challenges for a new era?" In.: J. Surkyn, P. Deboosere and J. van Bavel and (eds.) *Demographic challenges for the 21st Century. A state of art in demography.* Brussels: VUBPRESS, pp. 115-141.

Lundberg, S. and R. A. and Pollak. 2007. "The American family and family economics." Working Paper 12908, National Bureau of Economic Research, Cambridge, Massachusetts. http://www.nber.org/papers/w12908.

Lutz, W. and T. Sobotka. 2008. "Misleading policy messages from the period TFR: Should we stop using it?" Paper presented at the 2008 Annual Meeting of the Population Association of America, New Orleans, 17-19 April 2008.

Lutz, W., V. Skirbekk, and M. R. Testa. 2006. "The low fertility trap hypothesis. Forces that may lead to further postponement and fewer births in Europe." *Vienna Yearbook of Population Research* 2006: 167-192.

Manning, N. 2004. "Diversity and change in pre-accession Central and Eastern Europe since 1989." *Journal of European Social Policy* 14(3): 211-232.

Matsuo, H. 2001. "Is Japan a second demographic transition country? Observations based on union, first birth status and values in the Netherlands and Japan." Paper presented at workshop "The Second Demographic Transition in Europe," Bad Herrenalb, Germany, 23-28 June 2001. http://www.demogr.mpg.de/Papers/workshops/ 010623_paper23.pdf.

McDonald, P. 2000. "Gender equity, social institutions and the future of fertility". *Journal of Population Research* 17 (1): 1-15.

McLanahan, S. 2004. "Diverging destinies: How children are faring under the second demographic transition?" *Demography* 41(4): 607-627.

Micheli, G. 2004. "On the verge of familistic interpretation. Familism, moods and other alchemies." In.: G. Dalla Zuanna and G. Micheli (eds.) *Strong family and low fertility: A paradox?"* European Studies of Population, Vol. 14, Kluwer Academic Publishers, Dordrecht, pp. 127-160.

Mills, M. and H.-P. Blossfeld. 2005. "Globalization, uncertainty and the early life course. A theoretical framework." In: H.-P. Blossfeld, E. Klijzing, M. Mills and K. Kurz (eds.) *Globalization, Uncertainty and Youth in Society.* London/New York: Routledge Advances in Sociology Series, pp. 1-24

Možný, I. and T. Katrňák. 2005. "The Czech family". In.: B. N. Adams and J. Trost (eds.) *Handbook of World Families.* Thousand Oaks, California: Sage Publications Inc, pp. 235-261.

Muresan, C. 2007. "Family dynamics in pre- and post-transition Romania: a life-table description." *MPIDR Working paper* WP 2007-18, Max Planck Institute for Demographic Research, Rostock. www.demogr.mpg.de/Papers/Working/WP-2007-018.pdf

Muresan, C., Hărăgus, P.T., Hărăgus, M., and Schröder, C. 2008. Romania: Childbearing metamorphosis within a changing context, *Demographic Research* 19(23). http://www.demographic-research.org/Volumes/Vol19/23/

Myrskylä, M., H.-P. Kohler, and F. C. Billari. "Human development and low fertility." Paper presented at the 2008 Annual Meeting of the Population Association of America, New Orleans, 17-19 April 2008.

Neels, K. 2006. *Reproductive strategies in Belgian fertility.* NIDI/CBGS Publications No. 38, Brussels: CBGS.

OECD. 2005. *Education at a glance 2005.* Organisation for Economic Co-operation and Development, Paris.

Oláh, L., and Bernhardt, E. 2008. Sweden: Combining childbearing and gender equality. *Demographic Research* 19(28). http://www.demographic-research.org/Volumes/Vol19/28/

Pagnini, D. L. and R. R. Rindfuss. 1993. "The divorce of marriage and childbearing: Changing attitudes and behaviour in the United States." *Population and Development Review* 19(2): 331-347.

Perelli-Harris, B. 2008. Ukraine: On the border between old and new in uncertain times, *Demographic Research* 19(29). http://www.demographic-research.org/Volumes/Vol19/29/

Philipov, D. 2003. "Fertility in times of discontinuous societal change." In.: I. Kotowska, and J. Jóźwiak (eds.) *Population of Central and Eastern Europe. Challenges and Opportunities.* Statistical Publishing Establishment, Warsaw, pp. 665-689.

Philipov, D. 2006. "Portrait of the family in Europe." Chapter 2 in.: L. Hantrais, D. Philipov, and F. C. Billari (eds.) *Policy implications of changing family formation.* Population Studies, No. 49, Strasbourg: Council of Europe Publishing.

Philipov, D. and A. Jasilioniene. 2007. "Union formation and fertility in Bulgaria and Russia: a life table description of recent trends." *MPIDR Working paper* WP 2007-05, Max Planck Institute for Demographic Research, Rostock. www.demogr.mpg.de/Papers/Working/WP-2007-005.pdf

Pongrácz, M. 2002. "Birth out of wedlock." Working Papers on Population, Family and Welfare. Hungarian Central Statistical Office, Demographic research Institute, Budapest.

Pongrácz, M. and Z. Spéder. 2008. "Attitudes towards forms of partnership." In: Ch. Höhn, D. Avramov, and I. Kotowska (Eds.) *People, Population Change and Policies: Lessons from the Population Policy Acceptance Study – Volume 1.* Berlin: Springer, pp. 93-112.

Potančoková, M. 2007. "Konštrukcia plánovaného rodičovstva v období štátneho socializmu v bývalom Československu." [Construction of family planning in the era of state socialism in former Czechoslovakia]. *Gender-rovné příležitosti-výzkum* 8(2/2007). www.genderonline.cz.

Potančoková, M., Vaňo, B., Pilinská, V., and Jurčová, D. 2008. Slovakia: Fertility between tradition and modernity, *Demographic Research* 19(25). http://www.demographic-research.org/Volumes/Vol19/25/

Prioux, F. 2006. "Recent demographic developments in France." *Population-E* 61(4): 323-364.

Ravanera, Z. R. and F. Rajulton. 2004. "Social status polarization in the timing and trajectories to motherhood." Discussion Paper No. 04-06, Population Studies Centre, University of Western Ontario, London, Canada.

Reher, S. D. 1998. "Family ties in Western Europe: Persistent contrasts". *Population and Development Review* 24 (2): 203-234.

Rendall, M. S. and S. Smallwood. 2003. "Higher qualifications, first-birth timing, and further childbearing in Englands and Wales". *Population Trends* 111 (Spring 2003): 18-26.

RHS. 2005. *Reproductive Health Survey, Romania 2004. Summary Report.* Ministry of Health, World Bank, UNFPA, USAID, UNICEF.

Rindfuss, R. R., M. K. Choe, L. L. Bumpass, and N. O. Tsuya. 2004. "Social networkds and fertility change in Japan." *American Sociological Rewiew* 69: 838-861.

Rosina, A. and R. Fraboni. 2004. "Is marriage losing its centrality in Italy?" *Demographic Research* 11 (Article 6): 149-172. [www.demographic-research.org]

Rotariu, T. 2006. "Romania and the Second Demographic Transition. The traditional value system and low fertility rates." *International Journal of Sociology* 36(1):10-27.

Salles, A. 2006. "The effects of family policy in the former GDR on nuptiality and births outside marriage." *Population-E* 2006, 61(1-2): 141-152.

Smock, P. J. 2000. "Cohabitation in the United States: An appraisal of research themes, findings, and implications." *Annual Review of Sociology* 26: 1-20

Sobotka, T. 2003. "Re-emerging diversity: Rapid fertility changes in Central and Eastern Europe after the collapse of the communist regimes". *Population-E* 2003, 58 (4-5): 451-486.

Sobotka, T. 2004. *Postponement of childbearing and low fertility in Europe.* PhD Thesis, University of Groningen. Amsterdam: Dutch University Press.

Sobotka, T. 2005. "Childless societies? Trends and projections of childlessness in Europe and the Unites States" Paper presented at the 2005 PAA Annual Meeting Meeting, Philadelphia, 31 March-2 April 2005.

Sobotka, T. 2008. "Does persistent low fertility threaten the future of European populations?" In: J. Surkyn, P. Deboosere and J. van Bavel and (eds.) *Demographic challenges for the 21st Century. A state of art in demography.* Brussels: VUBPRESS, pp. 27-89.

Sobotka, T., K. Zeman, and V. Kantorová 2003. "Demographic shifts in the Czech Republic after 1989: A second demographic transition view". *European Journal of Population* 19 (3): 249–277.

Sobotka, T. and M. R. Testa. 2008. "Attitudes and intentions towards childlessness in Europe". In: Ch. Höhn, D. Avramov, and I. Kotowska (Eds.) *People, Population Change and Policies: Lessons from the Population Policy Acceptance Study – Volume 1.* Berlin: Springer, pp. 177-211.

Sobotka, T., Šťastná, A., Zeman, K., Hamplová, D., and Kantorová, V. 2008. Czech Republic: A rapid transformation of fertility and family behaviour after the collapse of state socialism, *Demographic Research* 19(14). http://www.demographic-research.org/Volumes/Vol19/14/

Spéder, Z. 2005. "The rise of cohabitation as first union and some neglected factors of recent demographic developments in Hungary." *Demográfia, English Edition* 48(2005): 77-103.

Stankuniene, V. and A. Maslauskaite. 2008. "Family transformations in the post-communist countries: Attitudes toward changes." In: Ch. Höhn, D. Avramov, and I. Kotowska

(Eds.) *People, Population Change and Policies: Lessons from the Population Policy Acceptance Study – Volume 1.* Berlin: Springer, pp. 113-138.

Stankuniene, V., and Jasilioniene, A. 2008. Lithuania: Fertility decline and its determinants, *Demographic Research* 19(20). http://www.demographic-research.org/Volumes/ Vol19/20/

Statistics Austria. 2006. *Demographisches Jahrbuch Österreichs 2005.* Vienna: Statistics Austria.

Statistics Austria. 1997. *Demographisches Jahrbuch Österreichs 1996.* Österreichisches Statistischen Zentralamt, Vienna.

Stropnik, N., and Šircelj, M. 2008. Slovenia: Generous family policy without evidence of any fertility impact, *Demographic Research* 19(26). http://www.demographic-research.org/Volumes/Vol19/26/

Thornton, A. and D. Philipov. 2007. "Developmental idealism and family and demographic change in Central and Eastern Europe." *European Demographic Research Papers* 3 / 2007. Vienna: Vienna Institute of Demography.

Thornton, A. and L. Young-deMarco. "Four decades of trends in attitudes toward family issues in the United States: The 1960s through the 1990s." *Journal of Marriage and Family* 63: 1009-1037.

Toulemon, L., Pailhé, A., Rossier, C. 2008. France: High and stable fertility, *Demographic Research* 19(16). http://www.demographic-research.org/Volumes/Vol19/16/

van Bavel, J. 2007. "Subreplacement fertility in the West before the baby boom (1900-1940). Current and contemporary perspectives." Paper presented at the 32nd Annual Meeting of the Social Science History Association, Chicago IL, November 18, 2007.

van de Kaa, D. J. 1987. "Europe's second demographic transition". *Population Bulletin* 42(1).

van de Kaa, D. J. 1994. "The second demographic transition revisited: Theories and expectations". In.: G. Beets et al. (eds.) *Population and family in the Low Countries 1993: Late fertility and other current issues.* NIDI/CBGS Publication, No. 30, Swets and Zeitlinger, Berwyn, Pennsylvania/Amsterdam, pp. 81-126.

van de Kaa, D. J. 1996. "Anchored narratives: The story and findings of half a century of research into the determinants of fertility." *Population Studies* 50(3): 389-432.

van de Kaa, D. J. 2001. "Postmodern fertility preferences: From changing value orientation to new behavior". In.: R. A. Bulatao, J. B. Casterline (eds.) *Global fertility transition.* Supplement to *Population and Development Review* 27, New York, Population Council, pp. 290-338.

van de Kaa, D. J. 2002. "The idea of a Second Demographic Transition in industrialized countries." Paper presented at the Sixth Welfare Policy Seminar of the National Institute of Population and Social Security, Tokyo, Japan, 29 January 2002. http://www.ipss.go.jp/webj-ad/WebJournal.files/population/2003_4/Kaa.pdf.

van de Kaa, D. J. 2004a. "The true commonality: In reflexive societies fertility is a derivative". *Population Studies* 58(1): 77-80.

van de Kaa, D. J. 2004b. "Demographic revolutions or transitions. A foreword." In: T. Frejka, and J.-P. Sardon (eds.) *Childbearing trends and prospects in low-fertility countries: A cohort analysis*, Dordrecht: Kluwer Academic Publishers, pp. x-xiv.

van Peer, C. and L. Rabušic. 2008. "Will we see an upturn in European fertility in the near future?" In: Ch. Höhn, D. Avramov, and I. Kotowska (Eds.) *People, Population*

*Change and Policies: Lessons from the Population Policy Acceptance Study –
Volume 1.* Berlin: Springer, pp. 215-241.

World Bank. 2007. *World development Indicators.* Database accessed at
http://web.worldbank.org

Zakharov, S. 2008. Russian Federation: From the first to second demographic transition,
Demographic Research 19(24). http://www.demographic-research.org/Volumes/
Vol19/24/

Appendix

Construction of the SDT indexes used in the analysis

Note that country-specific values of SDT1 and SDT2 indexes are displayed in Sobotka (2008, Table AP-1, pp. 86-87).

SDT1 index (behavioural dimension)

This index, composed for 34 countries, is based on the following indicators for 2004 (or the latest year available):

1) Mean age of mother at birth of first child (MAFB);
2) Sum of age-specific fertility rates below age 20, per 1000 women (TEENFERT);
3) Percentage of non-marital births (NONMAR);
4) Total first marriage rate (TFMR);
5) Mean age at first marriage (MAFM);
6) Total divorce rate (TDR).

Finally, the index is adjusted upwards by 0.5 if more than 10 per cent of co-residential unions were made up by cohabiting couples (data for 2001 based on Philipov 2005 and national data sources). Maximum, minimum and mean values of these indicators and the assigned SDT scores are displayed in table AP-2.

SDT2 index (attitudes and values dimension)

This index is based on the 1999/2000 results of the European Values Study, published in Halman (2001). It is based on the responses in 29 countries to the following questions and statements:

1) "…how important it is in your life: leisure time" (LEISURE, % "very important")
2) "How often do you spend time in church, mosque, or synagogue" (CHURCH, % "every week");
3) "Please use the scale to indicate how much freedom of choice and control you feel you have over the way your life turns out?" (CONTROL, mean value on the scale of 1 (=none control at all) to 10 (= a great deal of control));

4) "Do you think that a woman has to have children in order to be fulfilled or is this not necessary?" (NEED_KIDS, % responses "not necessary");
5) "Marriage is an outdated institution" (MARRIAGE, % "agree");
6) "A job is alright, but what women really want is a home and children" (F_HOME, % "agree strongly");
7) "One does not have the duty to respect and love parents who have not earned it by their behaviour and attitudes" (PAR_RESPECT, % "agree");
8) "Do you approve or disapprove abortion (…) where a married couple does not want to have any more children?" (ABORTION, % "approve").

Several questions were not asked in all the participating countries; the SDT2 index for these countries was based on the mean score of the responses to the remaining items. Maximum, minimum and mean values of these indicators and the assigned SDT scores are displayed in table AP-2.

Table AP-1: **Variables used for computing the SDT indexes: Mean, maximum, minimum and threshold values for selected SDT scores (0, 5, and 10)**

Variable	Values of SDT scores			Observed values			Mean SDT score
	SDT score=0	SDT score=5	SDT score=10	MIN	MAX	MEAN	
Index SDT1							
MAFB	<24	27	>30	23.29	29.30	26.60	4.3
TEENFERT	>180	90	0	26.0	209.3	84.4	5.3
NONMAR	0	30	>60	4.9	63.7	32.0	5.3
TFMR	>0.80	0.60	<0.40	0.405	0.826	0.577	5.6
MAFM	<23	27	>31	22.91	30.90	26.72	4.6
TDR	<0.15	0.35	>0.55	0.11	0.55	0.36	5.2
Index SDT2							
LEISURE	<16	32	>48	15.5	54.2	31.5	4.8
CHURCH	>30	15	0	3.1	34.2	14.8	5.2
CONTROL	<5.3	6.4	>7.5	5.4	7.6	6.7	6.2
NEED_KIDS	<5	45	>85	5.9	92.9	45.9	5.1
MARRIAGE	<6	20	>34	8.3	36.3	18.7	4.5
F_HOME	>35	20	<5	3.0	34.1	17.4	5.8
PAR_RESPECT	0	30	>60	13.5	67.3	29.6	4.9
ABORTION	<20	55	>90	15.2	85.1	56.9	5.3

Overview Chapter 7:
The rising importance of migrants for childbearing in Europe

Tomáš Sobotka[1]

Abstract

This contribution looks at the influence of immigration on childbearing trends in the countries of Western, Northern and Southern Europe, which have received relatively large numbers of immigrants during the last decades. It analyses the contribution of migrants to the total number of births and compares fertility rates of migrant women with the fertility rates of native women, pointing out huge diversity between migrant groups. It also discusses the evidence regarding the progressive 'assimilation' in migrants' fertility to the local fertility patterns and analyses the net impact of migrants on period fertility rates. This review reveals that migrant women typically retain substantially higher levels of period fertility than the 'native' populations, but this difference typically diminishes over time and with the duration of their stay in a country. Immigrants contribute substantially to the total number of births and their share of total births has increased in the last decade, exceeding in some countries one fifth of the recorded live births. However, the 'net effect' of the higher fertility of migrants on the period total fertility of particular countries remains relatively small, typically between 0.05 and 0.10 in absolute terms.

[1] Vienna Institute of Demography. E-mail: tomas.sobotka@oeaw.ac.at

1. Introduction

Immigration to Europe, especially to the European Union (EU), has surged in the last two decades due to a combination of multiple factors, including the general increase of mobility and easier international travel, the economic malaise in many post-communist countries after the collapse of state socialism, violent conflicts and instability in the Balkans and other areas. Also successful enlargement of the EU, which has progressed hand in hand with economic integration, has played a significant role. Migration and its various effects on the economy (including the overall economic performance, gross domestic product (GDP) growth, wages, employment and the labour market) and society are vigorously debated in the media on a daily basis. Overall, the economic and social effects of migration are difficult to assess and disagreement frequently exists among experts and researchers[2]. Migration involves various conflicts of interest which may contribute to an ambiguous assessment regarding the overall impact of immigration. For instance, the positive impact of immigration on the economic growth of a country may be counterbalanced by its negative impact on wages and employment prospects of some segments of the 'native' population, especially low-skilled workers (Boeri and Brücker 2005).

Migration constitutes a powerful component of demographic change, albeit one that is difficult to trace. After 1990 migration has become the main engine of population growth in many countries of Europe. It is gradually transforming European population in a manner unforeseen by various population projections (Coleman 2006). In 2004 the European Union (EU-25) recorded the highest population increase since 1972—0.54 percent—of which 0.38 percent was attributable to a positive migration balance (Eurostat 2006a, 2006b). Consequently, the EU has received larger migration streams since the early 2000s than the United States, which often serves as a model country of immigration. However, migration is also the most unstable and the least predictable component of population change (Alho et al. 2006). Despite the wealth of migration theories, projections of migration "continue to rely on ad-hoc assumptions based on little theory and virtually no definable methodology" (Howe and Jackson 2005: 1). Spain, which was until 1990 a country with negative migration balance, provides a telling example of the unexpected effects of migration on population change. Between 1999 and 2006 the total population of Spain rose by 4.0 million persons, i.e., by 10.2 percent, of which 9.3 percent was due to migration (Eurostat 2006a, Council of Europe 2006, Roig Vila and Castro Martín 2007; see also Spain chapter[*]).

---

[2] See Coleman and Rowthorn (2004) for an example of a debate on the economic costs and benefits of immigration to the United Kingdom.

[*] All country chapters referred to can be found online at: http://www.demographic-research.org/special/7/.

Besides contributing directly to population size and composition, migration has a broader demographic impact on each society, especially when immigrant populations have different levels and patterns of fertility, union formation and mortality. Most expert analyses and projections of population trends focus exclusively on the direct influence of migration on population size and composition and ignore the potentially important contribution of immigrants on birth rates and childbearing trends (country studies in Haug, Compton and Courbage 2002 are among important exceptions). At the same time, the wider public in many developed countries often believes that immigrants have high birth rates that may place the provision of welfare support to families under strain and may even eventually lead to an outnumbering of the native majority by a population of foreign origin. Immigrants might also be perceived as the main factor behind the recent rise in period fertility in a number of European countries (e.g., Héran and Pison 2007 for the case of France; see also below).

This contribution scrutinises contemporary evidence regarding the effects of immigration on childbearing trends in European countries. These effects have a growing relevance for the societies of Western, Northern, Southern, and recently also Central Europe. Focusing on these regions, I consider the contribution of migrants to the total number of births, compare fertility rates of migrant women with fertility of the native women and point out the heterogeneity between different migrant populations. Subsequently, I discuss the pace of 'assimilation' in migrants' fertility to local fertility patterns and the net impact of migrants on period fertility rates. In conclusion, this article lays emphasis on the multifaceted impact of migration on childbearing trends and population change. Given space limitations, lack of data and lack of comparative studies, this contribution focuses almost exclusively on women and does not discuss the effects of internal migration, short-term migration and illegal migration. It pays very little attention to the impact of emigration on fertility and also neglects immigrants' fertility in the post-communist countries of Central and Eastern Europe, where data availability is limited and larger-scale immigration either constitutes a very recent phenomenon or was an outcome of these countries being parts of larger state units (Czechoslovakia, Soviet Union and Yugoslavia).

2. Concepts and data limitations

Migration is linked to childbearing trends in a number of distinct ways. Considerable confusion therefore exists about the effects of migration on fertility. Several conceptual issues outlined below are of paramount importance for any understanding of these effects.

(1) Different definitions of what a migrant is are used by various statistical agencies. With respect to immigrants, the most common categorizations are those of foreign-born persons and persons with foreign citizenship. The latter category is problematic in statistics on migrants, as its size frequently depends more on national legislation on citizenship of a country of residence than on the size of immigration streams. There are vast differences between countries in the rate of *naturalisation* and the average period elapsing between immigration and naturalisation. Due to incomplete or missing records, there are also very few data on births to immigrant men, which means that statistics on the proportion of births with at least one immigrant parent is also usually unavailable. A study of the effects of immigration on fertility can be limited to the first generation of migrants, or it can also include the second and the third generation (see the Netherlands chapter).

(2) When assessing the effects of migration on fertility and population change, different estimates and assumptions should be made about the fertility and mortality of emigrants and immigrants. In practice, lack of data limits such empirical studies. Any analysis of the effects of migration on childbearing trends commonly takes differential fertility of immigrants into account, but usually ignores the potential fertility differentials due to emigration. This is because of the absence of information on childbearing patterns of emigrants and the impossibility of assessing how emigrants would have behaved if they had stayed in their country of origin (see Albania chapter). Practically all available studies focusing on European countries analyse the impact of legal migration and disregard the impact of illegal migration.

(3) Given these limitations, research on the effects of migration on fertility is usually confined to legally resident immigrant women. Several types of analysis can be distinguished. First, the effect of (im)migration on the total number of births can be analysed from the data on births by the country of origin of the mother and/or the father. Second, a comparative analysis of period and cohort fertility for different groups of migrants sheds light on their heterogeneity in childbearing patterns. Third, the *net migration effect* on fertility rates can be estimated when comparing the observed fertility rates with those that would have been achieved in the absence of (im)migration. Any analysis of migrants' period fertility rates is complicated by the interrelation between the events of migration and fertility, which distorts the commonly used period fertility measures. These are based on the assumption that fertility is a function of age, whereas immigrants' fertility rates are more closely linked to the timing of migration rather than their actual age (Toulemon 2004, Andersson 2004, Østby 2002, Alders 2000; see also France chapter).

3. Contribution of immigrants to the total number of births

The proportion of births to immigrant women provides a basic indication of the importance of immigrants for childbearing. This measure is a function of past immigration levels, the age composition of immigrants, and their fertility rates. In practice, most countries collect data on the proportion of births to women with foreign nationality (see also above). Since many women eventually obtain the nationality of their new host country, these statistics constitute a downward-biased approximation of immigrants' contribution to the total number of births in a country.

Table 1 summarises the percentage of births to immigrant or foreign-nationality women in eleven European countries with a recent history of sizeable migration streams. Births to immigrant women contribute considerably to the recorded total number of births in the analysed regions: well above one tenth of all births are attributable to immigrant women, even when the partial data on foreign nationals are considered. This share is typically higher than the proportion of immigrants, since migrant women tend to be younger and more fertile than the native population (see also below). Births to immigrant women currently account for around one fifth of all births in England and Wales, the Netherlands, Sweden and Germany (German data are for foreign nationals only), whereas in Switzerland women with foreign nationality contribute more than one quarter of the total number of births. When the second generation of immigrants is also considered, immigrant women account for more than one fifth of births in France (data pertain to 1998 and exclude French nationals born abroad) and more than a quarter of births in the Netherlands.

Almost all countries analysed in Table 1 have recorded a steady increase in the share of immigrant (or foreign-nationals) births since the mid-1990s, in part as a consequence of high immigration rates in the 1990s and the early 2000s. This trend has been most prominent in southern Europe, especially in Spain, where the proportion of births to mothers with foreign nationality rocketed from 3 percent in 1996 to 16 percent in 2006 (see also Roig Vila and Castro Martín 2007 and the chapters on Italy and Spain). In another 'high migration' region, England and Wales, the proportion of births to immigrant women rose from 13 to 22 percent between 1995 and 2006. The share of births to immigrant women is often strongly regionally differentiated, reflecting regional contrasts in the share of immigrant populations. For instance, in Italy, where 12.2 percent of children were born to foreign mothers in 2005, this indicator ranged from 3.3 percent in the islands and 3.7 percent in the south to 17.6 percent in the north-west and 18.6 percent in the north-east (ISTAT 2007). This share is highest in large cities, which traditionally serve as magnets for immigration. In many major European cities, the share of immigrant births approaches 50 percent (Coleman 2006: 427).

Table 1: Proportion of births to immigrant women and to parents of foreign nationality, selected years (different definitions)

	Period	Births to immigrant women (%)	Births to immigrant women, 1st + 2nd gen. (%)	Births to mothers with foreign nationality (%)	At least one parent foreign national (%)	Source
Austria	2000			13.5		Kytir 2006
	2005			11.7		Kytir 2006
Belgium (Flanders)	2003–2004	16.8[1]		12.4		VAZG 2007
Denmark	1999-2003	13.5		11.1		Statistics Denmark 2004
England and Wales	1980	13.3				Schoorl 1995
	1995	12.6				ONS 2006
	2005	20.8				ONS 2006,
	2006	21.9				ONS 2007
France	1991–98	12.4				Toulemon 2004
	1998		21[2]		14.5	Prioux 2005, Tribalat 2005
	2004	15		12.4 (2005)	18.2	Prioux 2005, Héran and Pison 2007
Germany	1980			15.0		Schoorl 1995
	1985			11.2		Schoorl 1995
	1995			16.2		Statistisches Bundesamt
	2004			17.6		2006
Italy	1999			5.4		ISTAT 2007
	2004			11.3		ISTAT 2007
	2005			12.2		ISTAT 2007
The Netherlands	1996	15.5	21.0[3]			CBS Statline 2006
	2005	17.8	25.5[3]			CBS Statline 2006
Spain	1996			3.3	4.5	
	2000			6.2	7.9	INE 2006 and 2007, Roig
	2004			13.7	16.9	Vila and Castro Martín
	2006			16.5		2007
Sweden	2005	19.5		11.8		Statistics Sweden 2006
Switzerland	1980			15.3		Coleman 2003
	2000			22.3		Coleman 2003
	2005			26.3		SFSO 2006

Note: Figures shown without decimal points are not available with higher precision.

[1] Births to women with other than Belgian nationality at the time of their birth. This share excludes immigrants born with Belgian nationality and births to women with unknown nationality at their birth (6.2 percent).

[2] When 'repatriate' women (i.e., French nationals born abroad) are included, births to immigrant women of the first and second generation made up 26.5 percent of all births in 1998 (Tribalat 2006, Figure 12).

[3] Births to the second generation of immigrants are defined as births to women born in the Netherlands, where one or both parents have immigrated to the Netherlands.

4. Differential fertility rates: immigrants vs. native women

Several contributions have argued that the commonly used period total fertility rate (TFR) cannot serve as a reliable indicator of the level of immigrants' fertility (Andersson 2004, Toulemon 2004). Schoorl (1995: 103) proposes that migrants' TFR reflects "various aspects of the migration process: selective migration and migration policies, disruption of the process of family formation due to migration, the degree to which migration is marriage migration, and—in time—adaptation or assimilation". This potential distortion in the TFR is particularly large for women with foreign nationality, who, depending on the process of naturalisation, constitute a select group of women with a relatively short duration of stay in the country. Thus, the closer immigration is linked to childbearing and the faster the process of naturalization, the more biased is the period TFR for foreign women. However, with the exception of alternative estimates of the TFR for France adjusted for age at entry and duration of stay (Toulemon and Mazuy 2003, Toulemon 2004, see also France chapter), there are no other readily available alternative indicators of immigrants' fertility rates. Despite its drawbacks, the period TFR gives a basic picture of the major trends in fertility of immigrants, differences between immigrants from various regions, and the overall impact of immigration on the observed TFR of national populations.

Tables 2a and 2b provide a summary of recent data on the period TFR by migration and nationality status in twelve countries of Western, Northern and Southern Europe. Whatever definition is used, immigrant women, when analysed together, have considerably higher fertility than native women. The TFR of all immigrant women typically ranges between 2.0 and 2.5 and is thus by 0.3-0.8 higher than the TFR of native women. Toulemon's (2004) estimates of the TFR in France, adjusted for age at immigration, also fit into this pattern, although these data show a strong reduction in fertility differentials between immigrant and native women (see France chapter). The more problematic data for foreign nationals depict higher variability in the TFR for foreign women, ranging from 1.9 (Switzerland in 1997) to 3.3 (France in 2004). In all cases, the TFR of foreign women also markedly exceeds the TFR of women with local nationality; for instance the TFR of foreign women in Italy and Flanders (Belgium) is twice as high as the TFR of women with Italian and Belgian nationality. Trends over time differ between countries, but typically indicate a gradual diminishing of differences between the fertility levels of immigrants and foreigners on one side and natives on the other (see the Netherlands chapter). However, a case of a complete convergence has not thus far been recorded (for an overview of trends, see Coleman 1994, Schoorl 1995 and the contributions in Haug, Compton and Courbage 2002).

Table 2a: Total fertility rate of native and immigrant women

Country	Period	TFR Native women	Immigrant women	Difference	Source
Denmark	1999–2003	1.69	2.43[1]	0.74	Statistics Denmark 2004
England and Wales	2001	1.6[2]	2.2	0.6	ONS 2006
France	1991–98	1.65	2.50	0.85	Toulemon 2004
	1991–98	1.70[3]	2.16[3]	0.46[3]	Toulemon 2004
The Netherlands	2005	1.65	1.97	0.31	CBS 2006
Norway	1997–98	1.76	2.42	0.66	Østby 2002
Sweden	2005	1.72	2.01	0.29	Statistics Sweden 2006

Table 2b: Total fertility rate of women with local and foreign nationality

Country	Period	TFR 'Native Nationals'	Foreign Nationals	Difference	Source
Austria	2001–5	1.29	2.03	0.74	Kytir 2006
Belgium	1995	1.49	2.13	0.64	Poulain and Perrin 2002
Flanders (Belgium)	2001–5	1.50	3.00	1.50	van Bavel and Bastiaenssen 2006
France	1999	1.72	2.80	1.08	Héran and Pison 2007
	2004	1.80	3.29	1.49	Héran and Pison 2007
Italy	2004	1.26	2.61	1.35	ISTAT 2006
Spain	2002	1.19	2.12	0.93	Roig Vila and Castro Martín 2007
Switzerland	1997	1.34	1.86	0.52	Wanner 2002

[1] Excluding immigrant women born with Danish nationality.
[2] Figures not available with a higher precision.
[3] Data adjusted for age at arrival to France and duration of stay in France.

5. The heterogeneity in immigrants' fertility

The overall differences in the TFR reported above hide a large heterogeneity between different groups of migrants. Migrants from certain countries and regions, such as Bangladesh, Morocco, Pakistan and parts of sub-Saharan Africa usually have a TFR far exceeding that of native populations in Europe. This pattern appears to be consistent for the first generation of migrants across different countries. In contrast, migrants from other regions of Europe and the Caribbean display a TFR similar to the natives (e.g., Coleman 1994).

Table 3 provides an illustration of some of these contrasts for a few European countries with statistics on the TFR of immigrants by country of origin. It shows the TFR of two high-fertility groups of migrants (Somalians and Pakistanis) compared with the TFR of women born in Turkey, Iran and Western Europe. The first two groups have a TFR that exceeds the TFR of the host country by a factor of two or more, ranging from 3.6 (Pakistani women in Denmark and Norway) up to 5.2 (Somali women in Denmark and Norway). Turkish women also have an elevated TFR level, which exceeds the TFR in their host country and frequently even the TFR of Turkey[3], but is well below the TFR of Somali, Pakistani, as well as Bangladeshi, Iraqi and Moroccan women (not shown here). European immigrants usually have a TFR close or somewhat below that of the host country. This also applies to women from Iran, who in the Netherlands and Sweden reached very low TFR levels, below 1.5.

Table 3: **TFR of immigrant women from Somalia, Pakistan, Turkey, Iran and Western Europe**

Country of residence	Period	Somalia	Pakistan	Turkey	Iran	(Western) Europe[3]	Source
Austria	2000–05[1]			2.96			Kytir 2006
Denmark	1999–2003	5.21	3.58		1.84	1.57	Statistics Denmark 2004
England and Wales	2001		4.7				ONS 2006
France[2]	1991–98			3.21		1.66	Toulemon 2004
The Netherlands	2005	4.4 (1999)		2.22	1.1 (1999)	1.45	CBS 2006; the Netherlands chapter
Norway	1997-8	5.2	3.59	3.09	1.92	2.02	Østby 2002
Sweden	2005	3.82		2.62	1.31	1.57	Statistics Sweden 2006

Country (region) of origin

[1] Women without Austrian nationality.
[2] Data adjusted for age at immigration and duration of stay in France.
[3] Denmark: EU-15 countries; France: EU-15 countries except Italy, Portugal and Spain; The Netherlands: 'western immigrants' (Europe, North America, Oceania, Indonesia and Japan); Norway: Western Europe; Sweden: EU-25 excluding Nordic countries.

---

[3] The TFR in Turkey shows a steadily declining trend over time, reaching 2.57 in 2000 and 2.19 in 2005 (Council of Europe 2006 and Eurostat 2006a).

These examples were selected to illustrate the heterogeneity in migrants' fertility that lies hidden in summary data for all immigrants in a country. They also show that the differences in fertility rates between ethnic or national groups cannot be explained by a single factor, such as religion. This is most clearly evident in the case of women coming from predominantly Muslim societies who, according to commonly held opinion, have fertility far above that of native women in European countries. Although some Muslim populations in Europe display the highest fertility and the slowest pace of fertility decline (e.g., Coleman 1994: 124; Østby 2002), the contrasting examples of very-high fertility of women from Somalia and Pakistan and low fertility of women from Iran and Indonesia (for the latter group in the Netherlands see Heering et al. 2002) point out that the pronatalist influence of religion, if any, is strongly modified by other factors, including woman's socio-economic position[4].

Four interrelated factors are frequently identified in order to explain higher fertility rates of some migrant groups.[5] First, the *selection hypothesis* emphasizes distinct social characteristics of immigrants (such as their educational level, income, level of integration, and rates of intermarriage) that may be conducive to higher fertility. Kahn (1994) reported that the higher fertility of immigrants in the United States was explained by their socioeconomic and demographic characteristics. Second, the *socialisation hypothesis (or 'culture' hypothesis)* emphasizes the effects of pronatalist culture, norms and values in the region of origin, which is mirrored in the reproductive behaviour of immigrants after their arrival to a new, low-fertility setting. Also relatively low fertility rates, typical of migrant groups coming from low-fertility countries, including migrants from European countries, from the Caribbean and many parts of South America, generally support the socialization hypothesis. Third, the *family formation hypothesis* accentuates the interrelatedness of migration and family formation among many groups of migrants. The frequent finding of elevated fertility of migrants during the first years after their arrival (Alders 2000, Østby 2002, Toulemon and Mazuy 2003, Andersson 2004, Andersson and Scott 2005) may be seen as an outcome of a common 'package' of migration, marriage, and childbearing (Milewski 2007; see also France chapter). It also suggests another selection effect: first-generation migrant women may form a distinct group immigrating mostly for the reasons of family formation and reunion (see Milewski 2007 for the case of West Germany).[6] The family

---

[4] Esposito (1998) stresses the importance of local context and cultural traditions in explaining the diversity in attitudes to and the actual prevalence of family planning across Muslim societies: "Islam has legitimated and reinforced traditional pronatalist believes and practices in areas where social conditions made large families desirable" (Esposito 1998: 513).

[5] See Forste and Tienda 1996, Abbasi-Shavazi and McDonald 2002, Kulu 2005, and Genereux 2007 for similar sets of explanations of ethnic and migrant differences in fertility.

[6] Alders (2000: 14) found that in the Netherlands the correlation between immigration and childbearing was particularly pronounced for women from Turkey and Morocco: 40 percent of women immigrating at age 20-

formation hypothesis contrasts with the *disruption hypothesis* that envisions lower fertility among recent migrants, linked to the disruption effect migration may have on partnership formation and childbearing.[7] Although such a disrupting effect of migration has not been found in the existing studies on immigrants' fertility in Europe, some supporting evidence for this hypothesis was found, for instance, among European migrants to Australia (Abbasi-Shavazi and McDonald 2002). Fourth, the *'minority status' explanation* can be proposed to explain both rapid fertility limitation among some groups of migrants as a way of achieving higher social mobility (Forste and Tienda 1996) and the persistence of higher fertility as a defensive response among the more disadvantaged communities with strong ethnic or religious consciousness and slow adaptation to local fertility ideals (Coleman 1994, Fargues 2000, McQuillan 2004).

Immigrants often differ from the native population in many fertility characteristics other than fertility rates. Several contributions in Haug, Compton and Courbage (2002) document an early start of childbearing among many groups of migrant women, especially those from Turkey (see also Italy chapter).[8] Foreign-born women also frequently display markedly lower levels of childlessness (see Garssen and Nicolaas 2006 and the Netherlands chapter) and high progression rates to third and higher-order births (see Austria chapter). This is also in part mirrored in their ideal family size, which remains high among migrants from Pakistan and northern Africa (Penn and Lambert 2002). A striking influence of the culture of the country of origin is demonstrated by vast differences in living arrangements, marriage patterns and non-marital fertility across migrant groups (see Sweden chapter for the case of Turkish young adults in Sweden). Even in societies where non-marital childbearing has become common, immigrants from the more culturally conservative societies realise childbearing exclusively within marriage (various chapters in Haug, Compton and Courbage 2002). In 2005, only two percent of children born in England and Wales to women originating from Bangladesh, India and Pakistan were non-marital, in contrast to 49 percent of children born to native-born mothers (ONS 2006). On the other hand, non-marital births are frequent among women from Latin America and from the Caribbean, in line with patterns in their countries of origin, suggesting again the

---

30 had a child in the calendar year after the year of their arrival. This pattern was not found for women from Suriname and the Netherlands Antilles.

[7] However, Milewski (2007: 861-862) points out that the 'disruption effect' may also explain elevated birth rates after migration, which may constitute a 'catching up' of childbearing that was postponed or interrupted in the period shortly before and during migration.

[8] De Valk and Liefbroer (2007, Table 2) show that both first and second-generation migrants from the main immigrant communities in the Netherlands (Turks, Moroccans, Surinamese and Antilleans) show a clear preference for an earlier age at motherhood than the native Dutch women and both generations of Turkish and Moroccan migrants preferred a markedly lower mean age at marriage for a woman (below 23) than the Dutch women did (26 years for the younger cohorts).

usefulness of the socialization hypothesis for explaining immigrants' childbearing behaviour. In Spain, a high proportion of non-marital births among the growing population of migrants from Latin America has largely contributed to the recent rapid rise in non-marital fertility in the whole country (see Spain chapter). Finally, immigrant women also display different patterns of contraceptive use and abortion. Immigrants from less developed societies frequently rely on ineffective means of contraception and on abortion. In the Netherlands, 60 percent of women undergoing abortion have an ethnic minority background (see the Netherlands chapter, Fokkema et al. 2008:770).

6. How rapid is the assimilation to local fertility patterns?

Because of the progressive assimilation of each subsequent generation of descendents of immigrants in their union formation and childbearing behaviour and, in a broader sense, their language and ethnic identity, any analysis of long-term effects of migration is very sensitive to assumptions on migrants' assimilation and on the emergence of mixed-origin populations (see Coleman 2006: 413-417).

Most studies find that, within a decade after their arrival, migrants' fertility rates decline to the level close to fertility rates among native women (Schoorl 1995; Toulemon and Mazuy 2004). Furthermore, over time immigrants' expectations about their future childbearing have been found to converge with the birth expectations of native women (Kahn 1994). However, some populations show a slower pace of convergence.[9] Women immigrating at a young age, sometimes called the '1.5 generation,' frequently display similar fertility rates to autochtonous women (Andersson 2004; Toulemon and Mazuy 2004). This 'assimilation' to local fertility patterns has also been reported in the incidence of early childbearing. Østby (2002: 43) found that women who arrived in Norway before age seven became mothers before age 22 much less frequently than women who arrived at a later age. The Sweden chapter highlights two non-demographic factors—educational attainment and exposure to Swedish society (as measured by neighbourhood composition)—which were important for an adaptation of family attitudes and behaviour of young adults from Poland and Turkey to the Swedish patterns. National welfare policies, employment patterns and other institutional factors constitute important mechanisms that facilitate an adjustment of migrants' fertility to 'local' fertility patterns. Andersson and Scott (2005) found a similar effect of labour market position on first birth intensity among different groups

---

[9] Østby (2002: 42) found that women immigrating to Norway from 'Muslim non-western countries' experience the slowest pace of fertility decline with respect to the duration of their stay. It is unclear to what extent this variable reflects the (pronatalist) influence of Islam and to what extent it reflects other cultural characteristics of specific immigrants' groups and their social composition.

of immigrants in Sweden: for immigrant and Swedish women alike, labour-market activity was positively linked with their propensity to have a first child.[10]

A cohort analysis gives another view on fertility assimilation across cohorts and generations of migrants. As the Netherlands chapter shows, younger cohorts of women from initially high-fertility groups usually display a marked decline in fertility when compared to their older counterparts (see also Alders 2000). This is in part a result of changes in reproductive norms and behaviour in their country of origin, but it is also a sign of an adaptation of their fertility to the conditions of the host country. Frequently, fertility of immigrants from high-fertility societies declines well below the fertility of women in their country of origin (see France chapter and Schoorl 1995). Due to a lack of data fertility patterns of the second and third generation of immigrants are relatively little researched. Dutch data suggest that the fertility level of the second generation of migrants is closer to that of the native women than to the first generation of migrants with the same ethnic origin. For instance, Turkish and Moroccan women from the second generation have much lower levels of cumulated fertility and substantially higher levels of childlessness at ages 25-35 than their first-generation migrant counterparts (Alders 2000, Garssen and Nicolaas 2006)[11].

---

[10] However, migrant women vastly differ in their labour market status: among childless women in Sweden aged 21-45, the percentage in the labour force having a job as the main source of income was 74 percent for Swedish-born women and 63 percent for migrant women, with a wide range from 10 percent (childless Somali women) to 75 percent (childless women from Finland; see Andersson and Scott 2005, Table 3 and Table A1). Also cross-country differences in the employment rate of migrant women aged 15-64 remain large, ranging from 40 percent in Belgium up to 64 percent in Greece in 2004 (Dumont and Liebig 2004: Figure 4). Despite a common trend of increasing employment rates of migrant women, reflecting in part their rising educational level and also an increase in the importance of work-related migration, migrant women in most countries still have lower employment rates than the 'native' women, especially when they come from non-OECD countries (Dumont and Liebig 2005, OECD 2007).

[11] Research on fertility trends among Mexicans in the United States of America (US) shows, however, that some populations may retain distinct fertility patterns over several generations. The third generation of Mexican-origin population in the US shows elevated fertility rates, with a pronounced peak at young ages (especially 20-24), when their fertility is close to that found among recent immigrants (and also among African-American women) and well above the fertility rates of non-Hispanic white women (Frank and Heuveline 2005). Since fertility rates in Mexico fell below the fertility of the Mexican-origin population in the US, Frank and Heuveline argue in favour of a 'racial stratification perspective' on childbearing behaviour and suggest that Mexican immigrants to the US are increasingly under the influence of 'unique structural factors' that encourage higher and earlier fertility among younger cohorts of Mexican-Americans.

7. The impact of migrants' fertility on total fertility rates

The aggregate net impact of migrants on observed trends and levels in period fertility appears to be relatively small, despite their fertility rates far exceeding those of the native population (see chapters on Austria, England and Wales, France, the Netherlands and Spain). In all eleven countries analysed in Table 4, fertility of immigrant (or foreign-national) women had a slight upward effect on the period TFR. This effect was of comparable size across countries and did not differ greatly when all immigrant women or only foreign-nationality women were analysed[12]: the period TFR shifted upwards by 0.05-0.10 (i.e., by 3-7 percent). In Switzerland, the net positive impact of foreign nationals on the TFR was greater and reached 0.14 in 1997, shifting the TFR upwards by 10 percent. The data for the Netherlands indicate that the inclusion of the second generation of immigrants (also used in the Netherlands chapter) considerably lowers the estimated impact of immigration on the TFR because their fertility rates frequently decline to or even below fertility rates of native women (see above).

This analysis indicates that immigration was not the main factor responsible for the recent upswing in the period TFR in some countries of Europe and that this upswing was mainly due to the rise in the TFR of the native population, probably associated with a slowing down of fertility postponement. The data for the Netherlands support this argument: Between 1996 and 2002, when the period TFR for all women increased from 1.53 to 1.73, the TFR among women born in the Netherlands rose even faster (from 1.47 to 1.69, data from CBS Statline 2006). In France, women with foreign nationality partly contributed to the rise of the period TFR between 1999 and 2004, but a larger part of this increase of 0.11 is attributable to the rise in the TFR among native French women by 0.08 (Héran and Pison 2007, Figure 1; see also Table 2b above).[13]

---

[12] The similarity of the two estimates of the net effect of immigrants' fertility is apparent in the case of France, where the data for all immigrant women in 1991-98 give the same net effect (+0.07) as the data for foreign-nationality women in 1990 and 1999 (Tables 4a and 4b). A possible explanation is that the selection effect, implying an elevated fertility of foreign-nationality women (as compared to all migrant women), is counterbalanced by their smaller population size, which is important for computing the overall effect on the TFR in a country.

[13] A decomposition of change in the period TFR in Italy and Spain between 1996 and 2004-2005 by Gabrielli, Paterno and Strozza (2007) distinguished between the effects of (1) an increased share of foreigners (estimating thus the direct impact of migration), (2) of the change in the TFR of foreign women, and (3) of the change in the TFR of 'native' women. In the case of Italy, the overall increase in the TFR of 0.11 was attributable to a mixture of all three factors, with the increase in the TFR of the 'native' women being slightly more important (38 percent) and the 'direct' effect of immigration accounting for 33 percent of the difference. In Spain, there was a negative effect of the TFR decline among foreign-born women in this period (changing the overall TFR by -0.04 in absolute terms), which was more than counterbalanced by a positive effect of an increase in the number of foreign women (+0.08) and an even larger positive effect of a change in the TFR of 'native' women (+0.125).

Table 4a: **'Net effect' of immigrant women on the observed period TFR**

		TFR			
Country	Period	All women	Native women	Net effect	Source
Denmark	1999–2003	1.760	1.685	0.075	Statistics Denmark 2004
England and Wales	1996	1.74	1.67	0.07	Coleman et al. 2002
France	1991–98	1.72	1.65	0.07	Toulemon 2004
The Netherlands	2000–2005	1.724	1.646	0.078	CBS Statline 2006
The Netherlands [1]	2000–2005	1.724	1.680	0.044	CBS Statline 2006
Norway	1997–98	1.81	1.76	0.05	Østby 2002 (Lappegård 2000)
Sweden	2005	1.769	1.716	0.053	Statistics Sweden 2006

Table 4b: **'Net effect' of women with foreign nationality on the observed TFR**

		TFR			
Country	Period	All women	Nationals	Net effect	Source
Austria	2000–2005	1.39	1.29	0.10	Kytir 2006
Belgium	1995	1.56	1.49	0.07	Poulain and Perrin 2002
Flanders (Belgium)	2001–2005	1.59	1.50	0.09	van Bavel and Bastiaenssen 2006
France	1990	1.78	1.71	0.07	Héran and Pison 2007
	1999	1.79	1.72	0.07	Héran and Pison 2007
	2004	1.90	1.80	0.10	Héran and Pison 2007
Italy	2004	1.33	1.26	0.07	ISTAT 2006
Spain	2002	1.27	1.19	0.08	Roig Vila and Castro Martín 2007
Switzerland	1997	1.48	1.34	0.14	Wanner 2002

[1] Including the second generation of immigrant women (mother born in the Netherlands, at least one of her parents born outside the Netherlands).

8. The multifaceted impact of migration on childbearing and population trends

Different studies often provide contrasting assessments about the actual and potential contribution of migration to fertility rates, total numbers of births, and also population growth and ageing. Although this partly reflects differences between countries, it is also a reflection of the fact that the evaluation of the importance of migration hinges critically on the specific questions asked. With some simplification, this review pertaining to Western, Northern and Southern Europe has shown that:

- Despite their relatively rapid demographic assimilation, immigrants usually have markedly higher levels of period fertility than the 'native' populations;
- This differential varies widely by country of origin;
- Immigrants contribute substantially to the total number of births;
- The 'net effect' of the higher fertility of immigrants on the total fertility of particular countries is relatively small.

An interaction between the numerical size of immigrants, their relatively young age structure (migration typically occurs at a young age) and their higher fertility implies that migration has a potentially strong and long-lasting impact on population growth and structure. Immigrants are therefore one of the few population groups that record significant rates of natural growth across Europe (Compton and Courbage 2002).

As a result, immigration has increasingly become perceived as a potential means to prevent population decline, sustain the size of the labour force, and slow down the pace of population ageing. As Feld (2005: 638) noted, the "debate on the role of immigration in Europe has been largely undermined by the fact that it has been saddled with a wide range of functions that should each be aiming at a different objective." A well-publicised United Nations (UN) report (UN, 2000) and a number of other studies (e.g., Coale 1988, Feld 2000 and 2005, Lutz and Scherbov 2003, Beaujot 2003 and Holzmann 2005) address these issues, some of them referring to the notion of 'replacement migration' (i.e., migration that 'makes up' for below-replacement fertility and thus enables countries to avoid population decline or even to prevent population ageing). Most studies show that any realistic level of migration cannot stop population ageing and can only have a relatively modest impact in slowing down this process. However, migration is likely to have a considerable (positive) effect on the size of the labour force (Feld 2000, Bijak et al. 2007) as well as on the total population size (UN 2000, Sobotka 2008).

Immigration levels have been consistently under-projected in historical forecasts in many European countries (Alders, Keilman, and Cruijsen 2007, Shaw 2007). The inclusion of recently recorded higher migration rates into population projections postpones the likely start of future population decline in the EU-15 countries, Norway, Iceland and Switzerland after the year 2050 (Alho et al. 2006). Recent research by Dalla Zuanna (2006), focusing on the industrial triangle of north-west Italy and including the effects of internal (south to north) migration, has shown that significant and continuous immigration may slow population ageing and prevent population decline, even in a region experiencing half a century of very low fertility. In addition, the higher fertility of migrants, typically not envisioned in projection scenarios, may further strengthen the importance of immigration for population trends. In the case of Mexicans in the United States, Jonsson and Rendall's (2004) estimates and projections show that the long-term contribution of immigrants to childbearing is frequently underestimated when conventional methods of analysis are used. They also suggest that "differences in the fertility of immigrants and the native born are likely to be the primary cause of any rejuvenation of the population induced by migration" (Jonsson and Rendall: 146) and that Mexican migration flows after 1981 may generate one additional working-age person for every four Americans in the retirement age by 2040. The open question remains whether European regions with long experience of low fertility can attract and accommodate migration streams necessary to achieve the relative stability in the size of their populations and labour force.

The importance of immigration for childbearing trends and population change in many European countries underlines the need to rethink the traditional concept of replacement-level fertility (Smallwood and Chamberlain 2005). Calot and Sardon (2001) suggest that the 'net replacement rates' which reflect both mortality and migration are preferable to the widely used 'net reproduction rates' and that the application of these measures may change the evaluation of future population prospects (see also Preston and Wang 2007 and Sobotka 2008). In addition, much research needs to be done on various effects of immigration that have an indirect influence on fertility. The Spain chapter outlines one such channel: it suggests that migration may reduce imbalances in the marriage market, and, through increased marriage rates and partnership formation, it may also have an additional positive effect on fertility. Another contribution on Spain (Roig Vila and Castro Martín 2007) proposes that immigrants in Spain also positively contribute to fertility by filling the domestic 'caring gap.' Their frequent employment in the care of children and the elderly partly substitutes inadequate childcare and social services and thus enables more Spanish women to have a child.

Finally, our knowledge about the impact of temporary and long-term emigration on fertility remains rudimentary at best. Three chapters that directly address this issue

(Albania, Lithuania and Slovakia chapters) suggest that temporary labour emigration, typical of these societies, has above all a disrupting effect on family formation, which contributes to the ongoing postponement of childbearing. Such disruption may be most pronounced when emigration streams are sex-specific, as was the case of Albania in the early 1990s: male-dominated emigration reduced women's exposure to pregnancy due to the lack of male partners staying in the country (see Albania chapter). The Lithuania chapter also points at other factors related to emigration: the destabilization of already created families, the weakening of ties between family members and adaptation to new trans-national lifestyles. The returning emigrants can be seen as conveyors of new ideas and behaviour related to family and fertility, which they adopted during their stay abroad (Fargues 2006). Such a reciprocal effect between circular migration and fertility in the country of origin constitutes an important area for further research.

9. Acknowledgements

Many thanks to Gunnar Andersson, Hill Kulu and four anonymous reviewers for their valuable comments on the previous draft of this article. The first version of this article was presented at the 4th International Conference of the EAPS working group on the "Second Demographic Transition" in Budapest, Hungary, 6-8 September 2007. Much of the work on this study was undertaken when the author was a guest researcher at the Max Planck Institute for Demographic Research in Rostock.

References

Abbasi-Shavazi, M. J., and P. McDonald. 2002. A comparison of fertility patterns of European immigrants in Australia with those in the countries of origin, *Genus* 58(1): 53–76.

Alders, M. 2000. *Cohort fertility of migrant women in the Netherlands.* Paper presented at the BSPS-NVD-URU Conference in Utrecht (the Netherlands), 31 August–1 September 2000.

Alders, M., N. Keilman, and H. Cruijsen. 2007. Assumptions for long-term stochastic population forecasts in 18 European countries, *European Journal of Population* 23(1): 33–69.

Alho, J., M. Alders, H. Cruijsen, N. Keilman, T. Nikander, and D. Q. Pham. 2006. New forecast: Population decline postponed in Europe, *Statistical Journal of the United Nations ECE* 23: 1–10.

Andersson, G. 2004. Childbearing after migration: fertility patterns of foreign-born women in Sweden, *International Migration Review* 38(2): 747–775.

Andersson, G., and K. Scott. 2005. Labour-market status and first-time parenthood: the experience of immigrant women in Sweden, 1981–97, *Population Studies* 59(1): 21–38.

Beaujot, R. 2003. *Effect of immigration on Canadian population: Replacement migration?* Discussion paper No. 03–03, London, Canada: University of Western Ontario. Population Studies Centre. http://sociology.uwo.ca/popstudies/dp/dp03-03.pdf.

Bijak, J., D. Kupiszewska, M. Kupiszewski, K. Saczuk, and A. Kicinger. 2007. Population and labour force projections for 27 countries, 2002–2052: impact of international migration on population ageing, *European Journal of Population* 23(1): 1–31.

Boeri, T., and H. Brücker. 2005. Why are Europeans so tough on migrants?, *Economic Policy* October 2005: 629–703.

Calot, G., and J.-P. Sardon. 2001. Fécondité, reproduction et replacement, *Population* 56(3): 337–396.

CBS. 2006. *CBS Statline.* Internet database of the Centraal Bureau voor de Statistiek (Statistics Netherlands). Voorburg. http://statline.cbs.nl.

Coale, A. C. 1988. Demographic effects of below-replacement fertility and their social implications, in K. Davis, M. S. Bernstam, and R. Ricardo-Campbell (Eds.) *Below-Replacement Fertility in Industrial Societies: Causes, Consequences, Policies.* Supplement to *Population and Development Review* 12,: 203–216.

Coleman, D. 2006. Immigration and ethnic change in low-fertility countries: a third demographic transition?, *Population and Development Review* 32(3): 401–446.

Coleman, D. 2003. Mass migration and population change, *Zeitschrift für Bevölkerungswissenschaft* 28 (2–4): 183–215.

Coleman, D. 1994. Trends in fertility and intermarriage among immigrant populations in Western Europe as measures of integration, *Journal of Biosocial Science* 26: 107–136.

Coleman, D., and R. Rowthorn. 2004. The economic effects of immigration into the United Kingdom, *Population and Development Review* 30(4): 579–624.

Coleman, D., P. Compton, and J. Salt. 2002. Demography of migrant populations: the case of the United Kingdom, in W. P. Haug, P. Compton and Y. Courbage (Eds.), *The Demographic Characteristics of Immigrant Populations.* Population Studies, No. 38, Strasbourg: Council of Europe Publishing, pp: 497–552.

Compton, P., and Y. Courbage. 2002. Synthesis report, in W. P. Haug, P. Compton, and Y. Courbage (Eds.), *The Demographic Characteristics of Immigrant Populations*. Population Studies, No. 38, Strasbourg: Council of Europe Publishing, pp: 553–592.

Council of Europe. 2006. *Recent Demographic Developments in Europe* 2005. Strasbourg: Council of Europe Publishing.

Dalla Zuanna, G. 2006. Population replacement, social mobility and development in Italy in the twentieth century, *Journal of Modern Italian Studies* 11(2): 188–208.

de Valk, H., and A. C. Liefbroer. 2007. Timing preferences for women's family-life transitions. Intergenerational transmission among migrants and the Dutch, *Journal of Marriage and Family* 69(1): 190–206.

Dumont, J.-C., and T. Liebig. 2005. *Labour market integration of immigrant women: overview and recent trends*. ROOM Document No. 3 prepared for the OECD and European Commission Seminar, Brussels, 26–27 September 2005. http://ec.europa.eu/ employment_social/employment_analysis/imm/imm_migrwom05_dum_lieb_en.pdf.

Esposito, J. L. 1998. Population ethics: Islamic perspectives, in W. T. Reich (Ed.), *The Ethics of Sex and Genetics*. USA, New York: Macmillan Reference, pp: 510–515.

Eurostat. 2006a. *Population in Europe 2005: First results. Statistics in Focus*. Population and Social Conditions 16/2006. Luxembourg: European Communities. http://epp. eurostat.cec.eu.int/cache/ITY_OFFPUB/KS-NK-06-016/EN/KS-NK-06-016-EN.PDF.

Eurostat. 2006b. *Population statistics. 2006 edition*. Luxembourg: Office for Official Publications of European Communities.

Fargues, P. 2000. Protracted national conflict and fertility change among Palestinians and Israelis in the twentieth century, *Population and Development Review* 26(3): 441–482.

Fargues, P. 2006. *The demographic benefit of international migration: Hypothesis and application to Middle Eastern and North African contexts*. World Bank Policy Research Working Paper 4050, November 2006.

Feld, S. 2000. Active population growth and immigration hypotheses in Western Europe, *European Journal of Population* 16(1): 3–40.

Feld, S. 2005. Labor force trends and immigration in Europe, *International Migration Review* 39(3): 637–662.

Fokkema, T., de Valk, H., de Beer, J., van Duin, C. 2008. The Netherlands: Childbearing within the context of a "Poldermodel" society, *Demographic Research* 19(21). http://www.demographic-research.org/Volumes/Vol19/21/

Forste, R., and M. Tienda. What's behind racial and ethnic fertility differentials?, in J. B. Casterline, R. D. Lee and K. A. Foote (Eds.), *Fertility in the United States. New patterns, new theories*. Supplement to *Population and Development Review* 22, New York, Population Council, pp: 109–133.

Frank, R., and P. Heuveline. 2005. A crossover in Mexican and Mexican-American fertility rates: evidence and explanations for an emerging paradox, *Demographic Research* 12(4): 77–104. http://www.demographic-research.org/volumes/vol12/4/

Garssen, J., and H. Nicolaas. 2006. Recente trends in de vruchtbaarheid van niet-Westers allochtone vrouwen, *Bevolkingstrends* 01–2006: 15–31.

Gabrielli, G., A. Paterno, and S. Strozza. 2007. *Dynamics, characteristics, and demographic behaviour of immigrants in some south-European countries*. Paper presented at an international conference on "Migration and Development," Moscow 13–15 September 2007.

Genereux, A. 2007. *A review of migration and fertility theory through the lens of African immigrant fertility in France.* MPIDR Working Paper WP 2007-008, Rostock: Max Planck Institute for Demographic Research.

Haug, W., P. Compton, and Y. Courbage (Eds.). 2002. *The Demographic Characteristics of Immigrant Populations.* Population Studies, No. 38, Strasbourg: Council of Europe Publishing.

Heering, L., H. de Valk, E. Spaan, C. Huisman, and R. van der Erf. 2002. The demographic characteristics of immigrant populations in the Netherlands, in W. P. Haug, P. Compton, and Y. Courbage (Eds.), *The demographic Characteristics of Immigrant Populations.* Population Studies, No. 38, Strasbourg: Council of Europe Publishing, pp: 245–298.

Héran, F., and G. Pison. 2007. Two children per woman in France in 2006: are immigrants to blame?, *Population and Societies* 432 (March 2007). http://www.ined.fr/fichier/t_ telechargement/7659/telechargement_fichier_en_publi_pdf2_pop.and.soc.english.432.pdf

Holzmann, R. 2005. *Demographic alternatives for aging industrial countries: Increased total fertility rate, labor force participation, or immigration.* IZA Discussion Paper No. 1885. Bonn: Institute for the Study of Labor.

Howe, N., and R. Jackson. 2005. *Projecting immigration. A survey of the current state of practice and theory.* A report of the CSIS Global Aging Initiative. Washington: CSIS. http://www.csis.org/media/csis/pubs/0504_howe_jacksonprojimmigration.pdf.

INE. 2006. *Vital Statistics 2005. Definitive data.* Madrid: Instituto National de Estadística. http://www.ine.es/inebase/cgi/um?M=%2Ft20%2Fe301&O=inebase&N=&L=1.

INE. 2007. *Movimiento natural de la población. Resultados provisionales 2006.* Madrid: Instituto National de Estadística. http://www.ine.es/inebase/cgi/um?M=%2Ft20%2Fe301%2Fprovi 06&O=pcaxis&N=&L=1.

ISTAT. 2006, 2007. *Natalità e fecondità della popolazione residente: caratteristiche e tendenze recenti. Anno 2004* [2005]. Roma: Instituto nazionale di statistica. http://www.istat.it.

Jonsson, S. H., and M. S. Rendall. 2004. Fertility contribution of Mexican immigration to the United States, *Demography* 41(1): 129–150.

Kahn, J. R. 1994. Immigrant and native fertility during the 1980s: adaptation and expectations for the future, *International Migration Review* 38(3): 501–519.

Kulu, H. 2005. Migration and fertility: Competing hypotheses re-examined, *European Journal of Population* 21(1): 51–87.

Kytir, J. 2006. Demographische Strukturen und Trends 2005, *Statistische Nachrichten* 2006(9): 777–790.

Lappegård, T. 2000. *Mellom to kulturer Fruktbarhetsmønstre blant innvandrerkvinner i Norge.* Reports 2000/25, Oslo: Statistics Norway. http://www.ssb.no/emner/02/02/10/rapp_ 200025/.

Lutz, W., and S. Scherbov. 2003. Can immigration compensate for Europe's low fertility? European Demographic Research Papers 1 (2003), Vienna: Vienna Institute of Demography.

McQuillan, K. 2004. When does religion influence fertility?, *Population and Development Review* 30(1): 25–56.

Milewski, N. 2007. *First child of immigrant workers and their descendants in West Germany: interrelation of events, disruption, or adaptation? Demographic Research* 17(29): 859–896. http://www.demographic-research.org.

OECD. 2007. *International Migration Outlook.* Paris: OECD (SOPEMI).

ONS. 2006. *Birth statistics. Review of the Registrar General on births and patterns of family building England and Wales, 2005*. Series FM1, No. 34. London Office of National Statistics. http://www.statistics.gov.uk/downloads/theme_population/FM1_34/FM1_no34 _2005.pdf

ONS. 2007. *Fertility rate is highest for 26 years*. News release, 7 June 2007. London: Office of National Statistics http://www.statistics.gov.uk/pdfdir/frc0607.pdf.

Østby, L. 2002. *The demographic characteristics of immigrant populations in Norway*. Reports 2002/22, Oslo: Statistics Norway.

Penn, R., and P. Lambert. 2002. Attitudes towards ideal family size of different ethnic/nationality groups in Great Britain, France and Germany, *Population Trends* 108: 49–58.

Poulain, M., and N. Perrin. 2002. The demographic characteristics of immigrant populations in the Belgium, in W. Haug, P. Compton, and Y. Courbage (Eds.), *The Demographic Characteristics of Immigrant Populations*. Population Studies, No. 38, Strasbourg: Council of Europe Publishing, pp: 57–130.

Preston, S., and H. Wang. 2007. Intrinsic growth rates and net reproduction rates in the presence of migration. *Population and Development Review* 33(4): 657-666.

Prioux, F. 2005. Recent demographic developments in France, *Population-E* 60(4): 371–414.

Roig Vila, M., and T. Castro Martín. 2007.Childbearing patterns of foreign women in a new immigration country: The case of Spain. *Population-E* 62(3): 351-380..

Schoorl, J. 1995. Fertility trends of immigrant populations, in S. Voets, J. Schoorl and B. de Bruijn (Eds.), *The Demographic Consequences of International Migration*. Proceedings of the symposium, NIAS, Wasenaar, 27–29 September 1990. Report No. 44, The Hague: NIDI, pp: 97–121.

SFSO. 2006. *Statistique du mouvement naturel de la population. Résultats définitifs 2005*. Neuchâtel: Swiss Federal Statistical Office. http://www.bfs.admin.ch/.

Shaw, C. 2007. Fifty years of United Kingdom national population projections: how accurate have they been?, *Population Trends* 128: 8–23.

Smallwood, S., and J. Chamberlain. 2005. Replacement fertility, what has it been and what does it mean?, P*opulation Trends* 119): 16–27.

Sobotka, T. 2008. Does persistent low fertility threaten the future of European populations?, Forthcoming in J. Surkyn, J. van Bavel and P. Deboosere (Eds.), *Demographic Challenges for the 21ˢᵗ Century. A State of Art in Demography*. Brussels; VUBPRESS, pp. 27-89.

Statistics Denmark. 2004. *Befolkningens bevægelser 2003. Vital statistics 2003*. Copenhagen: Danmarks Statistik.

Statistics Sweden. 2006. *Tabeller över Sveriges befolkning*. Statistiska centralbyrån Stockholm: Statistics Sweden.

Statistisches Bundesamt. 2006. *Statistisches Jahrbuch 2006*. Wiesbaden: Statistisches Bundesamt. http://www.destatis.de/jahrbuch/jahrbuch2006_downloads.htm.

Toulemon, L. 2004. Fertility among immigrant women: new data, new approach, *Population & Societies* 400 (April 2004): 1-4.

Toulemon, L., and M. Mazuy. 2004. *Comment prendre en compte l'âge à l'arrivée et la durée de séjour en France dans la mesure de la fécondité des immigrants?* Documents de travail 120, 2004, Paris: INED.

Tribalat, M. 2005. Fécondité des immigrées et apport démographique de l'immigration étrangère, in C. Bargouignan *et al.* (Eds.), *La population de la France. Évolutions démographiques depuis 1946. Vol. II.* CUDEP / IEDUB, Bordeaux, pp: 727–767.

UN. 2000. *Replacement migration. Is it a solution to declining and ageing populations?* New York: United Nations. http://www.un.org/esa/population/publications/migration/migration.htm.

Van Bavel, J., and V. Bastiaenssen. 2006. *De evolutie van de vruchtbaarheid in het Vlaamse Gewest tussen 2001 en 2005.* Interface Demography Working Paper 2006-1 Brussels: Vrije Universiteit Brussel.

VAZG. 2007. *Tables on births in Flanders provided by the Flemish Healthcare Agency.* (Vlaams Agentschap Zorg en Gezondheit); http://www.zorg-en-gezondheid.be/topPage.aspx?id=684.

Wanner, P. 2002. The demographic characteristics of immigrant populations in Switzerland, in W. Haug, P. Compton, and Y. Courbage (Eds.) *The Demographic Characteristics of Immigrant Populations.* Population Studies, No. 38, Strasbourg: Council of Europe Publishing, pp: 419–496.

Demographic Research: Volume 19, Article 10
research article

Overview Chapter 8:
The impact of public policies on European fertility

Jan M. Hoem [1]

Abstract

This chapter outlines the positions in the current debate about the possibility of using public policies to influence fertility. We note the polarization between, on the one hand, those who view public policies as obvious means for lifting the currently low fertility levels in Europe, in line with the role of economic policies in a modern society; and, on the other hand, those who feel that family policies are inefficient, and perhaps even unnecessary. We place the contributions of the national chapters of this book in this framework and describe the formidable methodological difficulties that face those who seek to investigate policy impacts on fertility behavior. While properly conducted empirical investigations have overcome such problems and have clearly demonstrated policy effects in specific circumstances, we conclude that, in general, national fertility is possibly best seen as a systemic outcome that depends more on broader attributes, such as the degree of family-friendliness of a society, and less on the presence and detailed construction of monetary benefits.

[1] Max Planck Institute for Demographic Research. E-mail: hoem@demogr.mpg.de

1. Introduction, the polarization of demographic opinion

The recent sharp decline in fertility and the subsequent stability of low-level fertility in many European countries have generated a new interest in identifying means to counteract further declines, and, if possible, to induce an increase in fertility back toward the replacement level. The discovery of these developments has served to concentrate people's minds, both in the media and among policymakers, on the national as well as the international level. (For a typical case from the press, see Süddeutsche Zeitung 2006. For national and international contributions, see, for example, the accounts in the chapters in this book on Austria, the Czech Republic or Italy, and papers from the European Commission 2005, 2006.) In many countries, it is possible to detect a re-awakened willingness to adopt instrumental considerations, and to pay less attention to the moral stance that once dominated the attitudes of policymakers in the shadow of past abuses by fascist and other authoritarian regimes. (See our chapters on Germany, Spain, Italy, and Romania. See also Prskawetz et al. 2006, Süddeutsche Zeitung 2006, Kühn and Palme 2005, and Auth and Holland-Cunz 2006.) There is now more talk about the need to prevent the rapid aging of the population, and less about how the unique sanctity of private life pre-empts policies that can increase fertility.

Many demographers are impatient with what they see as inadequately strong or inconsistent government policies. (See our chapters on Austria, Italy, Lithuania, and Poland.) Such impatience is interesting in view of the current polarization of opinion concerning the possibility of using fertility politics to affect childbearing behavior. A conviction that public policies can correct for recent fertility decreases (see below) has been countered with the argument that the types of pronatalist policies that would be considered acceptable in modern democratic societies are both expensive and ineffective. The latter opinion has actually long been held by many professional demographers. The futility of using public policies as a tool to raise long-run fertility in Europe (and elsewhere) has been asserted particularly eloquently by Paul Demeny (1986, 2003, 2005), who has, in addition, maintained in recent conference discussions that natural mechanisms of homeostasis will make deliberate pronatalist efforts unnecessary. The view that family policies have little impact has also been repeated most recently by Gauthier (2007, p. 339), who finds it difficult to understand why baby bonus schemes are so popular among governments, given her interpretation of the evidence she presents in an extensive literature review. In Gauthier's opinion, the effects of public policies tend to be small, and any effect they may have works on the *timing* of fertility (which she seems to regard as less important), rather than on *completed family size* (which many regard as the ultimate goal of family policies). Similarly, several chapters in this book maintain that public policies have influenced fertility only mildly, or have been quite inefficient. (See in particular the chapters on France, Russia, Slovakia, and the Ukraine.)

Western society would have been quite different if economists were equally timid in offering their opinions about the usefulness of *economic* policies. The pessimism shared by so many demographers flies in the face of such basic facts as the systematic differences in fertility levels and fertility trends in the various parts of Western Europe. (See Esping Andersen 1999, Lewis 1992, Gornick et al. 1997, Sainsbury 1999, Anttonen and Sipilä 1996, Castles 2003; for a recent overview, see Neyer 2003a.) One would assume that the higher fertility rates observed in France and in the Nordic countries are neither innate to these cultures nor a gift from heaven, but are somehow related to their deliberate public policies. French policies have long been explicitly pronatalist, as is made evident in the chapter on France included in this book. By contrast, the motivations behind corresponding policies in the Nordic countries have been formulated as considerations for social justice, gender equality and women's empowerment; they have also been seen as efforts to further diminish remaining differentials in income and wealth. The policies are pronatalist in effect, but not by stated intention. (See the chapter on Sweden in this book. Many of our chapters for countries in Central and Eastern Europe contain accounts of pronatalist policies that also go hand-in-hand with gender equality aspirations.) In both cases, the end product is a fertility rate (specifically, a total cohort fertility rate, CFR) that is high by European standards. Conversely, one would assume that the low fertility rates of the Mediterranean countries are, in part, a consequence of the lack of operational attention effectively paid to the need for systematic support of the family in a modern society, as is made clear in the corresponding chapters in this book. Automatic mechanisms of homeostasis are not easily visible, but, if they were present, would not public policies be a necessary part of any system to regulate fertility developments?

Typically, the gloomy view that dismisses the possibility of influencing fertility is not shared by economists like Björklund (2006), who claims that his results suggest that the policies "raised the level of fertility, shortened the spacing of births, and induced fluctuations in the period fertility rates". The pessimistic view also loses credibility as the weight of evidence, as interpreted by demographers like McDonald (2002, 2006) and others,[2] indicates that policies that are pronatalist in effect have indeed had an impact. It is possible that the contradictory readings of the facts may be rooted in different understandings of what aspects of fertility one should focus on, and which public policies one should count. A further issue is how an impact should be measured. We now turn to a discussion of such issues.

---

[2] For a further overview, see, for example, Neyer (2003b, Appendix). For additional contributions concerning the much-studied policy effects in Sweden and their contrasts with other countries, see Neyer (2006a), Neyer et al. (2006b) and Andersson (2005).

2. Methodological issues

Empirical investigations use a variety of data sources and a range of methodologies. Also, even well-founded empirical studies of policy effects are up against a number of difficulties. Let us spell out problematic issues connected to (1) *methodology*, (2) *endogeneity*, (3) the (im)possibility of providing *counterfactual examples* and (4) *context* as follows:

(1) The first major issue that the analyst of policy effects is confronted with is the choice of *statistical methodology*. This pertains both to the choice of dependent variable and to the selection of covariates when any "independent variables" are available. Here are some considerations:

(a) Despite the well-known weaknesses of a statistic like the period TFR as a temporal measure of the fertility level, this is used as the outcome variable in many investigations, in a tradition going back to the beginning of modern studies of the fertility-level/family-policy nexus. Conclusions about fertility effects could be firmer if more adequate statistics were used for analysis.

(b) When more complete statistics *are* available, fertility analysis is normally based on cohort data by preference, and statistics such as the cohort-based, age-accumulated completed fertility rate (CFR) are used. More complete analyses use age-partial CFRs (which are cohort-based, age-specific fertility rates cumulated up to strategically chosen ages, sometimes separately by birth order; see, for example, Frejka and Sardon 2004 and 2007).

(c) Moreover, demographers actually disagree about the absolute supremacy of cohort data over period data (Ní Bhrolcháin 1992). Period data reflect short-term effects, including policy effects of the kind the analyst is looking for, while cohort data are complementary and reflect longer-term developments. For example, the analysis of period data (Andersson 2005, Hoem 2005) has revealed that an ideologically motivated rigidity in the Swedish family policy rules has created great swings in Swedish fertility rates, while in Finland the swings may have been avoided through countervailing effects of a home care allowance (Vikat 2004). Because of the priority given to policies that induce mothers to avoid leaving their jobs even temporarily to work as homemakers, Sweden has not had such an allowance, except as a brief experiment during a short-lived center right government in the mid-1990s. Otherwise, motherhood benefits in Sweden have been closely linked to a woman's own labor income. In such a system, benefits fluctuate as incomes rise and fall, and fertility oscillates correspondingly. Such swings may have serious consequences for society: the school system, for example, would have to adjust to greatly varying cohort sizes. It has not been shown that such swings are related to the ultimate level of fertility for a birth cohort, but it is apparent that policy regulations do influence other aspects of fertility. It is important to note that policy impacts on fertility extend beyond the impact on ultimate cohort fertility. Indeed, exclusive concentration on the CFR may lead to a different fallacy, namely, to a fixation on the lifetime end product of childbearing (the "quantum of fertility"), and to a lack of attention to important timing effects.

(d) Ultimately, the causal structure of policy effects cannot be determined by aggregate statistics alone.[3] With aggregate statistics, the analyst is confined to aggregate-level variation in time and space, and that is far from enough for causal conclusions. If individual-level childbearing histories are available, the options are much wider. (See, for example, Kravdal 1996 and Hank and Kreyenfeld 2003, and many other more recent papers.) For example, analyses of individual-level data have demonstrated that so-called speed-premium effects have reduced birth intervals noticeably in Sweden.[4] (In classical demographic reasoning, this should work toward increasing aggregate ultimate fertility, or, at least, of helping to prevent a further decline.) A second case in point is the most thorough empirical paper on the effects of childcare availability that we have seen to date (Rindfuss et al. 2007), in which the authors suggest that there may be local factors that affect *both* fertility and childcare supply. They demonstrate that policy effects may even come out with the wrong sign if local confounders are not taken into account. The authors conclude that it is essential to pay attention to model specification when conducting studies of policy effects on fertility.

(2) The last paper mentioned illuminates the problem that, in principle, *endogeneity* may dog any investigation of cause-and-effect in demography. This means that even when a first-blush hypothesis posits that policies influence behavior, it may also be necessary to allow for the possibility of a causal influence in the reverse direction, i.e., for the possibility that demographic behavior may influence public policies. For example, policies might respond to an actual or anticipated trend in birth behavior. Thus, while it is commonly assumed that the availability and quality of public childcare influence childbearing behavior, it may instead be the case that regions with high levels of childbearing tend to develop more and better childcare institutions.[5] Politicians naturally cater to their constituencies, and regions with many children may be able to attract more political attention than other regions, with consequences for financial allocation. This may then, in turn, attract more families who want children. In principle, potential parents may migrate to take advantage of the availability of childcare facilities if they are unevenly allocated across locations. This would make

---

[3] For a concurring position, see, for example, Neyer and Andersson (2007).
[4] The latest contribution about this feature was given by Andersson, Hoem, and Duvander (2006).
[5] In this connection it is important to realize that the availability of care should not be measured by the absolute number of daycare slots, but by the provision *rate*. That rate standardizes for the number of children. Therefore one needs to argue that regions with high fertility expand public daycare over-proportionally. We are grateful to Michaela Kreyenfeld for underlining this distinction to us in a private communication.

such migration endogenous to fertility, and, presumably, it would work to exaggerate policy effects unless the role of migration as an intermediate process is accounted for in the analysis. Forgetting about two-way influences almost always results in biased conclusions.

Another example of the dangers of ignoring endogeneity has appeared in connection with regulations concerning non-marital births.[6] In 1998, the German government started allowing unmarried parents to have joint custody of their children; non-marital parenthood increased subsequently. It is unclear, however, whether the changed regulations caused non-marital fertility to increase, or whether the government just responded to the general trend in non-marital childbearing.

(3) A third difficulty inherent in any kind of demographic study is that the analyst rarely has any *counterfactuals* at hand to demonstrate effects. If a counterfactual is not available, it is impossible to know what would have happened if a policy had not been implemented, or if it had been formulated in a different manner. A pronatalist policy can, therefore, easily be judged ineffective when, in reality, the policy may have counteracted a fertility decline that would have occurred in its absence, in which case the policy should have been counted as a success. Fortunately, natural experiments do occur when, for example, neighboring populations are subject to closely similar economic trends but have different public policies, as was the case in the comparison between Sweden and Finland mentioned in item 1c above. Differentials between social groups in reaction to the Swedish speed premium may be another example. (See Andersson, Hoem, and Duvander, 2006, and their predecessors.) A further opportunity for comparison can be found in a before-and-after analysis when a major reform is introduced in a country, as when the three-year parental leave (the APE) for mothers of two children was introduced in France. (See the chapter on France in this book.) There may also be unexpected side effects of reforms made with quite different intentions, such as the peak in marriages following the Swedish widow's pension reform in 1989 (Hoem 1991), or the increase in marriages that occurred in France in 1996 after a change in the tax system for unmarried couples with children. The law was intended to discourage tax evasion among unmarried *couples* who had been making use of measures designed to support *single* parents. When the tax advantages these measures had once conferred disappeared for unmarried couples, marriages increased not only among the wealthy, but also among people who were not paying any income tax, and for whom there was no change at all in the amount of tax owed. It would be easy to underestimate the effect of a policy that was supposed to be limited to a targeted population.

(4) Finally, another difficulty that arises in conducting an empirical analysis is that family policies do not operate in a societal vacuum; the effect of a given policy may be

---

[6] We owe this example also to Michaela Kreyenfeld.

strongly dependent upon the social *context* in which it is implemented. Depending upon the policy constellation, economic trends in particular can interact closely with family policies in influencing fertility. By extension, fertility may be influenced by developments in areas well beyond those in the realm of core family policies. (In addition to economic policies, factors affecting fertility rates may include housing policies, gender policies, social equity, tax rules, school opening hours, and even the overall structure of the educational system, as mentioned by Hoem, Neyer, and Andersson 2006.) Public policies may even serve to change the context in which childbearing behavior operates, and may therefore also have an *indirect* impact on fertility. While each element may have only an incremental influence, together they may add up to something other than the constituent parts. Whether this "something other" is *more* than the parts depends upon how the elements fit into the social system (Neyer and Andersson 2007). As McDonald (2002, p. 442) has stated, "the effectiveness of any policy will depend on the broader setting. ... it is not so much the individual policies that matter as the nature of the society as a whole". Thus, in effectiveness studies, consideration of the whole policy package may be more relevant than attention to stand-alone policy details. An important consequence of this understanding is the recognition that these policies should not be evaluated only on the basis of their demographic consequences. For example, it may be shown that policy measures intended to increase fertility tend to encourage or discourage female labor force participation. Technically, studies of policy effects may need to contain context indicators, including indicators of public policies other than core family policies, otherwise biased conclusions may again be reached. Context indicators may be particularly important in international comparisons. (Gauthier and Hatzius 1997 courageously include indicators of a welfare state type in their extensive regression analysis.) A holistic approach is advisable regardless of the method of analysis one uses, whether it is a plain verbal description, hazard or linear regression, or yet another method. Neyer (2003a, 2006ab; also Neyer and Andersson 2007) has strongly emphasized the need to take into account both the policy context and the symbolic meaning of public policies, in addition to considering the specification of concrete policy parameters.

In a different take on these issues, McDonald (2006; also Sleebos 2003) has highlighted the need for insecurity reduction as part of a fertility recovery program, and posits that it is incumbent on governments to work toward achieving fertility recovery in its own right. (He thus picks up a thread from Hobcraft and Kiernan 1995, and Hobcraft 1996.) Such a program would include policies that promote healthy labor arrangements and economic stability. (It is notable how many of our chapters for countries in Central and Eastern Europe highlight economic insecurity as a fertility depressant.) An assessment of the efficiency of a program for insecurity reduction would indeed require a comprehensive approach to achieve reliable results.

3. Conclusion

By way of conclusion, let us consider what our reflections on research methodology can tell us about the likely efficacy of public policies as instruments to steer developments of ultimate fertility, deliberately or without intention. The evidence from France and the Nordic countries suggest that it should be possible to maintain a reasonably high ultimate fertility rate by a coordinated use of public policies in a range of interlocking areas (economic policy, employment policy, housing policy, gender policy, core family policy, and more) that are implemented in a spirit that furthers childbearing in general, and do not just consist of making more money available to married families in selected situations (Neyer and Andersson 2007; our chapter on Lithuania contains a particularly explicit call for focused and consistent policies). Fertility regulation will remain an ephemeral goal where such coordination is lacking. Generous arrangements for parental leave, child benefits, and childcare may be considered desirable in their own right, but such policies *alone* are unlikely to succeed in raising the fertility level on a grand scale; they must be embedded in a family-friendly culture deliberately nurtured by the state (McDonald 2002; Neyer and Andersson 2007). (For the same reasons, a culture that is friendly to working mothers would not hurt.) Developing such a culture takes time, so any government that wants to increase ultimate fertility needs to realize that it faces a long-term commitment to broadly conceived policies that go far beyond core family policies alone. Even *with* such policies in place, there is no guarantee that an increase in fertility will result. Given the difficulty of pinpointing policy effects, we cannot even be sure whether we will ever know in detail which particular policies are successful, and which are not. What we can observe may be the effect of a whole policy program. Since these kinds of limitations have seldom stopped states from implementing public policies in other fields, there should be no reason to be particularly reticent when policies in support of the family are designed.

4. Acknowledgement

Comments from three anonymous referees are gratefully acknowledged, as are discussions with Gerda Neyer and Michaela Kreyenfeld.

References

Andersson, G. 2005. *A study on policies and practices in selected countries that encourage childbirth: The case of Sweden.* Contribution to the Consultancy Study on Population Related Matters for the Government of Hong Kong Special Administrative Region. Also available as an MPIDR Working Paper. http://www.demogr.mpg.de/Papers/Working/wp-2005-005.pdf.

Andersson,G., J. M. Hoem, and A.-Z. Duvander. 2006. Social differentials in speed-premium effects in childbearing in Sweden, *Demographic Research* 14(4): 51–70.

Anttonen, A., and J. Sipilä. 1996. European social care services: is it possible to identify models?, *Journal of European Social Policy* 6(2): 87–100.

Auth, D., and B. Holland-Cruz. (eds.) 2006. *Grenzen der Bevölkerungspolitik. Strategien und Diskurse demographischer Steuerung.* Opladen: Verlag Barbara Budrich.

Björklund, A. 2006. Does family policy affect fertility? Lessons from Sweden, *Journal of Population Economics* 19(1): 3–24.

Castles, F. G. 2003. The world turned upside down: below replacement fertility, changing preferences and family-friendly public policy in 21 OECD countries, *Journal of European Social Policy* 13(3): 209–227.

Demeny, P. 1986. Pronatalist Policies in Low-Fertility Countries: Patterns, Performance, and Prospects. *Population and Development Review, Supplement: Below-Replacement Fertility in Industrial Societies: Causes, Consequences, Policies* 12: 335–358.

Demeny, P. 2003. Population Policy Dilemmas in Europe at the Dawn of the Twenty-First Century, *Population and Development Review* 29(1): 1–28.

Demeny, P. 2005. Policy challenges of Europe's demographic changes: from past perspectives to future prospects, in M. Macura, A. L. MacDonald and W. Haug (Eds.), *The New Demographic Regime. Population Challenges and Policy Responses.* New York/ Geneva: UNECE/ UNFPA, pp: 1–9.

Esping Andersen, G. 1999. *Social Foundations of Postindustrial Economies.* Oxford: Oxford University Press.

European Commission (Green Paper). 2005. *Confronting demographic change: a new solidarity between the generations.* Brussels.

European Commission (White paper) 2006. *The demographic future of Europe – from challenge to opportunity.* Brussels.

Frejka, T., and J.-P. Sardon. 2004. *Childbearing Trends and Prospects in Low-Fertility Countries: A Cohort Analysis.* European Studies of Population, Vol. 13. Dordrecht/ Boston/ London: Kluwer Academic Publishers.

Frejka, T., and J.-P. Sardon. 2007. Cohort birth order, parity progression ratio and parity distribution trends in developed countries, *Demographic Research* 16(11): 315–374. www.demographic-research.org.

Gauthier, A. H. 2007. The impact of family policies on fertility in industrialized countries: a review of the literature, *Population Research and Policy Review* 26:323–346.

Gauthier, A.-H., and J. Hatzius. 1997. Family benefits and fertility: an econometric analysis, *Population Studies* 51(3): 295–306.

Gornick, J. C., M. K. Meyers, and K. E. Ross. 1997. Supporting the employment of mothers: policy variation across fourteen Welfare States, *Journal of European Social Policy* 7(1): 45–70.

Hank, K., and M. Kreyenfeld. 2003. A multilevel analysis of child care and women's fertility decisions, *Journal of Marriage and the Family* 65(3): 584–596.

Hobcraft, J. 1996. Fertility in England and Wales: a fifty-year perspective, *Population Studies* 50(3): 485–524.

Hobcraft, J., and K. Kiernan. 1995. *Becoming a Parent in Europe, Evolution or Revolution in European Population.* Proceedings of the European Population Conference, Milano.

Hoem, J. M. 1991. To marry, just in case...: the Swedish widow's-pension reform and the peak in marriages in December 1989, *Acta Sociologica* 34: 127–135.

Hoem, J. M. 2005. Why does Sweden have such high fertility?, *Demographic Research* 13(22): 559–572.

Hoem, J. M., G. Neyer, and G. Andersson. 2006. Educational attainment and childlessness: the relationship between educational field, educational level, and childlessness among Swedish women born in 1955-59, *Demographic Research* 14(15): 331–380.

Kravdal, Ø. 1996. How the local supply of day-care centers influences fertility in Norway: a parity-specific approach, *Population Research and Policy Review* 15(3): 201–218.

Kühn, K., and J. Palme. 2005. *Elterngeld und Elternzeit (Föräldraförsäkring och föräldraledighet). Ein Erfahrungsbericht aus Schweden.* Studie der Prognos AG im Auftrag des (Deutschen) Bundesministeriums für Familie, Senioren, Frauen und Jugend.

Lewis, J. 1992. Gender and the development of welfare regimes, *Journal of European Social Policy* 2(3): 159–173.

McDonald, P. 2002. Sustaining fertility through public policy: the range of options, *Population (English Edition)* 57(3): 417–446.

McDonald, P. 2006. Low fertility and the state: the efficacy of policy, *Population and Development Review* 32(3): 485–510.

Neyer, G. 2003a. *Gender and Generations Dimensions in Welfare-State Policies.* MPIDR Working Paper. Rostock: Max Planck Institute for Demographic Research. http://www.demogr.mpg.de/papers/working/wp-2003-022.pdf.

Neyer, G. 2003b. *Family Policies and Low Fertility in Western Europe.* MPIDR Working Paper. Rostock: Max Planck Institute for Demographic Research. http://www.demogr.mpg.de/papers/working/wp-2003-021.pdf.

Neyer, G. (2006a), *Family policies and fertility in Europe: Fertility policies at the intersection of gender policies, employment policies and care policies.* MPIDR Working Paper. Rostock: Max Planck Institute for Demographic Research. http://www.demogr.mpg.de/papers/working/wp-2006-010.pdf.

Neyer, G., G. Andersson, J. M. Hoem, M. Rønsen, and A. Vikat. 2006b. Fertilität, Familiengründung und Familienerweiterung in den nordischen Ländern, in H. Bertram, H. Krüger, and C. K. Spieß (Eds.), *Wem gehört die Familie der Zukunft? Expertisen zum 7. Familienbericht der Bundesregierung.* Opladen: Verlag Barbara Budrich, pp: 207–233.

Neyer, G., and G. Andersson. 2007. *Consequences of family policies on childbearing behavior: effects or artifacts?* MPIDR Working Paper. Rostock: Max Planck Institute for Demographic Research. http://www.demogr.mpg.de/papers/working/wp-2007-021.pdf.

Ní Bhrolcháin, M. 1992. Period paramount? A critique of the cohort approach to fertility, *Population and Development Review* 18(4): 599–629.

Pritchett, L. H. 1994. Desired fertility and the impact of population policies, *Population and Development Review* 20(1): 1–55.

Prskawetz, A., I. Buber, T. Sobotka, and H. Engelhardt. 2006. Recent changes in family policies in Austria and Germany – a response to very low fertility, *Entre Nous* (63): 27–29. http://www.euro.who.int/document/ens/en63.pdf.

Rindfuss, R. R., D. Guilkey, S. P. Morgan, Ø. Kravdal, and K. B. Guzzo. 2007. Child care availability and first birth timing in Norway, *Demography* 44(2): 345–372.

Ringen, S. 1987. *The Possibility of Politics: A Study in the Political Economy of the Welfare State*. Oxford: Clarendon Press.

Sainsbury, D. 1999. *Gender and Welfare State Regimes*. Oxford: Oxford University Press.

Sleebos, J. 2003. *Low fertility rates in OECD countries: Facts and policy responses*. Working Paper No. 15. Paris: OECD Social, Employment and Migration

Süddeutsche Zeitung (13.10.2006), EU fördert Babywunsch. 62(236): 8.

Vikat, A. 2004. Women's labor force attachment and childbearing in Finland, *Demographic Research, Special Collection 3: Contemporary Research on European Fertility: Perspectives and Developments*. S3: 177–212. http://www.demographic-research.org/special/3/8/s3-8.pdf.

Book II of *Childbearing Trends and Policies in Europe* contains 9 Country Chapters

---

Albania:
Trends and patterns, proximate determinants and policies of fertility change

    http://www.demographic-research.org/volumes/vol19/11/

Arjan Gjonca
Arnstein Aassve
Letizia Mencarini

Austria:
Persistent low fertility since the mid-1980s

    http://www.demographic-research.org/volumes/vol19/12/

Alexia Prskawetz
Tomáš Sobotka
Isabella Buber
Henriette Engelhardt
Richard Gisser

Bulgaria:
Ethnic differentials in rapidly declining fertility

    http://www.demographic-research.org/volumes/vol19/13/

Elena Koytcheva
Dimiter Philipov

Czech Republic:
A rapid transformation of fertility and family behaviour after the collapse
of state socialism

    http://www.demographic-research.org/volumes/vol19/14/

Tomáš Sobotka
Anna Šťastná
Kryštof Zeman
Dana Hamplová
Vladimíra Kantorová

England and Wales:
Stable fertility and pronounced social status differences

    http://www.demographic-research.org/volumes/vol19/15/

Wendy Sigle-Rushton

France:
High and stable fertility

    http://www.demographic-research.org/volumes/vol19/16/

Laurent Toulemon
Ariane Pailhé
Clémentine Rossier

Germany:
Family diversity with low actual and desired fertility

    http://www.demographic-research.org/volumes/vol19/17/

Jürgen Dorbritz

Hungary:
Secular fertility decline with distinct period fluctuations

    http://www.demographic-research.org/volumes/vol19/18/

Zsolt Spéder
Ferenc Kamarás

Italy:
Delayed adaptation of social institutions to changes in family behaviour

    http://www.demographic-research.org/volumes/vol19/19/

Alessandra De Rose
Filomena Racioppi
Anna Laura Zanatta

Book III of *Childbearing Trends and Policies in Europe* contains 10 Country Chapters

---

Lithuania:
Fertility decline and its determinants

    http://www.demographic-research.org/volumes/vol19/20/

Vlada Stankuniene
Aiva Jasilioniene

The Netherlands:
Childbearing within the context of a "Poldermodel" society

    http://www.demographic-research.org/volumes/vol19/21/

Tineke Fokkema
Helga de Valk
Joop de Beer
Coen van Duin

Poland:
Fertility decline as a response to profound societal and labour market changes?

    http://www.demographic-research.org/volumes/vol19/22/

Irena Kotowska
Janina Józwiak
Anna Matysiak
Anna Baranowska

Romania:
Childbearing metamorphosis within a changing context

    http://www.demographic-research.org/volumes/vol19/23/

Cornelia Muresan
Paul-Teodor Haragus
Mihaela Haragus
Christin Schröder

Russian Federation:
From the first to second demographic transition

    http://www.demographic-research.org/volumes/vol19/24/

Sergei Zakharov

Slovakia:
Fertility between tradition and modernity

    http://www.demographic-research.org/volumes/vol19/25/

Michaela Potancokova
Boris Vano
Viera Pilinská
Danuša Jurcová

Slovenia:
Generous family policy without evidence of any fertility impact

    http://www.demographic-research.org/volumes/vol19/26/

Nada Stropnik
Milivoja Šircelj

Spain:
Short on children and short on family policies

    http://www.demographic-research.org/volumes/vol19/27/

Margarita Delgado
Gerado Meil
Francisco Zamora López

Sweden:
Combining childbearing and gender equality

    http://www.demographic-research.org/volumes/vol19/28/

Livia Sz. Oláh
Eva Bernhardt

Ukraine:
On the border between old and new in uncertain times

    http://www.demographic-research.org/volumes/vol19/29/

Brienna Perelli-Harris

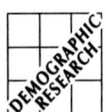

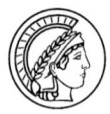

Demographic Research
www.demographic-research.org

first paper version printed August 2008